Ernst Schering Research Foundation Workshop
Supplement 2
Signal Transduction in Testicular Cells

Springer-Verlag Berlin Heidelberg GmbH

Ernst Schering Research Foundation
Workshop, Supplement 2

Signal Transduction in Testicular Cells

Basic and Clinical Aspects

V. Hansson, F.O. Levy, K. Taskén
Editors

With 59 Figures and 12 Tables

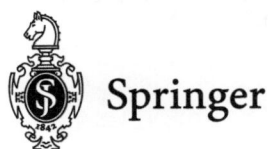 Springer

Series Editors: G. Stock and U.-F. Habenicht

ISBN 978-3-662-03232-9 ISBN 978-3-662-03230-5 (eBook)
DOI 10.1007/978-3-662-03230-5

Die Deutsche Bibliothek – CIP-Einheitsaufnahme
Schering-Forschungsgesellschaft <Berlin>:
Ernst Schering Research Foundation Workshop. – Berlin; Heidelberg; New York; Bar-
celona; Budapest; Hong Kong; London; Milan; Paris; Santa Clara; Singapore; Tokyo:
Springer.
NE:HST
Signal transduction in testicular cells: basic and clinical aspects ; with 12 tables / V.
Hansson ... ed. – Berlin; Heidelberg; New York; Barcelona; Budapest; Hong Kong; Lon-
don; Milan; Paris; Santa Clara; Singapore; Tokyo: Springer, 1996
(Ernst Schering Research Foundation Workshop; 1994, Suppl. 2)
ISBN 978-3-662-03232-9
NE: Hansson, Vidar [Hrsg.]; Schering-Forschungsgesellschaft <Berlin>:
Ernst Schering Research Foundation Workshop

CIP data applied for

© Springer-Verlag Berlin Heidelberg 1996
Originally published by Springer-Verlag Berlin Heidelberg New York
Softcover reprint of the hardcover 1st edition 1996
The use of general descriptive names, registered names, trademarks, etc. in this publication does not imply, even in the absence of a specific statement, that such names are
exempt from the relevant protective laws and regulations and therefore free for general
use. Product liability: The publishers cannot guarantee the accuracy of any information
about dosage and application contained in this book. In every individual case the user
must check such information by consulting the relevant literature.

Typesetting: Data conversion by Springer-Verlag
21/3135–5 4 3 2 1 0 – Printed on acid-free paper

Preface

The European Workshop on Molecular and Cellular Endocrinology of the Testis was organized for the first time at Geilo, Norway, 8–11 April 1980. Since then, these meetings have been held in Holland, France, Italy, England, Sweden/Finland (Åland), Germany, and Belgium. This year the circle has been closed: The 9th European Testis Workshop is back in the Norwegian mountains where it all started.

The Scientific Committee of the First European Testis Workshop included Dr. H.J. van der Molen (Rotterdam), Dr. V. Hansson (Oslo), Dr. B. Cooke (London), Dr. V. Monesi (Rome), Dr. E.M. Ritzén (Stockholm), and Dr. J.M. Saez (Paris). Since then, two of the founders have left the Scientific Committee. Dr. Monesi died suddenly on 29 December 1979, 3 1/2 months before the first workshop took place. Thus, in spite of being one of the founders, he never experienced a European Testis Workshop. Dr. Mario Stefanini, from the same research institute in Rome, replaced Dr. Monesi on the Scientific Committee. Another founder of this workshop series, Dr. H.J. van der Molen (Rotterdam), is one of the pioneers in research on molecular endocrinology of the testis in Europe. He left the Scientific Committee due to a change in his scientific career and was replaced by Dr. F.F.G. Rommerts, whose lectures on "Testomania" have been a characteristic feature of these meetings.

Later, the International Scientific Committee was complemented with scientists from other European countries. These include Dr. Ilpo Huhtaniemi (Turku, Finland), Dr. Eberhard Nieschlag (Münster, Germany), and Dr. Guido Verhoeven (Leuven, Belgium), who organized the 8th European Testis Workshop in Belgium 2 years ago.

These workshops are directed at scientists actively involved in testis research in Europe. However, the meetings are also open to non-Europeans, and this year, the program reflects the brilliance in science on both sides of the Atlantic. We know that "inbreeding" can lead to deterioration in ideas and the danger of losing new biological concepts and technical developments important for our research field. Therefore, in addition to bringing researchers in molecular endocrinology of the testis together, this workshop invites recognized experts in the more general fields of hormone action and molecular cell biology as main lecturers, the hope being that research on the testis will be viewed in a wider perspective, drawing on techniques and ideas from "unrelated" disciplines.

The chapters presented in these proceedings represent novel research on sex determination in mammals, molecular steroidogenesis, gene regulation, and various aspects of signal transduction. Furthermore, the inclusion of four chapters on the clinical aspects of testis research invites a more direct exchange of ideas between representatives of basic molecular research and more clinically oriented scientists. This book also contains several chapters on testis-specific gene expression and mechanisms for gene regulation specific for postmeiotic cells. Thus, molecular cell biology and molecular endocrinology have entered the field of testis research at high speed and the written contributions to this book highlight this.

We acknowledge the continuous support and assistance of E. Martin Ritzén, coorganizer of the meeting, and the International Scientific Committee of the European Testis Workshops, as well as the members of the Local Organizing Committee as listed below.

We also acknowledge the generous support and assistance of the Ernst Schering Research Foundation.

Hopefully, this workshop will be an opportunity for active scientists in Europe to meet international "forerunners" in the field in a relaxed setting and informal atmosphere. We also hope that this will improve collaboration and increase our knowledge on the molecular processes of testis functions.

V. Hansson, F.O. Levy, and K.Taskén

International Scientific Committee of the European Workshop on Molecular and Cellular Endocrinology of the Testis
Brian A. Cooke, London; Vidar Hansson, Oslo; Ilpo Huhtaniemi, Turku; Eberhard Nieschlag, Münster; Martin Ritzén, Stockholm; Focko F.G. Rommerts, Rotterdam; José Saez, Lyon; Mario Stefanini, Rome; Guido Verhoeven, Leuven.

Organizing Committee of the 9th European Workshop on Molecular and Cellular Endocrinology of the Testis
Vidar Hansson, Oslo; E. Martin Ritzén, Stockholm; Tore Jahnsen, Oslo; Rigmor Solberg, Oslo; Kjetil Taskén, Oslo; Winnie Eskild, Oslo; Finn Olav Levy, Oslo; Trine B. Haugen (Clinical Coordinator), Oslo.

Table of Contents

1   The Roles of the Cell-Selective Nuclear Receptor SF-1
    in Reproductive Function
    K.L. Parker, Y. Ikeda, and X. Luo 1

2   Regulation of Steroid Hormone Production
    M.R. Waterman 13

3   A Role for cAMP-Response Element Motifs
    in Transcriptional Regulation
    of Postmeiotic Male Germ Cell-Specific Genes
    Z. Sun and A.R. Means 29

4   Cyclic Nucleotide-Gated Channels in Sperm
    I. Weyand 53

5   CREM: A Transcriptional Master Switch
    Governing the cAMP Response in the Testis
    L. Monaco, F. Nantel, N.S. Foulkes, and P. Sassone-Corsi . . 69

6   Targeted Disruption of the Protein Kinase A System in Mice
    *G.S. McKnight, R.L. Idzerda, E.R. Kandel, E.P.Brandon,
    M. Zhuo, M. Qi, R. Bourtchouladze, Y. Huang, K.A. Burton,
    B.S. Skålhegg, D.E. Cummings, L. Varshavsky, J. V.Planas,
    K. Motamed, K.A. Gerhold, P.S. Amieux, C.R. Guthrie,
    K.M. Millett, M. Belyamani, and T. Su* 95

7   Posttranscriptional Regulation
     of Postmeiotic Gene Expression
     N.B. Hecht 123

8   Isolation and Culture of Immature Rat Type A
     Spermatogonial Stem Cells
     G. Dirami, N. Ravindranath, M.C. Jia, and M. Dym 141

9   Androgen Receptor in Transcriptional Regulation
     P.J. Kallio, T. Ikonen, A. Moilanen, H. Poukka,
     P. Reinikainen, J.J. Palvimo, and O.A. Jänne 167

10   The 3β-Hydroxysteroid Dehydrogenase/Isomerase
     Gene Family: Lessons from Type II 3β-HSD
     Congenital Deficiency
     F. Labrie, J. Simard, V. Luu-The, A. Bélanger, G. Pelletier,
     Y.Morel, F. Mebarki, R. Sanchez, F. Durocher, C. Turgeon,
     Y. Labrie, E. Rheaume, C. Labrie, and Y. Lachance 185

11   The Src Family of Protein Tyrosine Kinases
     C. Couture and T. Mustelin 219

12   Sperm–Zona Pellucida Interaction:
     A Model for Zona Receptor Kinase-Mediated Signaling
     P.M. Saling, D.J. Burks, and C.N. Tomes 247

13   The Use of Spermatids for Human Conception
     I. Aslam and S. Fishel 271

14   Evidence-Based Andrology:
     The Importance of Controlled Clinical Trials
     E. Leifke and E. Nieschlag 287

15   Molecular Genetics and Neurobiology
     of Kallmann's Syndrome
     P.-M.G. Bouloux, P. de Zoyza, V. Duke, and R. Quinton . . 307

16   The Polymorphisms of Gonadotropin Action:
     Molecular Basis and Clinical Implications
     I. Huhtaniemi, P. Pakarinen, A.-M. Haavisto, C. Nilsson,
     K. Pettersson, J. Tapanainen, and K. Aittomäki 319

Subject Index   343

Previous Volumes Published in this Series   353

List of Editors and Contributors

Editors

V. Hansson
Institute of Medical Biochemistry, University of Oslo,
P.O.Box 1112 Blindern, 0317 Oslo, Norway

F.O. Levy
Institute of Medical Biochemistry, University of Oslo,
P.O.Box 1112 Blindern, 0317 Oslo, Norway

K. Taskén
Institute of Medical Biochemistry, University of Oslo,
P.O.Box 1112 Blindern, 0317 Oslo, Norway

Contributors

K. Aittomäki
Department of Medical Genetics, University of Helsinki, 00290 Helsinki,
Finland

P.S. Amieux
Department of Pharmacology, University of Washington School of Medicine,
Seattle, WA 98195, USA

I. Aslam
Nottingham University Research Unit in Reproduction, Department of Obstetrics and Gynaecology, University Hospital, Queen's Medical Centre,
Nottingham, UK

A. Bélanger
MRC Group in Molecular Endocrinology, CHUL Research Center,
2705 Laurier Boulevard, Québec, Quebec G1V 4G2, Canada

M. Belyamani
Department of Pharmacology, University of Washington School of Medicine,
Seattle, W.A 98195, USA

P.-M.G. Bouloux
Centre for Neuroendocrinology, Department of Endocrinology, Royal Free
UCL School of Medicine, Rowland Hill Street, London NW3 2PF, UK

R. Bourtchouladze
Center for Neurobiology and Behavior, Howard Hughes Medical Institute,
College of Physicians and Surgeons of Columbia University,
722 West 168th Street, New York, NY 10032, USA

E.P. Brandon
Department of Pharmacology, University of Washington School of Medicine,
Seattle, WA 98195, USA

D.J. Burks
Joslin Diabetes Center, Harvard Medical School, One Joslin Place,
Boston, MA 02215, USA

K.A. Burton
Department of Pharmacology, University of Washington School of Medicine,
Seattle, WA 98195, USA

C. Couture
Division of Cell Biology, La Jolla Institute for Allergy and Immunology,
11149, North Torrey Pines Road, La Jolla, CA 92037, USA

D.E. Cummings
Department of Pharmacology, University of Washington School of Medicine,
Seattle, WA 98195, USA

G. Dirami
Department of Cell Biology, Georgetown University, 3900 Reservoir Road,
NW, Washington, DC, USA

V. Duke
Centre for Neuroendocrinology, Department of Endocrinology, Royal Free
UCL School of Medicine, Rowland Hill Street, London NW3 2PF, UK

F. Durocher
MRC Group in Molecular Endocrinology, CHUL Research Center,
2705 Laurier Boulevard, Québec, Quebec G1V 4G2, Canada

M. Dym
Department of Cell Biology, Georgetown University, 3900 Reservoir Road,
NW, Washington, DC, USA

S. Fishel
Nottingham University Research Unit in Reproduction, Department of Obste-
trics and Gynaecology, University Hospital, Queen's Medical Centre,
Nottingham, UK

N.S. Foulkes
Institut de Génétique et de Biologie Moléculaire et Cellulaire,
CNRS - INSERM, B.P. 163, 67404 Illkirch, Strasbourg, France

K.A. Gerhold
Department of Pharmacology, University of Washington School of Medicine,
Seattle, WA 98195, USA

C.R. Guthrie
Department of Pharmacology, University of Washington School of Medicine,
Seattle, WA 98195, USA

A.-M. Haavisto
Department of Physiology, University of Turku, 20520 Turku, Finland

N.B. Hecht
Tufts University, Department of Biology, Medford, MA 02155, USA

Y. Huang
Center for Neurobiology and Behavior, Howard Hughes Medical Institute,
College of Physicians and Surgeons of Columbia University, 722 West 168th
Street, New York, NY 10032, USA

I. Huhtaniemi
Department of Physiology, University of Turku, 20520 Turku, Finland

R.L. Idzerda
Department of Pharmacology, University of Washington School of Medicine,
Seattle, WA 98195, USA

Y. Ikeda
Departments of Medicine and Pharmacology and the Howard Hughes Medical
Institute, Duke University Medical Center, Durham NC 27710, USA

T. Ikonen
Institute of Biomedicine, Department of Physiology, University of Helsinki,
Siltavuorenpenger 20 J, 00014 Helsinki, Finland

O.A. Jänne
Institute of Biomedicine, Department of Physiology, University of Helsinki,
Siltavuorenpenger 20 J, 00014 Helsinki, Finland

M. C. Jia
Department of Cell Biology, Georgetown University, 3900 Reservoir Road,
NW, Washington, DC, USA

P.J. Kallio
Institute of Biomedicine, Department of Physiology, University of Helsinki,
Siltavuorenpenger 20 J, 00014 Helsinki, Finland

E.R. Kandel
Center for Neurobiology and Behavior, Howard Hughes Medical Institute,
College of Physicians and Surgeons of Columbia University,
722 West 168th Street, New York, NY 10032, USA

C. Labrie
MRC Group in Molecular Endocrinology, CHUL Research Center,
2705 Laurier Boulevard, Québec, Quebec G1V 4G2, Canada

F. Labrie
MRC Group in Molecular Endocrinology, CHUL Research Center,
2705 Laurier Boulevard, Québec, Quebec G1V 4G2, Canada

Y. Labrie
MRC Group in Molecular Endocrinology, CHUL Research Center,
2705 Laurier Boulevard, Québec, Quebec G1V 4G2, Canada

Y. Lachance
MRC Group in Molecular Endocrinology, CHUL Research Center,
2705 Laurier Boulevard, Québec, Quebec G1V 4G2, Canada

E. Leifke
Institute of Reproductive Medicine, University of Münster,
Steinfurter Straße 107, 48149 Münster, Germany

X. Luo
Departments of Medicine and Pharmacology and the Howard Hughes Medical
Institute, Duke University Medical Center, Durham NC 27710, USA

V. Luu-The
MRC Group in Molecular Endocrinology, CHUL Research Center,
2705 Laurier Boulevard, Québec, Quebec G1V 4G2, Canada

G.S. McKnight
Department of Pharmacology, University of Washington School of Medicine,
Seattle, WA 98195, USA

A.R. Means
Department of Pharmacology, Duke University Medical Center,
Durham, NC 27710, USA

F. Mebarki
INSERM U329 and Department of Pediatrics, Université de Lyon and Hôpital
Debrousse, Lyon Cedex 05, France

K.M. Millett
Department of Pharmacology, University of Washington School of Medicine,
Seattle, WA 98195, USA

A. Moilanen
Institute of Biomedicine, Department of Physiology, University of Helsinki,
Siltavuorenpenger 20 J, 00014 Helsinki, Finland

L. Monaco
Institut de Génétique et de Biologie Moléculaire et Cellulaire,
CNRS - INSERM, B.P. 163, 67404 Illkirch, Strasbourg, France

Y. Morel
INSERM U329 and Department of Pediatrics, Université de Lyon and Hôpital
Debrousse, Lyon Cedex 05, France

K. Motamed
Department of Pharmacology, University of Washington School of Medicine,
Seattle, WA 98195, USA

T. Mustelin
Division of Cell Biology, La Jolla Institute for Allergy and Immunology,
11149, North Torrey Pines Road, La Jolla, CA 92037, USA

F. Nantel
Institut de Génétique et de Biologie Moléculaire et Cellulaire,
CNRS - INSERM, B.P. 163, 67404 Illkirch, Strasbourg, France

E. Nieschlag
Institute of Reproductive Medicine, University of Münster,
Steinfurter Straße 107, 48149 Münster, Germany

C. Nilsson
Department of Biotechnology, University of Turku, 20520 Turku, Finland

P. Pakarinen
Department of Physiology, University of Turku, 20520 Turku, Finland

J.J. Palvimo
Institute of Biomedicine, Department of Physiology, University of Helsinki,
Siltavuorenpenger 20 J, 00014 Helsinki, Finland

K.L. Parker
Departments of Medicine and Pharmacology and the Howard Hughes Medical
Institute, Duke University Medical Center, Durham NC 27710, USA

G. Pelletier
MRC Group in Molecular Endocrinology, CHUL Research Center,
2705 Laurier Boulevard, Québec, Quebec G1V 4G2, Canada

K. Pettersson
Department of Biotechnology, University of Turku, 20520 Turku, Finland

J.V. Planas
Department of Pharmacology, University of Washington School of Medicine,
Seattle, WA 98195, USA

H. Poukka
Institute of Biomedicine, Department of Physiology, University of Helsinki,
Siltavuorenpenger 20 J, 00014 Helsinki, Finland

M. Qi
Department of Pharmacology, University of Washington School of Medicine,
Seattle, WA 98195, USA

R. Quinton
Centre for Neuroendocrinology, Department of Endocrinology, Royal Free
UCL School of Medicine, Rowland Hill Street, London NW3 2PF, UK

N. Ravindranath
Department of Cell Biology, Georgetown University, 3900 Reservoir Road,
NW, Washington, DC, USA

P. Reinikainen
Institute of Biomedicine, Department of Physiology, University of Helsinki,
Siltavuorenpenger 20 J, 00014 Helsinki, Finland

E. Rheaume
MRC Group in Molecular Endocrinology, CHUL Research Center,
2705 Laurier Boulevard, Québec, Quebec G1V 4G2, Canada

P.M. Saling
Department of Cell Biology, Duke University, Medical Center,
Durham, NC 27710, USA

R. Sanchez
MRC Group in Molecular Endocrinology, CHUL Research Center,
2705 Laurier Boulevard, Québec, Quebec G1V 4G2, Canada

P. Sassone-Corsi
Institut de Génétique et de Biologie Moléculaire et Cellulaire,
CNRS - INSERM, B.P. 163, 67404 Illkirch, Strasbourg, France

J. Simard
MRC Group in Molecular Endocrinology, CHUL Research Center,
2705 Laurier Boulevard, Québec, Quebec G1V 4G2, Canada

B.S. Skålhegg
Department of Pharmacology, University of Washington School of Medicine,
Seattle, WA 98195, USA

T. Su
Department of Pharmacology, University of Washington School of Medicine,
Seattle, WA 98195, USA

Z. Sun
Division of Molecular Pathogenesis, Skirball Institute of Biomolecular
Medicine, New York University Center, New York, NY 10061, USA ·

J. Tapanainen
Oulu University Central Hospital, 90220 Oulu, Finland

C.N. Tomes
Department of Cell Biology, Duke University, Medical Center,
Durham, NC 27710, USA

C. Turgeon
MRC Group in Molecular Endocrinology, CHUL Research Center,
2705 Laurier Boulevard, Québec, Quebec G1V 4G2, Canada

L. Varshavsky
Center for Neurobiology and Behavior, Howard Hughes Medical Institute,
College of Physicians and Surgeons of Columbia University,
722 West 168th Street, New York, NY 10032, USA

M.R. Waterman
Vanderbilt University School of Medicine, Department of Biochemistry,
Nashville, Tennessee 37232-0146, USA

I. Weyand
Forschungszentrum Jülich, Institut für Biologische Informationsverarbeitung,
Postfach 1913, 52425 Jülich, Germany

M. Zhuo
Center for Neurobiology and Behavior, Howard Hughes Medical Institute,
College of Physicians and Surgeons of Columbia University,
722 West 168th Street, New York, NY 10032, USA

P. de Zoyza
Centre for Neuroendocrinology, Department of Endocrinology, Royal Free
UCL School of Medicine, Rowland Hill Street, London NW3 2PF, UK

1 The Roles of the Cell-Selective Nuclear Receptor SF-1 in Reproductive Function

K.L. Parker, Y. Ikeda, and X. Luo

1.1	Introduction	1
1.2	Results	2
1.2.1	Isolation and Characterization of SF-1	2
1.2.2	Ontogeny of SF-1 Expression	3
1.2.3	The Mouse Gene Encoding SF-1 Is Essential for Adrenal and Gonadal Development	4
1.2.4	The *Ftz-F1* Gene also Acts at Other Levels of the Hypothalamic–Pituitary–Gonadal Axis	6
1.2.5	SF-1 Is the Essential Transcript Encoded by the *Ftz-F1* Gene	6
1.3	Discussion	8
1.4	Summary and Perspectives	9
References		10

1.1 Introduction

The cytochrome P450 steroid hydroxylases are expressed in a tissue-specific and developmentally regulated fashion (Miller 1988). Over the past several years, a major goal at our laboratory has been to define the molecular mechanisms that determine this regulation. As detailed below, each of these genes contains at least one copy of a shared regulatory element that interacts with a cell-selective, orphan nuclear receptor, steroidogenic factor 1 (SF-1). Recent studies have defined key roles of SF-1 in diverse endocrine processes that include adrenal and gonadal development, gonadotrope function, and development of the ventromedial hypothalamic nucleus. These studies collectively provide novel insights into mechanisms of endocrine development and reproductive function.

1.2 Results

1.2.1 Isolation and Characterization of SF-1

A number of elements that regulated the cytochrome P450 steroid hydroxylases had related AGGTCA sequences. The similar sequences of these steroidogenic regulatory elements suggested that the same regulatory protein interacted with these sequences to coordinate the expression of the steroid hydroxylases (Rice et al. 1991; Morohashi et al. 1992). Because the protein that formed this complex was restricted to steroidogenic cell lines, we designated it steroidogenic factor 1 (SF-1). When we isolated an SF-1 cDNA (Lala et al. 1992), several important features became apparent. First, SF-1 belonged to the nuclear hormone receptor family, a diverse group of structurally related proteins that mediate transcriptional activation by various steroid hormones, vitamin D, thyroid hormone, and retinoids (reviewed by Evans 1988). The SF-1 cDNA most closely resembled a cDNA isolated from embryonal carcinoma cells and designated embryonal long terminal binding protein (ELP) because it inhibited transcription of retroviral long terminal repeats (LTRs) (Tsukiyama et al. 1992). Isolation and characterization of genomic sequences encoding SF-1 ultimately revealed that both SF-1 and ELP arise from the same structural gene by alternative promoter usage and 3' splicing (Ikeda et al. 1993). The gene encoding these two transcripts was designated *Ftz-F1* because it also resembles the FTZ-F1 *Drosophila* nuclear receptor, which encodes two developmentally regulated isoforms and which regulates the *fushi tarazu* (*ftz*) homeobox gene (Lavorgna et al. 1991, 1993).

1.2.2 Ontogeny of SF-1 Expression

Based on the essential roles of steroid hormones in male sexual differentiation, we analyzed the developmental profile of SF-1 during mouse
embryogenesis. As summarized in Table 1, these analyses identified
several potential roles of SF-1 in steroidogenic organ development,
some of which were unanticipated (Ikeda et al. 1994). SF-1 transcripts
were present in the adrenal primordium, beginning at the earliest stages
of adrenal formation at approximately embryonic day 10.5 (E10.5).
Subsequently, as the chromaffin cell precursors migrated into the adrenal gland from the neural crest to form the medulla, SF-1 expression was
confined to the steroidogenic cells in the cortex. This expression of SF-1
from the earliest stages of adrenal differentiation suggested a key role in
adrenal development.

In the gonads, SF-1 was expressed in both male and female embryos
at very early stages of gonadogenesis, when the intermediate mesoderm
first begins to condense into the urogenital ridge (~E9). At this time,
male and female gonads are histologically indistinguishable and are
therefore termed indifferent or bipotential gonads. After ~ E12.5, as
morphologic sexual differentiation takes place, SF-1 transcripts were

Table 1. In situ hybridization analysis of the ontogeny of SF-1 expression in
mouse embryos

Adrenal gland
Expressed from earliest stages of development of adrenal primordium (E10.5)
As chromaffin cell precursors invade adrenal from neural crest at ~E13, ex-
pression localizes to outer, cortical region

Gonads
Expressed in indifferent gonad of both sexes from very early stages of gona-
dogenesis (~E9)
Expression in testis persists and increases coincidentally with sexual differentia-
tion (E12.5) in both Leydig and Sertoli cells
Expression in ovary decreases coincidentally with sexual differentiation
(E12.5)

Hypothalamus/pituitary
Expressed in retrochiasmatic ventral diencephalon (precursor to endocrine hy-
pothalamus)
Expressed in pituitary gonadotropes

expressed at even higher levels in the testes, but could no longer be detected in ovaries. Moreover, SF-1 was expressed in both compartments of the developing testes: the interstitial region, where fetal Leydig cells produce androgens, and the testicular cords, where fetal Sertoli cells synthesize Müllerian-inhibiting substance (MIS). The expression of SF-1 by Sertoli cells raised the possibility that SF-1's role in endocrine development extended beyond regulating the steroidogenic enzymes.

Intriguingly, SF-1 was also expressed in discrete regions of the retrochiasmatic ventral diencephalon and anterior pituitary (Ingraham et al. 1994). This region of the ventral diencephalon is the primordium of the endocrine hypothalamus, whereas the anterior pituitary includes the gonadotropes that produce gonadotropins, the predominant regulators of gonadal steroidogenesis. These findings again suggested that SF-1 also functions at additional levels of the hypothalamic–pituitary–steroidogenic tissue axis.

1.2.3 The Mouse Gene Encoding SF-1 Is Essential for Adrenal and Gonadal Development

To define the role of SF-1 in intact mice, we used targeted gene disruption to "knock out" the mouse *Ftz-F1* gene that encodes SF-1 (Luo et al. 1994). As shown in Fig. 1, our initial strategy abolished both ELP and SF-1 activity. In matings of heterozygous *Ftz-F1*-disrupted mice, -/- animals were born at the expected frequency of 1 in 4, establishing that neither ELP nor SF-1 is required for embryonic survival. All of these knockout mice died shortly after birth and had depressed corticosterone levels, consistent with the anticipated inability to make corticosteroids; they further had female external genitalia irrespective of genetic sex, consistent with the anticipated failure to produce testicular androgens. What we did not anticipate, however, was the complete absence of adrenal glands and gonads – a finding that revealed essential roles of the *Ftz-F1* gene in steroidogenic organ development. Developmental studies of *Ftz-F1*-disrupted embryos suggested that the earliest stages of intermediate mesodermal condensation to form the gonads were unimpaired, but that the SF-1 deficiency ultimately was associated with the induction of apoptosis in the adrenal glands and gonads and subsequent regression of the primary steroidogenic organs.

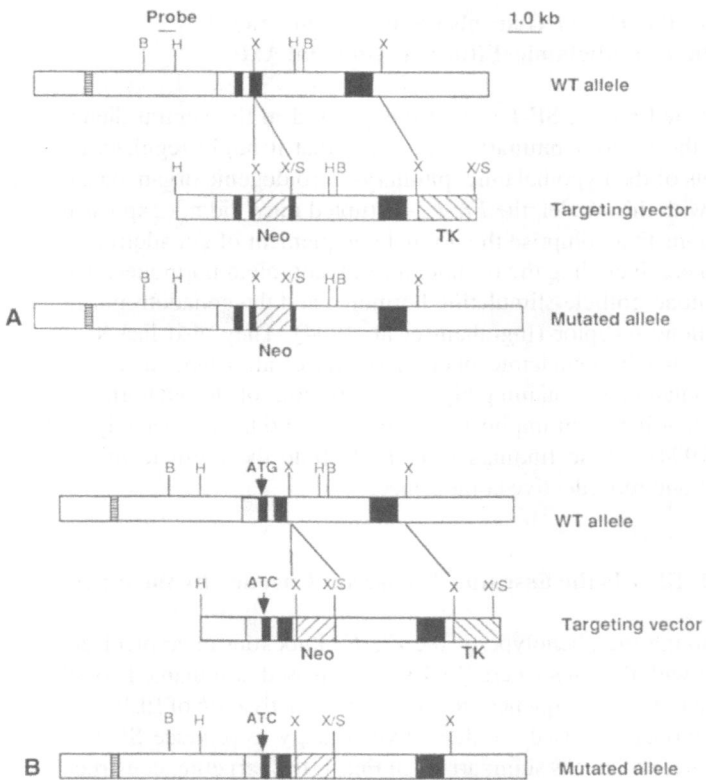

Fig. 1A,B. Alternative strategies for disrupting the mouse *Ftz-F1*gene.
A Schematic summary of the strategy used to disrupt the mouse *FTZ-F1*gene.
Solid areas indicate shared exons, *horizontally lined* areas denote steroidogenic factor 1 (SF-1)-specific exons, and *stippled areas* denote embryonal
long terminal binding protein (ELP)-specific exons. The Neo selectable marker and thymidine kinase (*TK*) gene were inserted into a plasmid containing
the indicated *Ftz-F1*genomic sequences. The *Neo* gene disrupts the second
zinc finger region required for DNA binding. Restriction endonuclease sites
include *B, Bgl*II; *X, Xho*I; *H, Hind*III; *E, Eco*47 III. The position of the probe
used for Southern blotting analyses is indicated. **B** Strategy for selective disruption of SF-1. The position of the initiator methionines for SF-1 is indicated;
in the targeting construct, the SF-1 *ATG* was changed to *ATC*, abolishing the
translation initiation site, while converting an internal methionine to isoleucine
(ATC) in the ELP coding sequence

1.2.4 The *Ftz-F1* Gene also Acts at Other Levels of the Hypothalamic–Pituitary–Gonadal Axis

As noted above, SF-1 was also expressed in the ventral diencephalon and the anterior pituitary, suggesting that it might regulate additional levels of the hypothalamic–pituitary–steroidogenic organ axis. Consistent with this model, the *Ftz-F1*-disrupted mice did not express multiple proteins that comprise the normal complement of gonadotrope-specific markers, including the α-subunit of glycoprotein hormones, luteinizing hormone, follicle-stimulating hormone, and the gonadotropin-releasing hormone receptor (Ingraham et al. 1994). They also lacked the ventromedial hypothalamic nucleus (Ikeda et al. 1995), a region of the hypothalamus containing high concentrations of steroid hormone receptors that has been implicated in female reproductive behavior (Pfaff et al. 1994). These findings further illustrate the intimate link between SF-1 and reproductive competence.

1.2.5 SF-1 Is the Essential Transcript Encoded by the *Ftz-F1* Gene

Although the phenotype of the *Ftz-F1* knockout mice precisely correlated with the sites where SF-1 was expressed, it remained possible that some of the consequences resulted from inactivation of ELP. To address this model, we used an alternative strategy to produce SF-1 selective knockout mice. As summarized in Fig. 1, this targeting construct altered the initiator methionine in the SF-1 transcript, which is an internal methionine in ELP. As a result, the essential site for SF-1 translation initiation is destroyed, whereas the ELP coding sequence is altered only by a conservative methionine to isoleucine mutation in a region that has no known function and that is not required for DNA binding (Luo et al. 1995). The phenotype of the SF-1 selective knockout mice resembled exactly that seen previously with the Ftz-F1 knockout mice, as exemplified by the gonadal and adrenal agenesis shown in Fig. 2, strongly indicating that SF-1 is the essential transcript encoded by the mouse *Ftz-F1*gene.

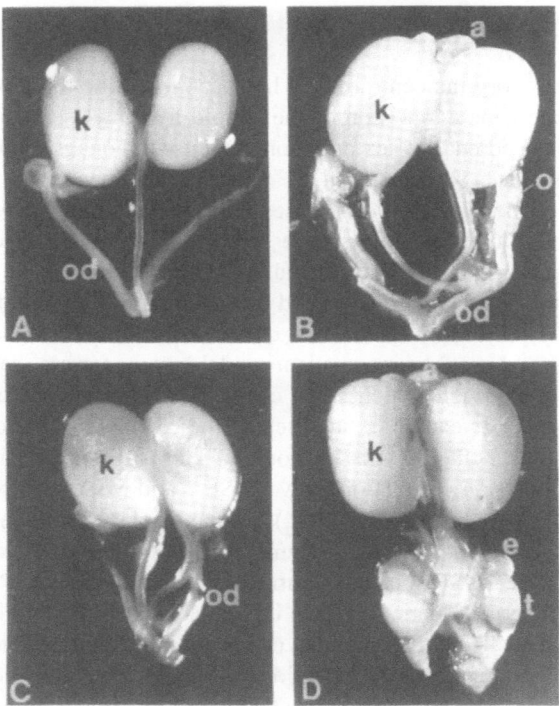

Fig. 2A–D. Steroidogenic factor 1 (SF-1)-specific knockout mice have adrenal and gonadal agenesis and female internal genitalia. The dissected genitourinary tracts of wild-type female (**B**) and male (**D**) and SF-1-deficient female (**A**) and male (**C**) mice are shown. Note the absence of adrenal glands and gonads in SF-1-deficient mice, and the oviducts in both males and females. *a*, adrenal gland; *k*, kidney; *o*, ovary; *t*, testis; *od*, oviduct. (From Luo et al. 1995)

1.3 Discussion

At our laboratory the central focus has been to define the mechanisms that regulate gene expression of the steroid hydroxylases, initially focusing on the adrenal cortex and more recently in gonads. In the course of these studies, we identified SF-1 and established it as a pivotal regulator of the steroid hydroxylases. Subsequent studies have shown unequivocally that SF-1 also makes essential contributions to adrenal and gonadal development (Luo et al. 1994) and to hypothalamic/pituitary function (Ikeda et al. 1995) and that SF-1 is the essential transcript encoded by the *Ftz-F1* gene (Luo et al. 1995). The *Ftz-F1*-disrupted animals should provide an excellent model system for ascertaining the target genes through which SF-1 exerts its actions in steroid organ development. For example, analyses of the 5'-flanking region of the gene encoding MIS identified a potential SF-1-response element and showed a temporal correlation between SF-1 and MIS gene expression (Shen et al. 1994; Hatano et al. 1994). If functional studies in intact mice ultimately support a role for this element in MIS gene expression, it will directly implicate SF-1 in both critical arms of male sexual development: androgen production by fetal Leydig cells and MIS production in fetal Sertoli cells. Following the cloning of the gene encoding the steroidogenic acute regulatory peptide (StAR), which plays a key role in delivering cholesterol to P450scc in the inner mitochondrial membrane, a potential SF-1 site was identified in its 5'-flanking region (Clark et al. 1995). The essential role of StAR in regulated steroidogenesis (Lin et al. 1995) and the presence of a potential SF-1 responsive sequence in the StAR 5'-flanking region suggest that StAR may be yet another target through which SF-1 regulates key events in endocrine development.

Another area of considerable interest will be to try to define the mechanisms that regulate the expression of the steroid hydroxylases in nonclassical sites of steroidogenesis. For example, P450scc is expressed in several sites, including the brain, placenta, and fetal gut, that do not express SF-1; moreover, we recently showed that P450scc expression was unimpaired in the *Ftz-F1*-disrupted mice (Keeney et al. 1995). Other transcriptional regulators therefore must determine expression of P450scc in nonclassical sites, and it will be of considerable interest to characterize these transcriptional regulators. At this time, it is tempting to speculate that those sites in which the steroid hydroxylases are regulated by SF-1 are sites that exhibit marked hormonal regulation of steroidogenesis, whereas the other sites are not predominantly regulated by trophic hormone. Further studies comparing and contrasting steroid hydroxylase regulation in these nonclassical sites should provide new insights into the regulation of the synthesis of steroids that play key roles in maintaining pregnancy and in neuronal function.

Another gene that may interact, either directly or indirectly, with SF-1 is the recently-described *DAX-1* gene. This gene was isolated by positional cloning from patients with congenital adrenal hypoplasia (Zanaria et al. 1994). These patients have an X-linked disorder characterized by adrenal hypoplasia and a subset of patients also exhibit hypogonadotrophic hypogonadism (Muscatelli et al. 1994), thus closely resembling the phenotype in the *Ftz-F1*-disrupted mice. Intriguingly, *DAX-1* encodes an orphan nuclear receptor that contains amino acids corresponding to the ligand-binding domain of nuclear receptors but lacks the zinc-finger DNA-binding domain typical of these transcriptional regulators. Perhaps most intriguingly, preliminary studies indicate that *DAX-1* is expressed in essentially all of the sites at which SF-1 is expressed, including the adrenal cortex, gonads, gonadotropes, and ventromedial hypothalamus (A. Swain and Y. Ikeda, unpublished observations). This striking colocalization further supports an intimate relationship between these two nuclear receptors, and further studies of their interactions will undoubtedly provide new insights into the complex events in endocrine development and differentiation.

1.4 Summary and Perspectives

Expression of the cytochrome P450 steroid hydroxylases is tissue-specific and developmentally regulated. Recent studies identified an orphan nuclear receptor, designated SF-1, that acts as a global regulator of the steroid hydroxylases and plays key roles in both developmental and cell-specific regulation. As analyzed by in situ hybridization, SF-1 expression in mouse embryos began at the earliest stages of adrenal and gonadal development, suggesting that SF-1 plays a key role in their differentiation. SF-1 expression was also seen in the embryonic pituitary gland and ventral diencephalon, suggesting additional roles within the hypothalamic–pituitary–steroidogenic organ axis. To examine SF-

1's role in vivo, we used targeted gene disruption to knock out the gene encoding SF-1. Analyses of these knockout mice established essential roles of SF-1 at multiple levels of endocrine development, including adrenal and gonadal differentiation, pituitary gonadotrope function, and formation of the ventromedial hypothalamic nucleus. These results indicate that SF-1 plays multiple roles in endocrine development that are essential for reproduction. A key area for further studies will be the identification and characterization of genes that act upstream and downstream of SF-1 in complex cascades of endocrine differentiation.

Acknowledgments. This work was supported by the Howard Hughes Medical Institute and the National Institutes of Health. We thank Dr. Douglas Rice, Dr. Andrea Mouw, and Dr. Deepak Lala for their key contributions to early studies of SF-1 and Dr. Beverly Koller for invaluable assistance in preparing the *Ftz-F1*-disrupted mice, and Dr. Barbara Clark and Dr. Douglas Stocco for invaluable collaboration in the analyses of StAR.

References

Clark BJ, Soo S-C, Caron KM, Ikeda Y, Parker KL, Stocco DM (1995) Hormonal and developmental regulation of the steroidogenic acute regulatory (StAR) protein. Mol Endocrinol 9:1346–1355

Evans RM (1988) The steroid and thyroid hormone receptor superfamily. Science 240:889–895

Hatano O, Takayama, K, Imai, T, Waterman, MR, Takakusu, A, Omura, T, Morohashi, K-I (1994) Sex-dependent expression of a transcription factor, Ad4BP, regulating steroidogenic P-450 genes in the gonads during prenatal and postnatal rat development. Development 120:2787–2797

Ikeda Y, Lala DS, Luo X, Kim E, Moisan M-P, Parker KL (1993) Characterization of the mouse FTZ-F1 gene, which encodes an essential regulator of steroid hydroxylase gene expression. Mol Endocrinol 7:852–860

Ikeda Y, Shen W-H, Ingraham HA, Parker KL (1994) Developmental expression of mouse steroidogenic factor 1, an essential regulator of the steroid hydroxylases. Mol Endocrinol 8:654–662

Ikeda Y, Luo X, Abbud R, Nilson JH, Parker KL (1995) The nuclear receptor steroidogenic factor 1 is essential for the formation of the ventromedial hypothalamic nucleus. Mol Endocrinol 9:478–486

Ingraham HA, Lala DS, Ikeda Y, Luo, X, Shen W-H, Nachtigal MW, Abbud R, Nilson JH; Parker KL (1994) The nuclear receptor SF-1 acts at multiple levels of the reproductive axis. Genes Dev 8:2302–2312

Keeney DS, Ikeda Y, Waterman MR, Parker KL (1995) Cholesterol side-chain cleavage cytochrome P450 gene expression in primitive gut of the mouse embryo does not require steroidogenic factor 1. Mol Endocrinol 9:1091–1098

Lala DS, Rice DA, Parker KL (1992) Steroidogenic factor I, a key regulator of steroidogenic enzyme expression, is the mouse homolog of fushi tarazu-factor I. Mol Endocrinol 6:1249–1258

Lavorgna G, Ueda H, Clos J, Wu C (1991) FTZ-F1, a steroid hormone receptor-like protein implicated in the activation of fushi tarazu. Science 252:848–851

Lavorgna G, Karim FD, Thummel CS, Wu C (1993) Potential role for a FTZ-F1 steroid receptor superfamily member in the control of Drosophila metamorphosis. Proc Natl Acad Sci USA 90:3004–3008

Lin D, Sugawara T, Strauss JF, Clark BJ, Stocco DM, Saenger P, Rogol A, Miller WL (1995) Role of steroidogenic acute regulatory protein in adrenal and gonadal steroidogenesis. Science 267:1828–1831

Luo X, Ikeda Y, Parker KL (1994) A cell specific nuclear receptor is required for adrenal and gonadal development and for male sexual differentiation. Cell 77:481–490

Luo X, Ikeda Y, Schlosser D, Parker KL (1995) Steroidogenic factor 1 is the essential transcript encoded by the mouse Ftz-F1 gene. Mol Endocrinol 9:1233–1239

Miller WL (1988) Molecular biology of steroid hormone biosynthesis. Endocr Rev 9:295–318

Morohashi K, Honda S, Inomata Y, Handa H, Omura T (1992) A common trans-acting factor, Ad4BP, to the promoters of steroidogenic P450s. J Biol Chem 267:17913–17919

Muscatelli F, Strom TM, Walker AP, Zanaria E, Recan D, Meindl A, Bardoni B, Guioli S, Zehetner G, Rabl W, Schwarz HP, Kaplan J-C, Camerino G, Meitinger T, Monaco AP (1994) Mutations in the DAX-1 gene give rise to both X-linked adrenal hypoplasia congenita and hypogonadotrophic hypogonadism. Nature 372:672–676

Pfaff DW, Schwartz-Giblin S, McCarthy MM, Kow L-M (1994) Cellular and molecular mechanisms of female reproductive behaviors. In: Knobil E, Neill JD (eds) The physiology of reproduction, 2nd edn. Raven, New York, pp 107–220

Rice DA, Mouw AR, Bogerd A, Parker KL (1991) A shared promoter element regulates the expression of three steroidogenic enzymes. Mol Endocrinol 5:1552–1561

Shen W-H, Moore CCD, Ikeda Y, Parker KL, and Ingraham HA (1994) Nuclear receptor steroidogenic factor 1 regulates MIS gene expression: a link to the sex determination cascade. Cell 77:651–661

Tsukiyama T, Ueda H, Hirose S, Niwa O (1992) Embryonal long terminal repeat-binding protein is a murine homolog of FTZ-F1, a member of the steroid receptor superfamily. Mol Cell Biol 12:1286–1291

Zanaria E, Muscatelli F, Bardoni B, Strom TM, Guioli S, Guo W, Lalli E, Moser C, Walker AP, McCabe ERB, Meitinger T, Monaco AP, Sassone-Corsi P, Camerino G (1994) An unusual member of the nuclear hormone receptor superfamily responsible for X-linked adrenal hypoplasia congenita. Nature 372:635–641

2 Regulation of Steroid Hormone Production

M.R. Waterman

2.1 Introduction 13
2.2 Regulation of Genes Encoding Enzymes Involved
in Sex Hormone Production 15
2.2.1 Developmental/Tissue Specific Regulation 16
2.2.2 Regulation by Peptide Hormones 18
2.3 Regulation of Enzymatic Activities 21
2.3.1 Cholesterol Side Chain Cleavage Activity 21
2.3.2 17α-Hydroxylase/17,20-Lyase Deficiency 22
2.4 Conclusions and Future Directions 24
References 25

2.1 Introduction

Genotypic sex programs gonadal sex, which in turn programs pheno-typic sex. This paradigm is obvious from the examination of individuals having forms of congenital adrenal hyperplasia in which sex hormone (testosterone, estrogen) production is reduced or blocked. In 46XY individuals, sex steroid production by the fetal testis (testosterone/dihy-drotestosterone) programs development of the male phenotype as well as maturation of the resultant male secondary sex characteristics necess-ary for reproduction. Without the timely production of testosterone the phenotype is female. In 46XX individuals, ovarian production of es-trogen does not control phenotypic sex, but does regulate sexual ma-turity and reproductive capacity. Without the production of estrogen the

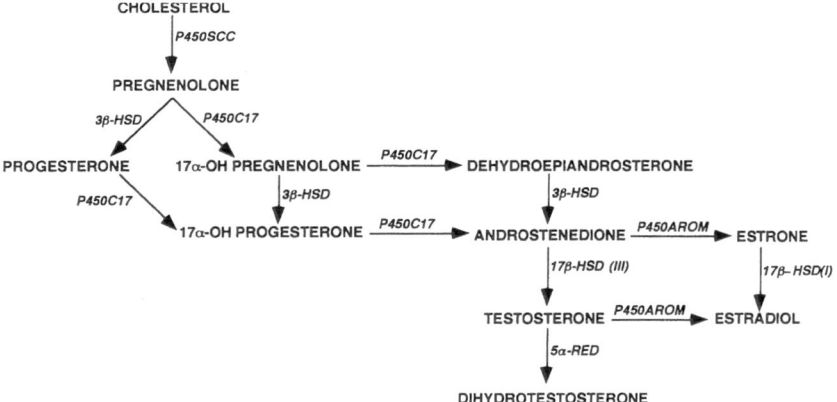

Fig. 1. Steroidogenic pathways in ovary and testis leading to sex steroid production. *P450scc,* cholesterol side chain cleavage cytochrome P450; *P450c17,* 17α-hydroxylase cytochrome P450; *3*β-HSD, 3β-hydroxysteroid dehydrogenase; *P450AROM,* aromatase cytochrome P450; *17*β-HSD, 17β-hydroxysteroid dehydrogenase; *5*α-RED, 5α-reductase

female phenotype remains immature and ovulation does not occur. Thus the 46XY karyotype programs testis development, but without testosterone production by the testis the male phenotype does not appear. The 46XX karyotype programs female gonadal sex and female phenotypic sex. Without sex hormone production, maturation of neither phenotype occurs. In both male and female, continued sex steroid production occurs throughout reproductive life.

Sex steroid production in theca and granulosa cells of the ovarian follicle and in testicular Leydig cells involves related pathways, whereby cholesterol is converted into sex hormones by a series of hemoprotein mixed-function oxidases and dehydrogenases (Fig. 1). The first step (cholesterol side chain cleavage leading to the production of pregnenolone) takes place in the mitochondrion while subsequent reactions occur in the endoplasmic reticulum. These pathways are closely related to the steroidogenic pathways in the adrenal cortex which lead to cortisol (glucocorticoid) and aldosterone (mineralocorticoid) production. Mutations in genes encoding the enzymes required for adrenal steroidogenesis lead to the group of genetic diseases collectively known as congenital adrenal hyperplasia. Mutations in the enzymes which overlap the adrenal steroidogenic pathways (P450scc, P450c17, 3β-hydroxysteroid dehydrogenase, HSD) lead to a variety of defects in the reproductive systems of both males and females, establishing for certain the importance of steroid hormone biosynthesis in human reproduction and development. This article will review the various mechanisms by which sex steroid hormone production is regulated. These mechanisms include transcriptional processes which regulate the levels of steroidogenic enzymes as well as factors which control the activities of these enzymes.

2.2 Regulation of Genes Encoding Enzymes Involved in Sex Hormone Production

Transcriptional regulation of genes encoding steroid hydroxylases is multifactorial and includes control of developmental expression, tissue-specific expression, and peptide hormone-dependent expression (Simpson and Waterman 1988). Developmental regulation assures that the orderly transition of gonadal sex to phenotypic sex and reproductive capacity occurs at properly staged times during human development. Tissue-specific regulation determines that genes encoding steroidogenic enzymes required for sex hormone biosynthesis are expressed in the gonads and not in other tissues. Regulation by peptide hormones derived from the anterior pituitary (luteinizing hormone, LH; follicle-stimulating hormone, FSH) serves the important role of assuring that optimal capacity for the synthesis of sex hormones is maintained in the gonads throughout reproductive life.

The great majority of studies on gene expression and sex steroidogenesis has focused on two steroid hydroxylases in these pathways, cholesterol side chain cleavage cytochrome P450 (P450scc) and 17α-hydroxylase cytochrome P450 (P450c17). This article will focus on regulation of CYP11A and CYP17, the genes which encode these two enzymes. While specific details concerning transcriptional control regulating the levels of P450scc and P450c17 will be described, it can be imagined that mechanisms regulating expression of genes encoding other enzymes in Fig. 1 will be similar at all levels; developmental, tissue specific, and cAMP-dependent. CYP11A(P450scc) is located on human chromosome 15 (Chung et al. 1986) while CYP17(P450c17) is on chromosome 10 (Matteson et al. 1986). These genes have been cloned in cows, mice, and rats, as well as in humans and the most detailed analysis of their transcriptional regulation by peptide hormones has been carried out using bovine genes. Furthermore, the most extensive study of the transcription of these genes has been executed in adrenocortical systems although it can be imagined that transcriptional regulation of these genes in Leydig cells, granulosa cells, and theca cells will be similar or identical to that in adrenocortical cells. Overall, general patterns of multifactorial regulation of genes encoding steroidogenic enzymes are emerging as outlined in this section.

2.2.1 Developmental/Tissue Specific Regulation

At present we cannot distinguish biochemically between developmental and tissue-specific regulation of CYP11A and CYP17. Each of the genes encoding the adrenal/gonadal steroid hydroxylases (P450scc, P450c17, 3β-HSD) and the ovarian steroid hydroxylase (P450arom), as well as the adrenal-specific steroid hydroxylases contain at least one binding site (Table 1) for the zinc-finger, orphan receptor, steroidogenic factor 1 (SF-1) (AD4BP) in their promoter regions (Lala et al. 1992; Morohashi et al. 1992). Detailed description of SF-1 and its distribution and function are found elsewhere in this volume. With reference to CYP11A and CYP17 expression, SF-1 expression in the genital ridge is observed by in situ hybridization prior to expression of the steroid hydroxylase genes (Ikeda et al. 1994). These observations strongly suggest that SF-1 plays an important role in both the developmental and tissue-specific expression of genes involved in testosterone and estrogen biosynthesis. It would not be surprising if all the genes in testis and ovary involved in sex hormone biosynthesis were activated transcriptionally at the same time by SF-1.

Disruption of the gene encoding SF-1 leads to the absence of adrenal glands and gonads and does not establish with certainty the role of SF-1 in turning on expression of genes involved in sex hormone biosynthesis (Luo et al. 1994). On the other hand, SF-1 expression remains high during fetal life in the mouse testis when testosterone production is essential for development of the male phenotype while SF-1 levels in

Table 1. Key DNA regulatory sequences in CYP11A and CYP17

SF-1   AGGTCA (consensus)
Found in all genes encoding steroidogenic enzymes in all species

CRS

		−118	−100
CYP11A (Bovine)	CRS1	ACTGAGTCTGGGAGGAGCT	
		−70	−50
	CRS2	GACCGCCCTGTCAGCTTCTCA	
		−243	−225
CYP17 (Bovine)	CRS1	TTGATGGACAGTGAGCAAG	
		−76	
	CRS2	TGAGCATTAACATAAAGTCAAGGAGAAGGT CAGGGG −40	

SF-1, steroidogenic factor 1; CRS, cAMP responsive sequences.

the fetal ovary are low throughout fetal life at a time when estrogen production is not required. Finally, certain cells in the hypothalamus express SF-1 but not any steroid hydroxylase genes, including CYP11A and CYP17 (Ikeda et al. 1995). Based on these observations it seems reasonable to propose that SF-1 is a key transcription factor required for initially turning on the expression of steroid hydroxylase genes in early fetal development, but that it is not the only regulator required for this function since these genes are not expressed in the hypothalamus when SF-1 is present. Of course, it is possible that a tissue-specific repressor blocks expression of these genes in the hypothalamus, the action of which cannot be overcome by SF-1.

Regarding tissue-specific expression it seems plausible at first glance that the same mechanisms which regulate developmental expression of CYP11A and CYP17 in testis and ovary also control tissue-specific expression. However, several examples of SF-1-independent expression of steroid hydroxylases (CYP11A in gut and skin (Keeney et al. 1995), CYP19 (aromatase) in brain (Lauber and Lichtensteiger 1994), CYP17 in stomach (Le Goascogne et al. 1995) suggest that there are multiple mechanisms which control tissue-specific expression of these genes. It is apparent that in the "factories" for production and distribution of sex hormones (testis and ovary), SF-1 plays a key role in both developmental and tissue-specific gene expression, probably in collaboration with other activators. In traditional nonsteroidogenic sites such as gut and brain, other regulatory systems which are SF-1-independent must be important.

2.2.2 Regulation by Peptide Hormones

More than 20 years ago it was demonstrated that hypophysectomy led to a decline in the levels of enzymes required for production of testosterone in rat testis (Purvis et al. 1973). Furthermore, the levels of these enzymes could be restored by treatment of hypophysectomized rats with pharmacological doses of human chorionic gonadotropin (hCG). This led to the conclusion that peptide hormones from the anterior pituitary regulate the levels of steroidogenic enzymes in testis just as they do in adrenal cortex. A similar study has not been carried out in ovary but it is believed that this paradigm holds true for enzymes required for estrogen production as well. Using primary cultures of bovine adrenocortical cells as an experimental system it has been established that several enzymes involved in the cortisol biosynthetic pathway, including P450scc and P450c17, are activated transcriptionally in a coordinate fashion by adrenocorticotropic hormone (ACTH; John et al. 1986). At present, detailed analysis of the factors required for peptide hormone-dependent transcriptional activation of genes encoding steroidogenic enzymes is underway, including CYP11A and CYP17 (Waterman 1994).

The action of peptide hormones to enhance steroid hydroxylase biosynthesis is mediated via cAMP. These peptide hormones (ACTH, LH, FSH) bind to their specific cell surface receptors in the adrenal gland, testis or ovary and activate adenylyl cyclase, leading to elevated levels of intracellular cAMP. Both acute (to be described later) and chronic actions on steroidogenic pathways result (Simpson and Waterman 1995). The chronic action is the enhanced transcription of genes encoding steroid hydroxylases and related enzymes which assures optimal steroidogenic capacity in the gonads throughout the reproductive lifespan. The great majority of investigation of the biochemical mechanisms of CYP11A and CYP17 transcription has focused on the action of ACTH in the adrenal gland. However, it seems clear that the action of LH and FSH in the gonads will utilize similar or identical mechanisms (Lauber et al. 1993). Because the mediator of transcription by peptide hormones is cAMP, it is expected that the mechanism of transcriptional regulation of these genes would be the same in all steroidogenic tissues, the only variables being the peptide hormones and their receptors. What is surprising, however, is that variation in these mechanisms seems to exist between genes and between species (Waterman 1994).

Common to all genes and species is the mechanism by which peptide hormones activate adenylyl cyclase, leading to elevated cAMP levels which in turn activate cAMP-dependent protein kinase. Variation in transcription between steroid hydroxylase genes and between species lies distal to this kinase. Because the SF-1-dependent developmental regulation appears to apply to all steroid hydroxylase genes and probably in all mammalian species and the transcription of these genes by cAMP is coordinated, it was expected that a common cAMP-dependent transcription mechanism would be present for all genes. As seen in Table 1 the cAMP-responsive sequences in bovine CYP11A and CYP17 are very different. The two elements in CYP11A bind the ubiquitous transcription factor Sp1 (Venepally and Waterman 1995). This transcription factor is not normally found to be involved in cAMP-dependent transcription although such a role for Sp1 has been reported in a few cases (Venepally and Waterman 1995). We have proposed that the cAMP-dependent transcription of CYP11A involving Sp1 is mediated through a cell-specific nuclear protein which in response to activation by cAMP interacts with Sp1 when the latter is bound to the CYP11A CRS elements. We believe that this unknown protein is not a DNA-binding protein but is activated by cAMP. Bovine CYP17 also contains two CRS elements but in this case they are distinct from one another (Lund et al. 1990). The proximal CRS (CRS2) binds two members of the nuclear receptor transcription factor superfamily, SF-1 and COUP-TF1 (Bakke and Lund 1995). These two factors compete for binding to CRS2; SF-1 being found to be the activator and COUP-TF the repressor. In a few other cases, SF-1 is reported to be involved in cAMP-dependent transcription of steroid hydroxylase genes in addition to its role in developmental/tissue-specific regulation, but the mechanism by which SF-1 plays this role remains unknown. The distal CRS in bovine CYP17 (CRS1) binds a complex of four nuclear proteins, two of which are found to be members of the Pbx homeodomain transcription factor family (Kagawa et al. 1994). Two spliced variants, Pbx1a and Pbx1b, bind to CRS1. These Pbx proteins contain a cAMP-dependent protein kinase phosphorylation site but have not yet been shown to be phosphorylated. Pbx1 was originally discovered as a result of a chromosomal translocation leading to pre-B cell acute lymphoblast leukemia (Kamps et al. 1990), and bovine CYP17 is the first cellular target identified for the Pbx gene family. It is apparent that Pbx binds to CRS1 as a complex with a partner which has not yet been identified.

Sequence analysis of the 5'-flanking region of CYP11A genes from human, rat, and mouse all indicate that Sp1-binding elements are present in the genes at approximately the same position as in bovine CYP11A (Venepally and Waterman 1995). Accordingly, it is assumed that peptide hormone-dependent transcription of CYP11A in the testis and ovary of many or all species involves Sp1 and an as yet to be identified nuclear protein which does not bind directly to DNA. Human CYP11A has also been found to have a consensus cAMP response binding element far upstream from the promoter (Inoue et al. 1991) which may participate with the Sp1 elements shown in Table 1 in optimizing the cAMP-responsive CYP11A transcription in human gonads. The 5'-flanking region of the CYP17 gene from other species does not reveal sequences closely related to bovine CRS1 and CRS2. It is possible that CYP17 in gonads of each species responds transcriptionally to cAMP via quite different mechanisms.

In summary, maintenance of optimal steroidogenic capacity in the testis and ovary of all species requires cAMP-dependent transcription of genes encoding steroid hydroxylases and perhaps other enzymes in the pathways leading to testosterone and estrogen biosynthesis. It is likely that different *cis* elements and transcription factors will be found to be associated with each gene in each pathway and that variation also exists between species. The reasons for the complexity and diversity associated with this essential aspect of reproduction in both males and females is not understood at the moment.

2.3 Regulation of Enzymatic Activities

It has now been experimentally established that, in addition to transcriptional regulation, the activities of the enzymes themselves in steroidogenic pathways require accessory proteins which can provide another level of regulation. The activities of both P450scc, a mitochondrial steroid hydroxylase, and P450c17, a microsomal steroid hydroxylase, are controlled by quite different mechanisms.

2.3.1 Cholesterol Side Chain Cleavage Activity

As indicated in the previous section, not only does cAMP mediate a chronic action on steroidogenic pathways but it also mediates an acute response (Simpson and Waterman 1988, 1995). The acute response results in mobilization of cholesterol to the vicinity of P450scc in the inner mitochondrial membrane. All mitochondrial membranes contain cholesterol, which influences their fluidity. In addition, steroidogenic mitochondria contain a separate pool of cholesterol which serves as substrate for P450scc, the first enzyme in all steroidogenic pathways (see Fig. 1). The supply of cholesterol in this steroidogenic pool is regulated by peptide hormones from the anterior pituitary via cAMP and cAMP-dependent protein kinase. The acute cAMP-dependent steroidogenic response has been known for 30 years (much longer than the chronic response has been known) and is inhibited by the protein synthesis inhibitor cycloheximide. The acute response is very rapid, such that increased production of pregnenolone in steroidogenic cells is detected within minutes of treatment with peptide hormone. The elevation of intracellular cAMP activates cleavage of cholesterol esters in lipid droplets and cholesterol is transported to mitochondria. This transporter is unknown although it is possible that sterol carrier protein 2 may serve this purpose (Jefcoate et al. 1992). In the presence of cycloheximide, cholesterol accumulates in the outer mitochondrial membrane, indicating that the cycloheximide-sensitive factor is required for transport of cholesterol from the outer mitochondrial membrane across the intermembrane space to the inner mitochondrial membrane where P450scc resides (Jefcoate et al. 1992). A protein required for this intramitochondrial transport of cholesterol has recently been discovered and is named steroidogenic acute regulatory protein (StAR) (Clark et al. 1994). How this protein functions remains unknown; perhaps it binds and transports cholesterol this distance or perhaps it serves to establish contact points between the two membranes, allowing cholesterol to diffuse from the outer membrane to the inner membrane.

Thus, the acute peptide hormone response is required for making substrate (cholesterol) available for steroidogenic pathways. Without this level of regulation, steroid hormone production would be predicted not to occur. This has now been found to be the case in congenital lipoid adrenal hyperplasia, one form of congenital adrenal hyperplasia in which mutations in StAR rather than in P450scc are present and lead to the absence of steroid hormone production (Lin et al. 1995).

2.3.2 17α-Hydroxylase/17,20-Lyase Deficiency

The 17α-hydroxylase (P450c17) plays two key roles in steroid hormone biosynthesis. In the adrenal cortex, 17α-hydroxylation of pregnenolone and/or progesterone is required for cortisol biosynthesis. In the testis and ovary the second activity catalyzed by P450c17 is the 17,20-lyase reaction which converts C21 steroids (17α-hydroxyprogesterone and/or 17α-hydroxypregnenolone) to C19 androgens, direct precursors for sex steroids. However, considerable species variation exists for the 17,20-lyase activity. The rat enzyme freely converts both 17α-hydroxyprogesterone and 17α-hydroxypregnenolone to their respective androgens (androstenedione and dehydroepiandrosterone; Fevold et al. 1989; see Fig. 1). Surprisingly, purified human P450c17 can only efficiently catalyze the conversion of 17α-hydroxypregnenolone to dehydroepiandrosterone and not that of 17α-hydroxyprogestone to androstenedione (Imai et al. 1993). As can be seen in Fig. 1, this inability to produce androstenedione would mean that any 17α-hydroxyprogesterone produced in testis and ovary would be a dead-end product and not be available for androgen synthesis. Because 3β-HSD is present in testis and ovary, significant production of 17α-hydroxyprogesterone is expected. It has recently been shown that the microsomal hemoprotein cytochrome b_5 interacts with human P450c17 and activates the conversion of 17α-hydroxyprogesterone to androstenedione (Katagiri et al. 1995). In the presence of cytochrome b_5, human P450c17 is equally efficient at

Table 2. Enhancement of human P450c17 activities by cytochrome b_5

Substrate	b_5	17α-Hydroxylase activity	17,20-Lyase activity	Hydroxylase/lyase
Pregnenolone	–	1.07	0.16	6.8
($\Delta5$)	+	2.58	1.98	1.3
Progesterone	–	2.89	0.04	80.4
($\Delta4$)	+	3.11	0.42	7.4

Activities presented as nanomoles of product per minute per nanomole P450.

androgen production in either pathway ($\Delta4$ or $\Delta5$) (Table 2). Human testis contains excess cytochrome b_5 compared to P450c17 (ratio=10:1) (Mason et al. 1973). Thus it would be predicted that because of the high level of cytochrome b_5 in testis, both the $\Delta4$ and $\Delta5$ steroidogenic pathways can lead to testosterone production. Evidence for this important role of cytochrome b_5 in testosterone production in human testis is found in one family where pseudohermaphroditism (male karyotype, female phenotype) is found to result from mutations in cytochrome b_5 (Hegesh et al. 1986; Giordano et al. 1994). This single case indicates that the activity of 3β-HSD in converting pregnenolone and 17α-hydroxypregnenolone to progesterone and 17α-hydroxyprogesterone exceeds the ability of P450c17 to convert 17α-hydroxypregnenolone to dehydroepiandrosterone in the developing testis. The absence of a functional form of cytochrome b_5 leads to a lack of androgen production at a crucial time in development and thus absence of male external genitalia. Had functional cytochrome b_5 been present in this family, 17α-hydroxyprogesterone would have been converted to androstenedione, leading to testosterone production and the male phenotype. Thus, in some species, including human, the action of cytochrome b_5 to interact with P450c17 enhances androgen production through the $\Delta4$ pathway and assures sufficient testosterone production for development of the male phenotype. Perhaps this role of cytochrome b_5 is important throughout reproductive life.

In this section we have seen that in addition to mechanisms which regulate developmental expression, tissue-specific expression, and optimal expression of genes encoding enzymes required for testosterone and estrogen biosynthesis, mechanisms controlling enzymatic activities exist within steroidogenic tissues. Besides the enzymes themselves, accessory proteins such as StAR and cytochrome b5 play essential roles in the biosynthesis of sex steroids in human tissues.

2.4 Conclusions and Future Directions

Coupling of gonadal sex with phenotypic sex and reproductive capacity is regulated by a complex array of mechanisms. Unlike many biochemical pathways (glycolysis, tricarboxylic acid cycle, cholesterol biosynthesis), steroid hormone biosynthetic pathways and their regulation show considerable variation from one mammalian species to another. Nevertheless, it is now clear that the developmental/tissue-specific regulation of genes encoding sterodogenic enzymes follows the same basic principles in steroidogenic tissues of most, if not all, species, SF-1 being essential for the presence of steroidogenic pathways in both testis and ovary. Factors that participate with SF-1 in both developmental and tissue-specific expression remain unknown. It is also unclear whether common factors partner with SF-1 in all steroidogenic genes in testis and ovary or whether different factors participate with SF-1 in each gene. These are questions waiting to be answered.

Peptide hormone-dependent regulation of optimal steroidogenic capacity in testis and ovary involves unique biochemical mechanisms for each gene. This cAMP-dependent process follows a common path up to the action of cAMP-dependent protein kinase and then diverges into gene-specific mechanisms. An obvious goal for future studies of sex steroid production in humans is to characterize at the biochemical level each of these gene-specific mechanisms and to determine whether they couple directly to developmental and tissue-specific regulatory systems.

An important new area of study in sex steroid production is the control of enzymatic activities by accessory proteins such as StAR and cytochrome b5 and the biochemical basis by which these proteins function in steroidogenic pathways. While we now have a general view of regulation of steroidogenic pathways in testis and ovary, both at the transcriptional level and the enzymatic level, the biochemistry of these various regulatory systems remains to be elucidated.

Acknowledgments. The author acknowledges the efforts of his many colleagues who have participated in studies on steroidogenesis, particularly his friend and confidant, Evan Simpson. Support of USPHS grant DK28350 is also appreciated.

References

Bakke M, Lund J (1995) Mutually exclusive interactions of two nuclear orphan receptors determine activity of a cyclic adenosine 3',5'-monophosphate-responsive sequence in the bovine CYP17 gene. Mol Endocrinol 9:327–339

Chung B-C, Matteson KJ, Voutilainen R, Mohandas TK, Miller WL (1986) Human cholesterol side-chain cleavage enzyme, P450scc: cDNA cloning, assignment of a gene to chromosome 15, and expression in the placenta. Proc Natl Acad Sci USA 83:8962–8966

Clark BJ, Wells J, King S, Stocco DM (1994) The purification, cloning and expression of a novel LH-induced mitochondrial protein in MA-10 mouse Leydig tumor cells: characterization of the steroidogenic acute regulatory protein (StAR). J Biol Chem 269:28314–28322

Fevold HR, Lorence MC, McCarthy JL, Trant JM, Kagimoto M, Waterman MR, Mason JI (1989) Rat testis $P450_{17\alpha}$: characterization of a full-length cDNA encoding a unique steroid hydroxylase capable of catalyzing both $\Delta4$ and $\Delta5$-17,20-lyase reactions. Mol Endocrinol 3:968-976

Giordano SJ, Kaftory A, Steggles AW (1994) A splicing mutation in the cytochrome b_5 gene from a patient with congenital methemoglobinemia and pseudohermaphrodism. Hum Genet 93:568–570

Hegesh E, Hegesh J, Kaftory A (1986) Contribution of cytochrome b_5. N Engl J Med 314:757–761

Ikeda Y, Shen W-H, Ingraham HA, Parker KL (1994) Developmental expression of mouse steroidogenic factor-1, an essential regulator of steroid hydroxylases. Mol Endocrinol 8:654–662

Ikeda Y, Luo X, Abbud R, Nilson JH, Parker KL (1995) The nuclear receptor steroidogenic factor 1 is essential for the formation of the ventromedial hypothalamic nucleus. Mol Endocrinol 9:478–486

Imai T, Globerman H, Gertner J, Kagawa N, Waterman MR (1993) Expression and purification of functional human 17α-hydroxylase/17,20-lyase ($P450_{17\alpha}$) in Escherichia coli: use of this system for study of a novel form of combined 17α-hydroxylase/17,20-lyase deficiency. J Biol Chem 268:19681–19689

Inoue H, Watanabe N, Higashi Y, Fujii-Kuriyama Y (1991) Structures of regulatory regions in the human cytochrome P450scc (desmolase) gene. Eur J
Biochem 195:563–569

Jefcoate CR, McNamara BC, Artemenko I, Yamazaki T (1992) Regulation of
cholesterol movement to mitochondrial cytochrome P450scc in steroid hormone synthesis. J Steroid Biochem Molec Biol 43:751–767

John ME, John MC, Boggaram V, Simpson ER, Waterman MR (1986) Transcriptional regulation of steroid hydroxylase genes by ACTH. Proc Natl
Acad Sci USA 83:4715–4719

Kagawa N, Ogo A, Takahashi Y, Iwamatsu A, Waterman MR (1994) A
cAMP-responsive sequence (CRS1) of CYP17 is a cellular target for the
homeodomain protein Pbx1. J Biol Chem 269:18716–18719

Kamps MP, Murre C, Sun X-H, Baltimore D (1990) A new homeobox gene
contributes the DNA binding domain of the t(1;19) translocation protein in
pre-B ALL. Cell 60:547–555

Katagiri M, Kagawa N, Waterman MR (1995) The role of cytochrome b_5 in
the biosynthesis of androgens by human $P450_{c17}$. Arch Biochem Biophys
317:343–347

Keeney DS, Ikeda Y, Waterman MR, Parker K (1995) Cholesterol side-chain
cleavage cytochrome P450 gene expression in primitive gut of the mouse
embryo does not require steroidogenic factor-1. Mol Endocrinol 9:1091–
1098

Lala DS, Rice DA, Parker KL (1992) Steroidogenic factor 1, a key regulator of
steroidogenic enzyme expression, is the mouse homolog of Fushi tarazu
factor 1. Mol Endocrinol 6:1249–1258

Lauber ME, Lichtensteiger W (1994) Pre- and postnatal ontogeny of aromatase cytochrome P450 messenger ribonucleic acid expression in the male
rat brain studied by in situ hybridization. Endocrinology 135:1661–1668

Lauber ME, Kagawa N, Waterman MR, Simpson ER (1993) cAMP-dependent
and tissue specific expression of genes encoding steroidogenic enzymes in
bovine luteal and granulosa cells in primary culture. Mol Cell Endocrinol
93:227–283

Le Goascogne C, Sananes N, Eychenne B, Gouezou M, Baulieu E-E, Robel P
(1995) Androgen biosynthesis in the stomach: expression of cytochrome
P450 17α-hydroxylase/17,20-lyase messenger ribonucleic acid and protein,
and metabolism of pregnenolone and progesterone by parietal cells of the
rat gastric mucosa. Endocrinology 136:1744–1752

Lin D, Sugawara T, Strauss JF, Clark BJ, Stocco DM, Saenger P, Rogol A,
Miller WL (1995) Role of steroidogenic acute regulatory protein in adrenal
and gonadal steroidogenesis. Science 267:1828–1831

Lund J, Ahlgren R, Wu D, Kagimoto M, Simpson ER, Waterman MR (1990)
Transcriptional regulation of the bovine CYP17 ($P450_{17α}$) gene. Identifica-

tion of two cAMP regulatory regions lacking the consensus CRE. J Biol Chem 265:3304-3312

Luo X, Ikeda Y, Parker KL (1994) A cell-specific nuclear receptor is essential for adrenal and gonadal development and sexual differentiation. Cell 77:481–490

Mason JI, Estabrook RW, Purvis JL (1973) Testicular cytochrome P-450 and iron-sulfur protein as related to steroid metabolism. Ann N Y Acad Sci 212:406–419

Matteson KJ, Picado-Leonard J, Chung B-C, Mohandas TK, Miller WL (1986) Assignment of the gene for adrenal P450c17 (steroid 17α-hydroxy-lasse/17,20-lyase) to human chromosome 10. J Clin Endocrinol Metab 63:789–791

Morohashi K, Honda S, Inomata Y, Handa, H, Omura T (1992) A common trans-acting factor, Ad4-binding protein, to the promoters of steroidogenic P450s. J Biol Chem 267:17913–17919

Purvis JL, Canick JA, Latif SA, Rosenbaum JH, Hologgitas J, Menard RH (1973) Lifetime of microsomal cytochrome P450 and steroidogenic enzymes in rat testis as influenced by human chorionic gonadotropin. Arch Biochem Biophys 159:39–49

Simpson ER, Waterman MR (1988) Action of ACTH to regulate the synthesis of steroidogenic enzymes in adrenal cortical cells. Annu Rev Physiol 50:427-440

Simpson ER, Waterman MR (1995) Steroid hormone biosynthesis in the adrenal cortex and its regulation by adrencorticotropin. In: DeGroot LJ (ed) Endocrinology, 3rd edn. Grune and Stratton, New York, pp 1630–1641

Venepally P, Waterman MR (1995) Two Sp1-binding sites mediate cAMP-induced transcription of the bovine CYP11A gene through the protein kinase A signaling pathway. J Biol Chem 270:25402-25410

Waterman MR (1994) Biochemical diversity of cAMP-dependent transcription of steroid hydroxylase genes in the adrenal cortex. J Biol Chem 269:27783–27786

3 A Role for cAMP-Response Element Motifs in Transcriptional Regulation of Postmeiotic Male Germ Cell-Specific Genes

Z. Sun and A.R. Means

3.1	Introduction	30
3.2	Calspermin mRNA Is Generated from the Calmodulin Kinase IV Gene in Postmeiotic Germ Cells	34
3.3	Identification of the Calspermin Promoter	36
3.4	Regulation of Expression of the Calspermin Gene Requires the CREs	40
3.5	CREMτ Binding to the CREs Stimulates Transcription of the Calspermin Gene	41
3.6	CREMτ Is the Transcription Factor Primarily Responsible for Activation of the Calspermin Gene in Testis	42
3.7	CREMτ Phosphorylated by CaM Kinase IV Stimulates Calspermin Promoter Activity	42
3.8	The First Intron of the Calspermin Gene Is Required for the Stimulatory Effect of CREMτ	43
3.9	Mechanism of Activation of Postmeiotic Germ Cell-Specific Genes	44
References	....	48

3.1 Introduction

Spermatogenesis is a series of complex developmental events by which diploid spermatogonia in the testis divide and differentiate into haploid spermatozoa (Russell et al. 1990). Stem cells divide mitotically to produce spermatogonia which either commit to the spermatogenic pathway or remain as stem cells. Cells committed to spermatogenesis undergo several mitotic divisions, and all the subsequent daughter cells of an individual stem cell remain interconnected by cytoplasmic bridges forming a cohort of cells. Subsequently, these associated and synchronous cells enter into meiosis and produce haploid spermatids. Unique morphological changes occur in the haploid cells, including remodeling and condensation of the nucleus, assembly of a flagellum, and formation of the acrosome. These differentiation events are dependent upon the temporally ordered expression of groups of gene products (Erickson 1990; Hecht 1990).

Results from isolated testicular cells confirm that postmeiotic germ cells are very active in RNA synthesis. Two-dimensional gels of in vitro translation products from mRNA purified from isolated spermatocytes and spermatids showed that there are twice as many spermatid-specific gene products as spermatocyte-specific gene products (Fujimoto and Erickson 1982), and there are few common proteins. Erickson et al. (1980) have shown that mRNAs for protamine and phosphoglycerate kinase-2 increase after meiosis (Erickson et al. 1980). Comparing some specific mRNAs in several cDNA libraries made from cells at different developmental stages in spermatogenesis also revealed that clones for some specific mRNAs increased or first appeared after meiosis (Thomas et al. 1989). The above results not only indicated that postmeiotic germ cells are active in RNA synthesis, but also revealed that many genes are transcribed only in postmeiotic cells. A number of postmeiotic-specific genes have been cloned. However, the lack of permanent cell lines or a system that supports complete spermatogenesis in vitro has slowed progress to characterize the molecular mechanisms involved in germ cell-specific transcription.

In the absence of an appropriate cell line, transgenic mice have been employed to evaluate regulatory regions of genes expressed only subsequent to late meiosis. Such studies identified a 2.4-kb DNA fragment sufficient for tissue-specific expression of the protamine 1 gene (Peschon et al. 1987). The 2.4-kb DNA fragment flanking the mouse protamine 1 gene was linked to a 237-bp DNA fragment of SV40 which served as a reporter. Mice carrying the transgene were identified, and expression of the transgene relative to the endogenous protamine gene was determined. The pattern of transgene expression was parallel to that of the endogenous gene during spermatogenesis. Upon further analysis in transgenic mice, the *cis*-acting sequences required for testis-specific protamine expression were located to a 880-bp DNA fragment just upstream of the transcription initiation site (position +1) (Zambrowicz et al. 1993). Various portions of this 880-bp DNA fragment were fused upstream of a human growth hormone (hGH) reporter gene containing 83 bp of the hGH promoter. These constructs retained the hGH TATA box element but eliminated the protamine TATA box element. Although the 83 bp of the hGH promoter itself did not target gene expression in testis, transgenic mice bearing the protamine 113-bp DNA fragment from nucleotide −150 to nucleotide −37 displayed testis-specific transcription of hGH gene. Transgenic mice were also employed to study the promoter of testis-specific angiotensin-converting enzyme (ACE) which is expressed at the same time as protamine in spermatogenesis. A 698-bp DNA fragment immediately upstream from the transcription start site of testis ACE targets LacZ reporter gene expression to round spermatids (Langford et al. 1991). Deletion analyses in transgenic mice revealed that 91 bp of this promoter fragment was sufficient for testis-specific expression of the reporter gene (Howard et al. 1993). In similar studies employing transgenic mice, an 859-bp DNA fragment 5' to the transcription start site of the mouse protamine 2 gene was found to be sufficient to specify transcription of a c-myc reporter gene to haploid spermatids (Stewart et al. 1984, 1988), a 323-bp region 5' to the testis-specific PGK-2 coding region was found to contain information essential for testis-specific and cell type-specific expression of a CAT reporter gene (Robinson et al. 1989) and a 796-bp DNA fragment containing 543 bp 5' to the transcriptional start site of testis-specific β4-galactosyltransferase directed expression of a β-galactosidase reporter gene exclusively to the pachytene spermatocytes and round spermatids of transgenic mice (Shaper et al. 1994).

In order to identify *cis*-acting sequences that regulate postmeiotic gene expression, sequence homologies present in the promoters described above have been studied. It was found that there are cyclic AMP

Table 1. The sequences of CRE motifs found in different testis-specific promoters

Testic-specific genes	Reference	Sequence of CRE motifs
Protamine 1	Johnson et al. 1988	TGACTTCA
Protamine 2	Johnson et al. 1988	ACAGGTCA
Transition protein 1	Heidaran et al. 1989	TGACGTCA
PGK-2	Robinson et al. 1989	AGAAGTCA
Tpx-1a	Mizuki et al. 1992	AGACGTCA
Tpx-1b	Mizuki et al. 1992	ATACGTCA
Thymosin	Lin et al. 1991	GCTGGTCA
ACE	Howard et al. 1993	TGAGGTCA
β4-Galactosyltransferase	Shaper et al. 1994	GACGTCG and GTACGTCA
RT7	van der Hoorn and Tarnasky 1992	TGAGGTCA
Calspermin	Sun et al. 1995a	TGACCTCA and TGATGTCA

CRE, cAMP response element; ACE, angiotensin-converting enzyme.

response element-like motifs in most of these promoters (Table 1). For example, there is a cAMP-response element (CRE) motif in the 113-bp protamine 1 promoter which was sufficient to target gene expression to haploid germ cells. This CRE could form a specific DNA–protein complex in a bandshift assay with adult testis nuclear extract, but not with nuclear extracts prepared from somatic tissues such as liver or day 12 testis which does not express protamine. A point mutation in the CRE motif abolished the binding of the testis-specific factor (Zambrowicz and Palmiter 1994). Deletion of the DNA fragment containing the CRE motif almost eliminated reporter gene expression in the testis of transgenic mice (Zambrowicz et al. 1993), suggesting that the CRE motif played a critical role in regulation of protamine gene expression. In fact, all protamine genes studied so far contain a CRE that is located in a similar position (Oliva and Dixon 1991).

The CRE motif in the 91-bp fragment of the testis-specific ACE promoter was protected from DNase I digestion in nuclear extract prepared from adult testis but not from liver (Howard et al. 1993). In an in vitro transcription assay supplemented by testis nuclear extract, this

91-bp promoter supported the highest level of transcription (Howard et al. 1993) and the transcription activity was reduced 70% by mutation of the CRE or addition to the reaction of an oligonucleotide containing the CRE sequence (Zhou et al. 1995). Similar results were obtained from studies of promoters of other postmeiotic genes. CRE motifs in the protamine 2 promoter and RT7 promoter formed specific DNA–protein complexes in adult testis nuclear extract (Johnson et al. 1991; van der Hoorn and Tarnasky 1992) and, in both cases, deletion of the CRE motifs resulted in greatly reduced promoter activity in in vitro transcription assays (Bunick et al. 1990; Delmas et al. 1993). Therefore, CRE motifs are not only conserved in the promoters of many postmeiotic germ cell-specific genes, but are also required for transcriptional activity of those promoters.

It is well known that the CRE binding protein (CREB) transcription factor binds to CREs and stimulates transcription from promoters that contain these elements (Foulkes et al. 1992; Quinn 1993; Yamamoto et al. 1988). Since CREB is expressed at constant, relatively low levels in a range of tissues and cells, it cannot account for testis specific activation of these postmeiotic genes. However, there is another CRE binding transcriptional activator, CRE modulatory protein (CREMτ), which is expressed only in adult testis (Foulkes et al. 1992). There are several isoforms of CREM; CREMα, CREMβ, CREMγ, and CREMτ. Under most circumstances only CREMτ is a transcriptional activator; the other three are transcriptional repressors. During spermatogenesis, the CREMα, β, and γ transcripts are present at low levels in premeiotic germ cells. From the prophase of meiosis, the activator, CREMτ, is transcribed exclusively and accumulates to high levels (Foulkes et al. 1992). Although spermatocytes contain abundant CREMτ mRNA, the CREMτ protein is not detected until the haploid round spermatid stage. Interestingly, the appearance of CREMτ protein corresponds to the appearance of transcripts of several other postmeiotic-specific proteins, such as protamine, RT7, and ACE. The CRE elements in the promoter regions of these genes have been shown to bind bacterially expressed CREMτ protein (Delmas et al. 1993). Moreover, CREMτ antibody reduced activity of the RT7 promoter in in vitro transcription assays supported by testis nuclear extracts (Delmas et al. 1993). These data suggested that transcriptional activation of postmeiotic germ cell-specific genes with CRE motifs in the promoters could require CREMτ.

A testis-specific factor called Tet-1 was also shown to bind to an 11-mer oligonucleotide sequence containing a CRE motif present in the protamine 1 promoter (Tamura et al. 1992). However, Zambrowicz and Palmiter (1994) have shown that residues 5' to the CRE element were required for binding of the factor present in testis nuclear extract but were not involved in Tet-1 binding. These authors concluded that Tet-1 probably was not involved in CRE-mediated transcription of the protamine 1 gene and suggested that CREMτ might represent such a factor, although this possibility was not tested directly.

The function and regulation of testis-specific Ca^{2+}/calmodulin binding proteins during spermatogenesis has been a special interest at our laboratory. Calcium is involved in the cellular actions of luteinizing hormone (LH) and follicle-stimulating hormone (FSH), the regulation of cell proliferation, acquisition of sperm motility, and the actual fertilization process. Most of the Ca^{2-}requiring events are mediated by the intracelluar Ca^{2+} receptor, calmodulin. The specificity of cellular responses to the Ca^{2+}/calmodulin signal is usually determined by the specific target proteins present in the cells. Therefore, one obvious approach to examine the function of calmodulin during spermatogenesis is to identify testis-specific targets of the Ca^{2+}/calmodulin complex. Calspermin is one of the most abundant Ca^{2+}/calmodulin-binding proteins in sperm and is expressed only in postmeiotic germ cells (Ono et al. 1984, 1985). Interestingly, when the gene was cloned, two CRE motifs were found to be present at −50 and −70 bp relative to the calspermin transcription initiation site (Means and Cruzelagui 1993). We have utilized calspermin as a model gene to study the importance of CRE motifs in the regulation of expression of postmeiotic germ cell-specific genes in mammalian testis.

3.2 Calspermin mRNA Is Generated from the Calmodulin Kinase IV Gene in Postmeiotic Germ Cells

The 1.1-kb full-length calspermin cDNA was cloned from a rat testis cDNA library (Ono et al. 1989). This cDNA hybridized to a single 1.1-kb mRNA in spermatids but also recognized a 2.0-kb mRNA present in early-stage spermatocytes and brain. The 2.0-kb cDNA was also cloned and found to encode a Ca^{2+}/calmodulin-dependent protein ki-

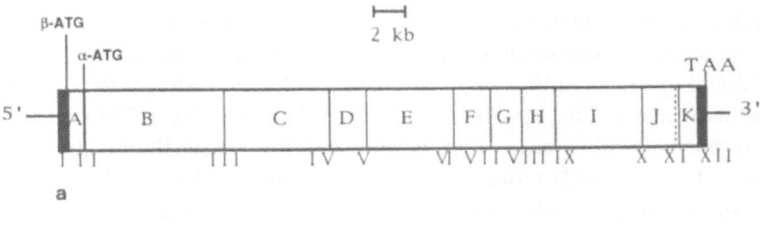

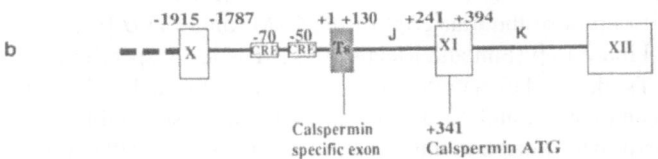

Fig. 1a,b. Schematic representation of the calmodulin (CaM) kinase IV and calspermin gene. **a** Genomic structure of the CaM kinase IV and calspermin gene. Exons are indicated by *Roman numerals* and introns are indicated by *captial letters*. CaM kinase IV is encoded by 12 exons. CaM kinase IVα is initiated in exon II, whereas the initiation of the β form is in exon I. Calspermin is encoded by three exons, two of them are shared with CaM kinase IV (exons XI and XII). The calspermin-specific exon is located within intron J and is indicated by the *dotted line*. **b** Calspermin gene structure. Exons are indicated by *boxes*, and the *shaded box* is the testis-specific calspermin exon (*Ts*); *+1* is the calspermin transcription initiation site. The *numbers* indicate the positions of the intron and exon junctions. Two CRE motifs are located at −50 and −70 relative to the transcriptional intiation site

nase (CaM kinase IVα) in which the calspermin sequence constitutes the entire 169 amino acid carboxyl terminal portion of the molecule, including the CaM-binding domain (Means et al. 1991; Jones et al. 1991; Ohmstede et al. 1991). The CaM kinase IV cDNA was used to obtain genomic DNA that was found to encode both kinase and calspermin mRNAs. The organization of about 42 kb representing the entire genomic fragment encoding this gene is shown in Fig. 1a. Exons II to XII encode the α-form of the kinase. Sakagami and Kondo (1993) cloned a β-form of CaM kinase IV mRNA which is the same as the α-form except for a unique 28 amino acid N-terminal extension. By in situ hybridization, they also showed that the α and β forms of the kinase mRNA were expressed differently in mature and developing rat brains. The predicted translation initiation codon for the β-form of the kinase is 530 bp upstream of the kinase translation initiation codon of the α-form as indicated in Fig. 1a. The first eight amino acids of CaM kinase IVβ are encoded by exon I, which is separated from exon II, encoding the rest of the unique N-terminal 20 amino acids of β and the ATG for α by a 445-bp intron A. Therefore, two isoforms of CaM kinase IV would be generated by alternative usage of exon I. We identified a transcriptionally active promoter element within intron A, and this promoter functions to produce the transcript of the CaM kinase IVα but not that for CaM kinase IVβ (Sun and Means 1995). The testis-specific calspermin exon Ts (denoted by a dotted line in Fig. 1a) is located within the intron between exons X and XI. Primer extension analysis confirmed that the calspermin transcription initiation site was the start site of exon Ts in the penultimate intron of the kinase gene. Exon Ts encodes the 5' untranslated region of calspermin mRNA, and the translation initiation ATG is represented as Met-306 of the kinase in exon XI (Fig. 1b). Therefore, the entire 169 amino acids of calspermin are identical to the carboxyl end of the kinase. Whereas calspermin mRNA is detected only in adult testis and its expression is developmentally regulated, the CaM kinase IV transcript is detected in several other somatic tissues as well as in testis (Means et al. 1991). Thus it became of interest to elucidate the mechanism by which the testis specific calspermin transcript was generated from the complex CaM kinase IV gene.

3.3 Identification of the Calspermin Promoter

Germ cell-specific transcripts are generated in testis by a number of mechanisms, including alternative splicing and alternative promoter usage. In order to distinguish which mechanism was utilized to produce the calspermin message, we analyzed the 1.8-kb intron immediately upstream of the testis-specific exon (Ts) for the presence of potential transcription factor binding sites. Two CRE motifs at nucleotides −50 and −70 relative to the transcriptional initiation site were identified (Sun et al. 1995a). Whereas the consensus CRE element is an inverted repeat sequence TGACGTCA, the −50 element in the calspermin gene is TGACCTCA and the −70 element is TGATGTCA. Since CRE motifs

Table 2. Calspermin promoter activity as a function of DNA length

Promoter constructs	CAT activity
pCATbasic	1±0.12
–80/+50	14±1.8
–80/+180	14±1.5
–80/+200	15±2.0
–80/+241	30±4.3
–80/+300	59±8.6
–80/+321	75±9.1
–80/+361	76±10.3
–200/+361	24±4.2
–300/+361	22±3.1
–400/+361	20±3.0
–500/+361	11±1.4
–1200/+361	5±0.8
–1900/+361	2±0.3

NIH3T3 cells were transfected with 10 μg of DNA containing different portions of the calspermin promoter ligated to CAT. The left panel of the table indicates the 5' and 3' terminal nucleotide of each promoter construct relative to the transcriptional initiation site of the calspermin gene (+1). CAT activity is expressed as the ratio of that obtained from the construct to be tested relative to pCAT basic which is a promoterless CAT construct. The results shown are the mean values of at least three independent experiment + S.E.M.

are found in many promoters of genes specifically expressed in postmeiotic germ cell (Delmas et al. 1993), we postulated that the DNA fragment containing the two CRE motifs served as a testis-specific promoter for the calspermin gene.

To determine whether the region containing both putative CREs functioned as a promoter, different segments of DNA upstream of the calspermin gene were linked to a CAT reporter gene (Sun et al. 1995a). The ability of each construct to direct expression of the CAT gene was analyzed following transfection of the chimeric genes into NIH3T3 cells. The results are summarized in Table 2. The DNA fragment from nucleotide –80 to nucleotide +50 had basal promoter activity. However, the highest promoter activity was obtained from the –80 to +361 DNA fragment, suggesting that an active promoter element is harbored in this

DNA fragment which also contains the 111-bp calspermin first intron from +130 to +242. The promoter activity was not significantly changed by deletion of sequences 3' to the intron region (–80/+321, –80/+300), but the deletions close to (construct –80/+242), or into the intron sequences (constructs –80/+200 and –80/+180) greatly reduced CAT activity, suggesting that the intron sequence was required for maximum promoter activity. Extensions of the promoter from –80 to –1900 progressively reduced CAT activity, and the greatest reduction resulted from extension from –80 to –200. Based on these experiments, we postulated that the negative regulatory elements between –80 and –200 contribute to the silencing of the calspermin gene in somatic tissues.

The putative calspermin promoter was identified in NIH3T3 fibroblast cells, thus direct evidence that this promoter could function in testis was required. Since a suitable germ cell line was unavailable, an in vitro transcription system was used to analyze promoter activity in testis nuclear extract (Sun et al. 1995b). The promoter region used in the in vitro assay extended from –200 to +361 of the calspermin promoter, a region which contains the negative regulatory elements between –80 and –200, both CRE motifs, and the intron. This promoter appropriately initiated transcription in testis nuclear extract and produced a transcript of the predicted size. This in vitro transcription activity was totally inhibited by α-amanitin, an RNA polymerase II inhibitor, showing that the calspermin transcript generated in vitro was the product of RNA polymerase II activity. These data implied that the promoter identified in NIH3T3 cells also functions in testis.

To test whether the –200 to +321 fragment of the calspermin promoter was sufficient to direct testis-specific gene expression in vivo, transgenic mice were generated (Sun et al. 1995b). The –200 to +321 region of the calspermin promoter was linked to a LacZ reporter gene as shown in Fig. 2a, and expression of β-galactosidase in different tissues of transgenic mice and nontransgenic littermates was measured as shown in Fig. 2b. Testis from the transgenic mice was the only tissue analyzed that expressed an elevated level of β-galactosidase activity. Immunohistochemical studies localized β-galactosidase protein primarily in the elongating spermatids and in cells from later stages of postmeiotic germ cell development. Therefore, the transgene was targeted to testis and specifically to cell types that express the endogenous calspermin gene. Expression of the transgene was also examined as a function

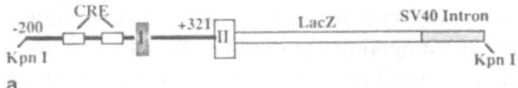

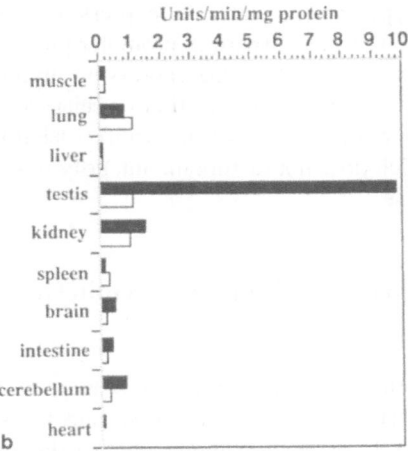

Fig. 2. a Structure of the construct used to generate transgenic mice. The −200 to +321 region of the calspermin promoter was linked to a LacZ reporter gene. *CRE*, cAMP-response element. **b** β-Galactosidase activity from various tissues. *Black bars* indicate β-galactosidase activity from tissues of postpubertal transgenic mice. *White bars* indicate β-galactosidase activity from tissues of nontransgenic littermates of the same age

of postnatal development. The first cycle of spermatogenesis begins at birth and is completed at about day 34 (Russell et al. 1990). Spermatogonia constitute the predominant germ cell population in 6 to 8-day-old mice. Leptotene and zygotene spermatocytes appear at day 10, pachytene spermatocytes at day 14, round spermatids at day 19–20, and elongating spermatids at day 23–25 (Bellve et al. 1977). Analysis of β-galactosidase transgene activity in testes from transgenic mice of different postnatal ages showed there was no significant β-galactosidase activity before day 19. The first obvious increase in β-galactosidase activity occurred between days 22 and 24, correlating with the first appearance of elongating spermatids. β-Galactosidase activity continued to increase until day 35 when the first cycle of spermatogenesis was completed. This expression pattern was entirely compatible with that of the endogenous calspermin gene. These results indicate that the −200 to +321 region of the calspermin gene is sufficient to confer a developmental and cell type-specific pattern of expression during spermatogenesis. Identification of the calspermin promoter provides a useful reagent for study of testis-specific gene expression. In addition, it should now be possible to examine the function of calspermin during spermatogenesis by generating mice with a specific deletion of the calspermin promoter which does not disrupt the integrity or expression of the CaM kinase IV gene.

3.4 Regulation of Expression of the Calspermin Gene Requires the CREs

The two CRE motifs in the calspermin promoter were protected from DNase I digestion in NIH3T3 cell nuclear extract and testis nuclear extract (Sun et al. 1995a). In order to examine whether this protection was sequence specific, several point mutations were created to disrupt the inverted repeat structure of the CRE-motifs. The −50 CRE was changed from TGACCTCA to AGTCCTGA, and the −70 CRE was changed from TGATGTCA to TCATGACT. Mutation of the CREs prevented protection in testis nuclear extract, whereas both wild-type CREs were protected. In addition, oligonucleotides based on either the −50 CRE or the −70 CRE effectively competed for protection of both CREs in a similar DNase I footprint assay. Therefore, both CREs of the calspermin promoter bind factors present in testis nuclear extract in a sequence-specific manner.

The promoter constructs containing these mutated CREs were transfected into NIH3T3 cells and studied in an in vitro transcription system to test the function of the CREs in regulation of calspermin promoter activity (Sun et al. 1995a, b). Mutation of either or both CRE resulted in greatly reduced promoter activity in both NIH3T3 cells and testis nuclear extract. Similar results were obtained from promoter constructs in which the CREs were deleted. These results suggested that both CREs bind transcription factors and stimulate transcription from the calspermin promoter in NIH3T3 cells and in testis.

3.5 CREMτ Binding to the CREs Stimulates Transcription of the Calspermin Gene

Mutations in the −50 CRE or the −70 CRE which prevented protection from DNase I digestion in testis nuclear extract also abolished binding of purified CREMτ, suggesting that CREMτ is able to bind to both CREs of the calspermin promoter in a sequence-dependent manner. In a bandshift assay in testis nuclear extract, oligonucleotides representing either CRE formed a DNA–protein complex which comigrated with a complex consisting of purified CREMτ and the corresponding CRE-containing oligonucleotide. This band disappeared if the CREMτ in testis nuclear extract was depleted using CREMτ antibody. These data suggested that both CREs of the calspermin promoter specifically bind purified CREMτ and the CREMτ present in testis nuclear extract.

In order to determine whether CREMτ had an effect on calspermin promoter activity in vivo, the −80 to +361 calspermin promoter construct containing both CRE-motifs was cotransfected into NIH3T3 cells with expression vectors encoding CREMτ and protein kinase A (PKA) (Sun et al. 1995a). The promoter activity was increased eightfold when expression vectors encoding CREMτ and PKA were cotransfected, whereas cotransfection of CREMτ or PKA alone did not result in stimulation of transcription. Similar levels of activation were achieved by cotransfection of CREB and PKA expression vectors. Deletion of both CREs resulted in the loss of the CREMτ stimulatory effect, suggesting that phosphorylated CREMτ physically binds to the CREs and stimulates transcription from the calspermin promoter. A requirement for transcription from the calspermin promoter was identified in testis nuclear extract using a specific CREMτ antibody (Sun et al. 1995b). As the amount of the CREMτ antibody added to the nuclear extract was increased, the transcription product produced from the calspermin promoter decreased. These results suggest that transcription from the calspermin promoter in testis requires CREMτ that is present in the nuclear extract.

3.6 CREMτ Is the Transcription Factor Primarily Responsible for Activation of the Calspermin Gene in Testis

Whereas the calspermin promoter (−80/+361) exhibited very high activity in NIH3T3 cells, it was totally inhibited when the length of the DNA 5' of the promoter was extended to 2.1 kb (−1.9 kb/+361). However, promoter activity of the 2.1-kb fragment was restored by cotransfection of the genes encoding CREMτ and PKA, but not by PKA and CREMα, which is generally a transcriptional inhibitor of the CREM family (Sun et al. 1995a). This result suggested that CREMτ was sufficient to restore activity to an otherwise inactive calspermin promoter in heterologous cell lines of somatic origin. A similar result was obtained with skin fibroblasts prepared from transgenic mice (Sun et al. 1995b). The β-galactosidase transgene was normally expressed only in testis of transgenic mice and not in other cells, including skin fibroblasts. However, β-galactosidase activity was restored in primary cultures of these fibroblasts by ectopic expression of CREMτ and CaM kinase IV. Ectopic expression of CREMτ did not result in expression of the endogenous calspermin gene, suggesting that, although CREMτ was sufficient to activate the calspermin transgene in somatic cells, the accessibility of the promoter region to the transcription factor was also an important determinant in cell-specific gene expression.

3.7 CREMτ Phosphorylated by CaM Kinase IV Stimulates Calspermin Promoter Activity

In vitro studies have shown that CREB can be phosphorylated by CaM kinase II and CaM kinase IV (Dash et al. 1991; Sun et al. 1994; Matthews et al. 1994), and that CREMτ can be phosphorylated by CaM kinase II. Cotransfection of CaM kinase IV and CREMτ in NIH3T3 cells resulted in an eightfold stimulation of calspermin promoter activity, which is the same level of stimulation achieved by cotransfection of PKA and CREMτ (Sun et al. 1995a). In contrast to CaM kinase IV, CaM kinase IIα did not stimulate calspermin promoter activity when cotransfected with CREMτ. Similar results were obtained by cotransfection of CREB and CaM kinase IV or CaM kinase IIα. Therefore, CaM kinase IV, but not CaM kinase IIα, can replace PKA to phosphorylate CREMτ and transcriptionally activate the calspermin gene. Since calspermin and CaM kinase IV transcripts are derived from one gene, and both proteins bind calmodulin, these results suggest the potential for the existence of an autoregulatory loop, as will be discussed later.

Phosphorylation on Ser-117 in the KID domain of CREMτ is essential for its transcription activation function (de Groot et al. 1993). Both PKA and CaM kinase II can phosphorylate this site in vitro. Our studies indicate that phosphorylation of this residue can also be catalyzed by CaM kinase IV, which is consistent with the result that phosphorylation of the equivalent site (Ser-133) of CREB by CaM kinase IV leads to its activation (Cruzalegui and Means 1993; Sun et al. 1994). PKA and CaM kinase IV phosphorylate CREB at Ser-133 only, whereas CaM kinase II can phosphorylate an additional residue, Ser-142 (Sun et al. 1994). Phosphorylation of this additional site blocks the activation of CREB by phosphorylation of Ser-133. When Ser-142 is mutated to alanine, CREB can be activated as a transcription factor by PKA, CaM kinase IV, and CaM kinase II since the only site phosphorylated is Ser-133. CREMτ has a Ser at position 126 which is in the same context as Ser-142 in CREB and de Groot et al. (1993) present evidence that Ser-126 of CREMτ is phosphorylated in vivo. Therefore, we predict that like CREB, CREMτ could be phosphorylated by CaM kinase IIα at two sites which would block activation of CREMτ.

3.8 The First Intron of the Calspermin Gene Is Required for the Stimulatory Effect of CREMτ

Transfection studies in NIH3T3 cells showed that maximal promoter activity was obtained from the −80 to +361 DNA fragment containing the 111-bp intron. Deletion, inversion of the intron, or internal deletion of the entire intron from the −80/+361 promoter not only resulted in markedly reduced promoter activity, but also eliminated the stimulatory effect of CREMτ. Thus, the first intron of the calspermin gene is required for the stimulatory effect of CREMτ on the promoter (Sun and Means 1995). Furthermore, results from our footprint and bandshift assays suggested that CREMτ could still physically bind to the CRE motifs in the absence of the intron (Sun et al. 1995a). In addition, CREMτ stimulated transcription when the intron was moved upstream of the transcription initiation site, but CREMτ lost its effect when the orientation of the intron was reversed. Therefore, the intron was required for CREMτ to activate calspermin promoter activity in a position-independent but orientation-dependent manner. A region within the intron was protected from DNase I digestion in NIH3T3 cell nuclear extract, suggesting that there are some factors binding to the intron. By deletion analysis we have found that the shortest DNA fragment that still facilitates CREMτ to stimulate transcription is the entire 111-bp intron.

3.9 Mechanism of Activation of Postmeiotic Germ Cell-Specific Genes

CRE motifs are conserved and functionally important in the promoters of many postmeiotic-specific genes. Based on the available data and our studies of transcriptional regulation of the calspermin gene, we postulate that CREMτ functions as a master transcription factor responsible for transcriptional activation of all genes that contain a CRE in their promoters and are expressed at a similar time during spermatogenesis.

Both CREB and CREMτ transcriptionally activate the calspermin gene with the same efficiency and are present in male germ cells, albeit at different developmental stages. CREB predominates in premeiotic cells which contain only the transcriptional repressor isoforms of CREM, α, β, and γ (Foulkes et al. 1991). These isoforms are not only incompetent to activate the calspermin promoter when cotransfected with PKA (Sun et al. 1995a), but also heterodimerize with CREB and inhibit its transactivation function (Laoide et al. 1993). CREMτ transcripts are first detected in late meiosis and arise from an alternative splicing event that generates exclusively the activator form of the protein from the CREM gene (Foulkes et al. 1992). The production of CREMτ has been suggested to be controlled by FSH, although how FSH acting in Sertoli cells could rapidly stimulate expression of a gene in spermatids remains an open and provocative question (Foulkes et al. 1993). CREMτ protein accumulates to very high levels in postmeiotic cells where the calspermin transcript is detected (Delmas et al. 1993; Means et al. 1991). A repressor isoform of CREM, CREM(C-G), has been reported to be expressed during spermatogenesis, but CREM(C-G) protein is limited to the elongated spermatid stage when general transcription has already terminated (Walker et al. 1994). Whereas CREB also exists in adult testis, the concentration is much lower than that of CREMτ in postmeiotic cells (Delmas et al. 1993). In addition, truncated forms of CREB containing neither nuclear translocation signals nor DNA binding domains are generated by alternative splicing mechanisms (Waeber and Habener 1992; Waeber et al. 1991). Therefore, CREMτ is the only transactivation-competent form of CRE binding protein in spermatids and is present at much higher levels than those of CREB in most other tissues (Delmas et al. 1993; Howard et al. 1993; Mellstrom et al. 1993). We postulate that the high levels of CREMτ in postmeiotic germ cells result in activation of the CRE-containing promoters of postmeiotic specific genes.

In addition to the availability of abundant CREMτ, the accessibility of the CRE-containing promoters to CREMτ also determines the state of postmeiotic gene expression. We found that cotransfection of CREMτ and CaM kinase IV results in activation of a β-galactosidase transgene in skin fibroblasts from transgenic mice, but does not result in expression of the endogenous calspermin in NIH3T3 cells or other cells of somatic origin (Sun et al. 1995b). Since the transgene likely integrates at random sites in the genome, its promoter may exist in a transcriptionally permissible environment, whereas the endogenous calspermin gene promoter may not be accessible to CREMτ produced from the transfected CREMτ gene. One of the mechanisms which determines the accessibility of promoters to transcription factors is DNA methylation (Cedar 1988). Methylation inhibits gene expression by interfering with transcription factor binding to DNA. Studies on the DNA methylation patterns of some testis-specific genes reveals good correlation between undermethylation and gene expression. The testis-specific histone 2B (Choi and Chae 1991), TP1 (Trasler et al. 1990), and PGK2 (Ariel et al. 1991) genes are undermethylated in testis and more methylated in somatic tissues where they are not expressed. We speculate that the postmeiotic gene promoters are exposed during meiosis by chromatin reorganization and/or demethylation. With the subsequent appearance of abundant CREMτ in postmeiotic cells, transcription can be activated from these promoters.

Interactions between transcription factors are the basis for transcriptional regulation (Mitchell and Tjian 1989). Interactions between CRE-

binding factors and other transcription factors have been postulated
(Imai et al. 1993; Delegeane et al. 1987; Sun and Maurer 1995). Our
studies show that the 111-bp first intron of the calspermin gene is
required for enhancement of transcription of this gene by CREMτ, via
the CRE motifs, in a position-independent but orientation-dependent
manner (Sun and Means 1995). CREMτ binds to CRE motifs but, in the
absence of the intron, it does not stimulate transcription from the calspermin promoter. Since a region in the intron was protected from
DNase I digestion in a footprint assay, we postulate that these factors
bind to the intron and interact with CREMτ in a spatially and direction-
ally specific manner. These interactions presumably stabilize the transcription initiation complex or are otherwise required for CREMτ function. Reversal of the orientation of the intron could lead to the disruption
of these spatial and directional interactions with CREMτ, explaining the
orientation dependence of the intron. Chrivia et al. (1993) identified a
coactivator of CREB, CREB binding protein which interacts with
CREB in a phosphorylation-dependent manner. We speculate that
CREMτ may have a similar coactivator which can mediate the interactions between CREMτ and intron-binding factors. The correct orientation of the intron could position intron-binding factors in the proper
conformation necessary to interact with this putative coactivator.

Based on the available data, we propose a model for the mechanism
of activation of genes specifically expressed in postmeiotic germ cells
that are regulated by CREs (Fig. 3). There are three requirements for
activation of the calspermin gene as well as other postmeiotic germ
cell-specific genes: First, abundance of CREMτ; second, a kinase that
can phosphorylate CREMτ; and third, accessibility of the calspermin
promoter region. During meiosis, CREMτ transcripts are generated and
accumulate to high levels in response to FSH (Foulkes et al. 1993;
Delmas et al. 1993). We postulate that reorganization of chromatin
occurs during meiosis and results in exposure of the calspermin promoter region (maybe by demethylation). Both PKA and CaM kinase IV
can phosphorylate CREMτ, and since both kinases exist in testis, either
could be responsible for the phosphorylation of CREMτ. However,
since CaM kinase IV is expressed earlier than CREMτ during spermatogenesis, we postulate that CaM kinase IV initially phosphorylates
CREMτ, which then participates in the activation of postmeiotic-specific genes such as calspermin which contains CRE motifs in their

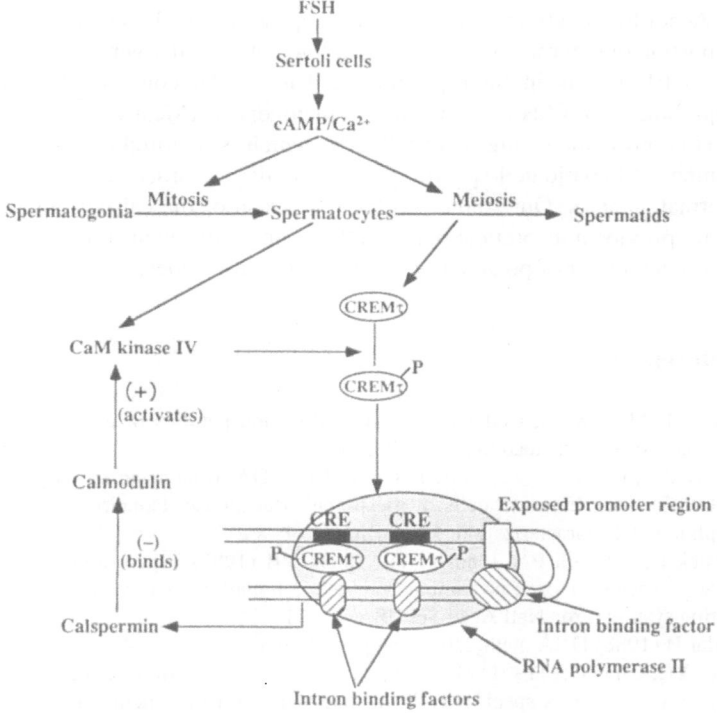

Fig. 3. Model for transcriptional regulation of the calspermin gene. *FSH*, follicle-stimulating hormone; *CaM*, calmodulin; *CRE*, cAMP-response element; *CREM*, CRE modulator; *P-CREM*, phosphorylated CREM

promoters. Calspermin binds calmodulin which is needed for activation of CaM kinase IV. The relatively high concentration of calspermin which results from activation of the gene by phosphorylated CREMτ could sequester calmodulin and thus reduce CaM kinase IV activity. With reduced CaM kinase IV activity the level of phosphorylated CREMτ would decrease and result in a concomitant decrease in transcription of the calspermin gene. In theory, transcription of the calspermin gene could be regulated by this "autoregulatory" loop. Such a mechanism could buffer these cells from an excess of calmodulin, which is generally inhibitory to differentiation at high concentrations (Epstein et al. 1989).

According to our model, the sudden appearance of abundant CREMτ in postmeiotic germ cells activates haploid cell-specific genes that contain CRE motifs in their promoters. This model could explain the requirement for FSH to complete spermatogenesis (Means et al. 1976). FSH controls the synthesis of CREMτ, which is required to activate a number of haploid cell-specific genes essential for proceeding through spermatogenesis. Our studies on the regulation of the calspermin promoter provide a theoretical but testable common mechanism for activation of a number of postmeiotic germ cell specific genes.

References

Ariel M, Mccarrey J, Cedar H (1991) Methylation patterns of testis-specific genes. Proc Natl Acad Sci USA 86:2317–2321

Bellve AR, Cavicchia JC, Millette CF, O'Brien DA, Bhatnagar YM, Dym M (1977) Spermatogenic cells of the prepubertal mouse. Isolation and morphological characterization. J Cell Biol 74:68–85

Bunick D, Johnson PA, Johnson TR, Hecht NB (1990) Transcription of the testis-specific mouse protamine 2 gene in a homologous in vitro transcription system. Proc Natl Acad Sci USA 87:891–895

Cedar H (1988) DNA methylation and gene activity. Cell 53:3–4

Choi YC, Chae CB (1991) DNA hypomethylation and germ cell-specific expression of testis-specific H2B histone gene. J Biol Chem 266:20504–20511

Chrivia JC, Kwok RP, Lamb N, Hagiwara M, Montminy MR, Goodman RH (1993) Phosphorylated CREB binds specifically to the nuclear protein CBP. Nature 365:855–859

Cruzalegui FH, Means AR (1993) Biochemical characterization of the multifunctional Ca^{2+}/calmodulin-dependent protein kinase type IV expressed in insect cells. J Biol Chem 268:26171–26178

Dash PK, Karl KA, Colicos MA, Prywes R, Kandel ER (1991) cAMP response element-binding protein is activated by Ca^{2+}/calmodulin-as well as cAMP-dependent protein kinase. Proc Natl Acad Sci USA 88:5061–5065

de Groot RP, Hertog JD, Vandenheede JR, Goris J, Sassone-Corsi P (1993) Multiple and cooperative phosphorylation events regulate the CREM activator function. EMBO J 12:3903–3911

Delegeane AM, Ferland LH, Mellon PL (1987) Tissue-specific enhancer of the human glycoprotein hormone alpha-subunit gene: dependence on cyclic AMP-inducible elements. Mol Cell Biol 7:3994–4002

Delmas V, van der Hoorn F, Mellstrom B, Jegou B, Sassone-Corsi P (1993) Induction of CREM activator proteins in spermatids: down-stream targets and implications for haploid germ cell differentiation. Mol Endocrinol 7:1502–1514

Epstein PN, Christenson MA, Means AR (1989) Chicken calmodulin promoter activity in proliferating and differentiated cells. Mol Endocrinol 3:193–202

Erickson RP (1990) Post-meiotic gene expression. TIG 6:264–269

Erickson RP, Kramer JM, Rittenhouse J, Salkeld A (1980) Quantitation of mRNAs during mouse spermatogenesis: protamine-like histone and phosphoglycerate kinase-2 mRNAs increase after meiosis. Proc Natl Acad Sci USA 77:6086–90

Foulkes NS, Borrelli E, Sassone-Corsi P (1991) CREM gene: use of alternative DNA-binding domains generates multiple antagonists of cAMP-induced transcription. Cell 64:739–749

Foulkes NS, Mellstrom B, Benusiglio E, Sassone-Corsi P (1992) Developmental switch of CREM function during spermatogenesis: from antagonist to activator. Nature 355:80–84

Foulkes NS, Schlotter F, Pevet P, Sassone-Corsi P (1993) Pituitary hormone FSH directs the CREM functional switch during spermatogenesis. Nature 362:264–267

Fujimoto H, Erickson RP (1982) Functional assays for mRNA detect many new messages after male meiosis in mice. Biochem Biophys Res Commun 108:1369–1375

Hecht NB (1990) Regulation of "haploid expressed genes" in male germ cells. J Reprod Fertil 88:679–693

Heidaran MA, Kozak CA, Kistler WS (1989) Nucleotide sequence of the Stp-1 gene coding for rat spermatid nuclear transition protein 1 (TP1): homology with protamine P1 and assignment of the mouse Stp-1 gene chromosome 1. Gene 75:39–46

Howard T, Balogh R, Overbeek P, Bernstein KE (1993) Sperm-specific expression of angiotensin-converting enzyme (ACE) is mediated by a 91 base pair promoter containing a CRE like element. Mol Cell Biol 13:18–27

Imai E, Miner JN, Mitchell JA, Yamamoto KR, Granner DK (1993) Glucocorticoid receptor-cAMP response element-binding protein interaction and the response of the phosphenolpyruvate carboxykinase gene to glucocorticoids. J Biol Chem 268:5353–5356

Johnson P, Peschon JJ, Yelick PC, Palmiter RD, Hecht NB (1988) Sequence homologies in the mouse protamine 1 and 2 genes. Biochim Biophys Acta 950:45–53

Johnson PA, Bunick D, Hecht NB (1991) Protein binding regions in the mouse and rat protein-2-genes. Biol Reprod 44:127–34

Jones DA, Glod J, Silson-Shaw D, Hahn WE, Sikela JM (1991) cDNA sequence and differential expression of the mouse Ca^{2+}/calmodulin-dependent protein kinase IV gene. FEBS Lett 289:105–109

Langford KG, Shai SY, Howard TE, Kovac MJ, Overbeek PA, Bernstein KE (1991) Transgenic mice demonstrate a testis-specific promoter for angiotensin-converting enzyme. J Biol Chem 266:15559–15562

Laoide BM, Foulkes NS, Schlotter F, Sassone-Corsi P (1993) The functional versatility of CREM is determined by its modular structure. EMBO J 12:1179–1191

Lin SC, Morrison-Bogorad M (1991) Cloning and characterization of a testis-specific thymosin b10 cDNA. J Biol Chem 266:23347–23353

Matthews RP, Guthrie CR, Wailes LM, Zhao X, Means AR and McKnight GS (1994) Calcium/calmodulin-dependent protein kinase types II and IV differentially regulated CREB-dependent gene expression. Mol Cell Biol 14:6107–6116

Means AR, Cruzalegui F (1993) Differential gene expression from a single transcription unit during spermatogenesis. Rec Prog Horm Res 48:79–97

Means AR, Fakunding JL, Huckins C, Tindall DJ, Vitale R (1976) Follicle-stimulating hormone, the Sertoli cell, and spermatogenesis. Rec Prog Horm Res 32:477–527

Means AR, Cruzalegui F, LeMagueresse B, Needleman D, Slaughter GS, Ono T (1991) A novel Ca^{2+}/calmodulin-dependent protein kinase and a male germ cell-specific calmodulin-binding protein are derived from the same gene. Mol Cell Biol 11:3960–3971

Mellstrom B, Naranjo JR, Foulkes NS, Lafarga M, Sassone-Corsi P (1993) Transcriptional response to cAMP in brain: specific distribution and induction of CREM antagonists. Neuron 10:655–665

Mitchell PJ, Tjian R (1989) Transcriptional regulation in mammalian cells by sequence-specific DNA binding proteins. Science 245:371–378

Mizuki N, Sarapata DE, Garcia-Sanz JA, Kasahara M (1992) The mouse male germ cell-specific gene Tpx-1: molecular structure, mode of expression in spermatogenesis, and sequence similarity to two non-mammalian genes. Mammalian Genome 3:274–280

Ohmstede C, Bland MM, Merrill BM, Sahyoun N (1991) Relationship of genes encoding Ca^{2+}/calmodulin-dependent protein kinase Gr and calspermin: a gene within a gene. Proc Natl Acad Sci USA 88:5784–5788

Oliva R, Dixon G (1991) Vertebrate protamine genes and the histone-to-protamine replacement reaction. Prog Nucleic Acid Res Mol Biol 40:25–94

Ono T, Koide Y, Arai Y, Yamashita K (1984) Heat-stable calmodulin binding protein in rat testis. J Biol Chem 259:9011–9016

Ono T, Koide Y, Yamashita K (1985) Establishment of an efficient purification method and further characterization of 32 K calmodulin-binding protein in testis. J Biochem (Tokyo) 98:1455–1461

Ono T, Slaughter GR, Cook RG, Means AR (1989) Molecular cloning, sequence and distribution of rat calspermin, a high affinity calmodulin-binding protein. J Biol Chem 264:2081–2087

Peschon JJ, Behringer RR, Brinster RL, Palmiter RD (1987) Spermatid-specific expression of protamine 1 in transgenic mice. Proc Natl Acad Sci USA 84:5316–5319

Quinn GP (1993) Distinct domains with cAMP response element-binding protein (CREB) mediate basal and cAMP-stimulated transcription. J Biol Chem 268:16999–17009

Robinson MO, McCarrey JR, Simon MI (1989) Transcriptional regulatory regions of testis-specific PGK2 defined in transgenic mice. Proc Natl Acad Sci USA 86:8437–8441

Russell LD, Ettlin RA, Sinha Hakim AP, Clegg ED (1990) Histological and histopathological evaluation of the testis. Cache River, Clearwater

Sakagami H, Kondo H (1993) Cloning and sequencing of a gene encoding the b polypeptide of Ca^{2+}/calmodulin-dependent protein kinase IV and its expression confined to the mature cerebellar granule cells. Mol Brain Res 19:215–218

Shaper NL, Harduin-lepers A, Shaper JH (1994) Male germ cell expression of murine beta-4-galactosyltransferase. J Biol Chem 269:25165–25171

Stewart TA, Bellve AR, Leder P (1984) Transcription and promoter usage of the myc gene in normal somatic and spermatogenic cells. Science 226:707–710

Stewart TA, Hecht NB, Hollingshead PG, Johnson PA, Leong JL, Pitts SL (1988) Haploid specific transcription of protamine-myc and protamine T anigen fusion genes in transgenic mice. Mol Cell Biol 8:1748–1755

Sun P, Maurer RA (1995) An inactivating point mutation demonstrates that interaction of cAMP response element binding protein (CREB) with the CREB binding protein is not sufficient for transcriptional activation. J Biol Chem 270:7041–7044

Sun Z, Means AR (1995) An intron facilitates activation of the calspermin gene by the testis specific transcription factor CREMτ. J Biol Chem 270:20962–20967

Sun P, Enslen H, Myung PS, Maurer RA (1994) Differential activation of CREB by Ca^{2+}/calmodulin-dependent protein kinases type II and type IV involves phosphorylation of a site that negatively regulates activity. Genes Dev 8:2527–2539

Sun Z, Sassone-Corsi P, Means AR (1995a) Calspermin gene transcription is regulated by two cyclic AMP response elements contained in an alternative promoter in the calmodulin kinase IV gene. Mol Cell Biol 15:561–71

Sun Z, Means RL, LeMagueresse B, Means AR (1995b) Organization and analysis of the complete rat calmodulin dependent protein kinase IV gene. J Biol Chem 270:29507–29514

Tamura T, Makino Y, Mikoshiba K, Muramatsu M (1992) Demonstration of a testis-specific trans-acting factor Tet-1 in vitro that binds to the promoter of the mouse protamine 1 gene. J Biol Chem 267:4327–4332

Thomas KH, Wilkie TM, Tomashefsky P, Bellve AR, Simon MI (1989) Differential gene expression during mouse spermatogenesis. Biol Reprod 41:729–739

Trasler JM, Hake LE, Johnson PA, Alcivar AA, Millette CF, Hecht NB (1990) DNA methylation and demethylation events during meiotic prophase in the mouse testis. Mol Cell Biol 10:1828–1834

van der Hoorn FA, Tarnasky HA (1992) Factors involved in regulation of RT7 promoter in a male germ cell-derived in vitro transcription system. Proc Natl Acad Sci USA 89:703–707

Waeber G, Habener JF (1992) Novel testis germ cell-specific transcript of the CREB gene contains an alternatively spliced exon with multiple in-frame stop codons. Endocrinology 131:2010–2015

Waeber G, Meyer TE, Lesieur M, Hermann HL, Gerard N, Habener JF (1991) Developmental stage-specific expression of cyclic adenosine 3',5'-monophosphate response element-binding protein CREB during spermatogenesis involves alternative exon splicing. Mol Endocrinol 5:1418–1429

Walker WH, Sanborn BM, Habener JF (1994) An isoform of transcription factor CREM expressed during spermatogenesis lacks the phosphorylation domain and represses cAMP-induced transcription. Proc Natl Acad Sci USA 91:12423–12427

Yamamoto KK, Gonzalez GA, Biggs WH, Montminy MR (1988) Phosphorylation-induced binding and transcriptional efficacy of nuclear factor CREB. Nature 334:494–498

Zambrowicz BP, Harendza CJ, Zimmermann JW, Brinster RL, Palmiter RD (1993) Analysis of the mouse protamine 1 promoter in transgenic mice. Proc Natl Acad Sci USA 90:5071–5075

Zambrowicz BP, Palmiter RD (1994) Testis-specific and ubiquitous proteins bind to functionally important regions of the mouse protamine-1 promoter Biol Reprod 50:65–72

Zhou Y, Delafontaine P, Martin BM, Bernstein KE (1995) Identification of two positive transcriptional elements within the 91 bp promoter for mouse testis angiotensin converting enzyme (testis ACE). Dev Gen 16:201–209

4 Cyclic Nucleotide-Gated Channels in Sperm

I. Weyand

4.1   Introduction 53
4.2   Cyclic Nucleotides as Internal Messengers in Sperm 55
4.3   CNG Ion Channels 56
4.4   CNG Channels in Sperm 58
4.5   Function of CNG Channels in Sperm 61
4.6   Summary 64
References 64

4.1 Introduction

The successful encounter and fusion of gametes are a premise for the development of a new organism by sexual reproduction. This is achieved by a complex series of interactions between the motile sperm and the egg. Although our knowledge of these interactions is now expanding rapidly, many molecular mechanisms are still unknown, in particular because the details of fertilization vary considerably among species. Several stages of sperm–egg interactions can be distinguished during fertilization (Fig. 1). Prior to sperm–egg contact, sperm are directed towards the egg by signals either secreted by the egg itself or by the female reproductive tract. Chemoattraction of sperm has been well documented in species with external fertilization, for example, in many marine invertebrates (e.g., Miller 1985; Ward et al. 1985), whereas chemoattraction of vertebrate sperm is still a matter of discussion (Ma-

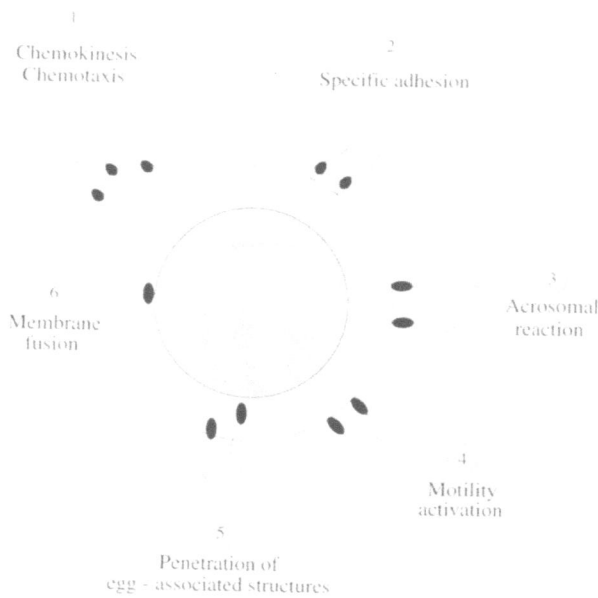

Fig. 1. The main stages of sperm–egg interaction. An egg is shown surrounded by its extracellular matrix. Acrosome-intact sperm arrive at the egg in response to chemoattractive signals (*1*). Sperm specifically bind to the extracellular matrix (*2*), and undergo the acrosomal exocytosis induced by signals from the matrix (*3*). Sometimes, acrosome-reacted sperm show changes in motility which may help to penetrate the extracellular matrix (*4*). After penetration of the matrix (*5*), the plasma membranes of the sperm and the egg interact and then fuse (*6*), resulting in egg activation. After Ward and Kopf (1993)

kler et al. 1995). However, recent studies argue for factors being involved in chemoattraction of human sperm (Ralt et al. 1991, 1994). A subsequent stage of sperm–egg interaction involves binding of sperm to the extracellular glycoprotein matrix of the egg. After binding, sperm undergo acrosomal exocytosis induced by signals from the extracellular matrix and subsequently penetrate the egg matrix. The plasma membranes of the sperm and the egg interact with each other and fuse; finally, the egg becomes activated. A detailed description of the different stages of fertilization is beyond the scope of this article and the reader is referred to other reviews (e.g., Ward and Kopf 1993; Myles 1993; Foltz and Lennarz 1993).

4.2 Cyclic Nucleotides as Internal Messengers in Sperm

In recent years, a growing body of experimental evidence suggests that cyclic nucleotides play an important role in sperm motility, chemoattraction, capacitation, and acrosomal exocytosis. (Maturational processes of sperm in the female reproductive tract which are poorly understood are collectively called capacitation.) Although a multitude of publications emphasize the role of cyclic nucleotides as internal messengers in both vertebrate and invertebrate sperm, we still know relatively little about the cyclic nucleotide signaling pathways when compared with our understanding of similar pathways in vertebrate photoreceptor cells or olfactory sensory neurons (OSNs). In particular, the sequence of intracellular events, their time course, and the coupling with other signaling pathways, for example, Ca^{2+} metabolism, are still poorly understood. It has become clear that sperm behavior can be affected by a bewildering variety of factors. Moreover, vertebrate sperm represent a heterogenous population of cells that are in different stages with respect to morphology, age, motility behavior, and the ability to respond to external stimuli. Besides, due to their morphology, investigations of signaling pathways in sperm with biophysical techniques are demanding, and direct molecular biology approaches are cumbersome for lack of poly(A)$^+$ RNA in sperm.

Twenty-five years ago, Garbers et al. (1971) showed that cyclic nucleotides or phosphodiesterase inhibitors can stimulate sperm motility. Many subsequent studies have confirmed these basic observations both for vertebrates and invertebrates (for reviews, see Garbers and Kopf 1980; Tash 1990; Morisawa 1994). The motility-stimulating effect of cAMP has been attributed to the phosphorylation of flagellar proteins, for example, dynein, by cAMP-dependent protein kinase (Tash 1990). Not only motility, but also capacitation, hyperactive motility, and acrosomal exocytosis are associated with changes in the intracellular concentration of cyclic nucleotides. Numerous studies have identified cAMP as the cyclic nucleotide in question (for review, see Fraser and Monks 1990). In contrast, convincing evidence for enzymes regulating the concentration of cGMP is still lacking in vertebrate sperm (Gray et al. 1976), and consequently cGMP has received little attention as internal messenger. In the guinea-pig, however, cGMP regulates acrosomal exocytosis most probably via a cGMP-induced Ca^{2+} influx into sperm (Santos-Sacchi and Gordon 1980).

For invertebrate sperm, cGMP is much more accepted as internal messenger. For example, chemoattraction of sea urchin sperm utilizes a cGMP-signaling pathway (Garbers 1989). Peptides secreted from sea urchin eggs specifically bind to membrane receptors of sperm. Subsequently, the intracellular concentrations of both cGMP and cAMP and of Ca^{2+} are elevated (Hansbrough and Garbers 1981; Schackmann and Chock 1986; Cook et al. 1994). One of the membrane receptors has been identified as a guanylyl cyclase (Shimomura et al. 1986), and a cGMP-specific phosphodiesterase has been also demonstrated in sea urchin sperm (Toowicharanont and Shapiro 1988). But even in sea urchin sperm, the sequence of intracellular events, the cellular targets, and the precise physiological function of cGMP are still enigmatic. In general, cellular targets of cyclic nucleotides are cAMP- or cGMP-dependent protein kinases and cyclic nucleotide-gated (CNG) ion channels.

4.3 CNG Ion Channels

CNG channels were first discovered in vertebrate photoreceptor cells (Fesenko et al. 1985; Haynes and Yau 1985) and OSNs (Nakamura and Gold 1987), where they transduce the respective stimulus into electrical signals. They are either nonselective cation or selective K^+ channels (del Pilar Gomez and Nasi 1995) that are opened by the binding of cAMP or cGMP to an intracellular binding site (for reviews, see Zufall et al. 1994; Yau 1994; Kaupp 1995). Several distinct CNG channels have been discovered by molecular cloning and electrophysiological techniques in a variety of neuronal and non-neuronal cells (for review, see Kaupp 1995). However, except for CNG channels in sperm (Weyand et al. 1994), little is known about the precise site of expression in non-neuronal tissue.

CNG channels form hetero-oligomeric complexes consisting of several distinct, yet homologous (so-called α and β) subunits. In verte-

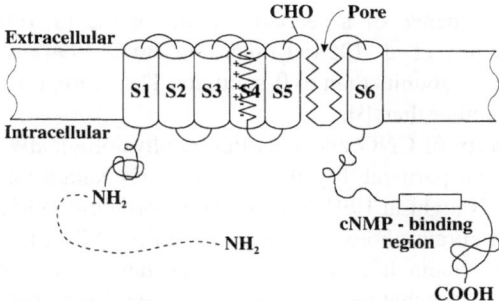

Fig. 2. The transmembrane topology of cyclic nucleotide-gated (CNG) channel α-subunit. CNG channel α-subunits carry six membrane-spanning segments (*S1–S6*), including a residual voltage-sensor (*S4*) motif. The topology model is consistent with the intracellular localization of the amino and carboxyl termini (Molday et al. 1991), and N-glycosylation (CHO) of the rod photoreceptor α-subunit (Wohlfart et al. 1992). The amino terminus of the rod photoreceptor α-subunit is cleaved post-translationally (Molday et al. 1991). After Henn et al. (1995)

brates, three distinct genes encoding α-subunits have been identified. The respective gene products are expressed either in OSNs (Dhallan et al. 1990; Ludwig et al. 1990; Goulding et al. 1992), or in rod (Kaupp et al. 1989; Bönigk et al. 1993), or in cone (Bönigk et al. 1993; Weyand et al. 1994) photoreceptor cells. These three α-subunit genes seem to be expressed in other tissues as well. For example, cDNA clones encoding the cone α-subunit have been isolated from testis (Weyand et al. 1994), kidney (Biel et al. 1994), and pineal gland (Bönigk et al., unpublished data).

The transmembrane topology of the α-subunit is now reasonably well understood (Henn et al. 1995; Fig. 2). The α-subunits carry six membrane-spanning segments, with the amino and carboxy termini and the cyclic nucleotide-binding domain located intracellularly. When heterologously expressed, the α-subunits form functional channels by themselves. In contrast, the β-subunits do not form functional channels by themselves, but confer on the respective α-subunits specific properties that are more characteristic of the native channels (Chen et al. 1993; Liman and Buck 1994; Bradley et al. 1994; Körschen et al. 1995). [The amino acid sequence of a second subunit of the rat olfactory CNG channel (Bradley et al. 1994; Liman and Buck 1994) is much more similar to all α-subunits than to β-subunits. Therefore, this subunit may represent α_2 rather than β].

One property of CNG channels that is physiologically important is their substantial permeability for Ca^{2+} ions (Nakatani and Yau 1988; Perry and McNaughton 1991; Picones and Korenbrot 1995; Frings et al. 1995). In vertebrate photoreceptor cells and in OSNs, the Ca^{2+} influx through CNG channels represents an important constituent of several Ca^{2+} feedback mechanisms (for reviews, see Koch 1994; Shepherd 1994). Ca^{2+} controls the cyclic nucleotide-signaling pathways by regulating synthesis or hydrolysis of cyclic nucleotides and by decreasing the ligand sensitivity of CNG channels via a Ca^{2+}/calmodulin-dependent mechanism. In the rod photoreceptor CNG channel, the β-subunit is responsible for regulating the ligand sensitivity by Ca^{2+}/calmodulin (Hsu and Molday 1993; Körschen et al. 1995), whereas in the olfactory channel, the α-subunit itself acts as sensor for Ca^{2+}/calmodulin (Liu et al. 1994).

The activity of other ion channels, in particular voltage-activated K^+ channels, is also modulated by the binding of cyclic nucleotides. However, these cyclic nucleotide-modulated (CNM) channels do not require cyclic nucleotides to open. The primary structures of a few CNM channels (e.g., *eag* K^+ channels) are known (Warmke and Ganetzky 1994; Ludwig et al. 1994), and the genetic and functional relationships between CNM and CNG channels are currently examined.

4.4 CNG Channels in Sperm

The best characterized CNG channel in sperm is the channel in bovine sperm. The primary structure, the cellular localization, and the principal electrophysiological properties of the CNG channel α-subunit have now been unraveled (Weyand et al. 1994; Spoormaker et al., manuscript in preparation). It is unknown whether CNG channels exist in invertebrate sperm as well. However, for sea urchin a cGMP-modulated K^+ channel has been postulated as a component of a signaling pathway controlling chemoattraction of sperm (Cook et al. 1994). Future work is required to demonstrate such a channel and its biological function.

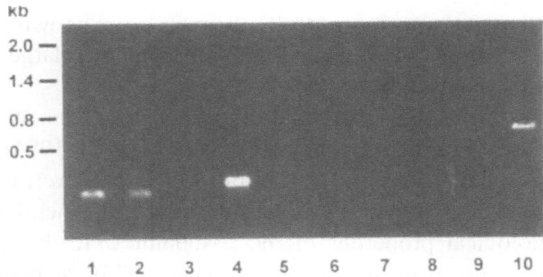

Fig. 3. Analysis of amplified polymerase chain reaction (PCR) fragments. PCR was carried out on cDNA from bovine testis (*lanes 1, 3, 5*) and retina (*lanes 2, 4, 6*) with gene-specific primers for *c*CNGCα (*lanes 1, 2*), *r*CNGCα (*lanes 3, 4*) and *o*CNGCα (*lanes 5, 6*). The testis tissue exclusively contained transcripts of *c*CNGCα, whereas the retina contained transcripts of both *c*CNGCα and *r*CNGCα. *Lanes 7–9*, negative controls; PCR with the gene-specific primers but without cDNA. *Lane 10*, positive control for *o*CNGCα-specific primers; cloned olfactory cDNA (Ludwig et al. 1990) was used as a template

The primary structure of the channel α-subunit was determined by cloning of cDNA from testis. The amino acid sequence is similar but distinct from the α-subunits expressed in rod photoreceptors (*r*CNGCα) and OSNs (*o*CNGCα). Surprisingly, the testis channel α-subunit is also expressed in cone photoreceptors, and in fact has been designated cone CNG channel α-subunit (*c*CNGCα). Polymerase chain reaction (PCR) analysis showed that testis tissue exclusively expresses transcripts of *c*CNGCα, whereas the retina expresses transcripts of both *c*CNGCα and *r*CNGCα (Fig. 3). Immunohistochemistry on bovine testis indicates postmeiotic expression of the CNG channel, and ejaculated sperm display α-subunit-specific immunoreactivity in the postacrosomal region and the tail. In Western blots of sperm membrane proteins the α-subunit behaves as a protein with a molecular mass (M_W) of ~ 70 kDa. The α-subunit heterologously expressed in human embryonic kidney (HEK 293) cells has a M_W of ~ 82 kDa which is virtually identical to the M_W value expected from the deduced amino acid sequence. These results suggest that the α-subunit in sperm may also exist in a proteolytically processed form as has been previously described for rod and cone α-subunits (Molday et al. 1991; Bönigk et al. 1993). While the physiological function of processing of CNG channels is not known, posttranslational modifications of α-subunits in general may enlarge the functional diversity of CNG channels.

Patch-clamp recording demonstrated that CNG channels are functionally expressed in sperm membranes (Weyand et al. 1994). The low success rate of patch-clamping sperm precluded, however, a thorough electrophysiological characterization of the native channel. Instead, the electrophysiological properties of the α-subunit were determined by heterologous expression in *Xenopus* oocytes. cGMP activates the α-subunit at $\geq$ 100-fold lower concentrations than cAMP. Mean values for half-maximal activation were ~ 8 μM for cGMP and ~ 1.7 mM for cAMP, suggesting that sperm rely on cGMP as the physiological ligand of the channel.

It is not surprising that the α-subunit is much more sensitive for cGMP , considering the role of cGMP as internal messenger in cone photoreceptor cells (Haynes and Yau 1985). The cGMP selectivity requires that cGMP also seriously be considered as a cellular messenger in vertebrate sperm, and that the proteins and regulatory mechanisms that control the cGMP concentration be identified.

The low channel density suggests that the principal function of CNG channels in sperm might be rather to control Ca^{2+} influx than to electrically excite the cell. In fact, Frings et al. (1995) recently showed that the heterologously expressed cCNGCα is 20-fold more permeable to Ca^{2+} than rCNGCα. Attempts to detect a CNG channel-mediated Ca^{2+} influx in intact sperm failed so far (Weyand et al. 1994), and this important piece of information still needs to be provided.

Compared to the heterologously expressed α-subunit, the single-channel conductance of the native CNG channel is smaller and its gating behavior is faster. These differences suggested that the sperm α-subunit, like the rod CNG channel, requires an additional subunit to exhibit native properties. In fact, we have identified a β-subunit of the CNG channel in sperm by cloning cDNA and immunocytochemical studies (Weiner et al. unpublished data). Remarkably, only the posterior part of the sperm tail displays both α- and β-subunit-specific immunoreactivity. These results suggest that homo- and hetero-oligomeric channels may coexist in sperm.

The β-subunit of the rod CNG channel, when coexpressed with the α-subunit, changes blockage by extracellular Ca^{2+} (Körschen et al.

1995). It probably also influences Ca^{2+} permeability, although that has not yet been shown. If so, an asymmetric distribution of homo- and hetero-oligomeric channels could lead to a Ca^{2+} gradient along the tail and the postacrosomal region of the sperm. In fact, oscillating changes of $[Ca^{2+}]_i$ have been demonstrated to occur in hamster sperm during hyperactive motility (Suarez et al. 1993). Interestingly, the flagellar-beating pattern of hyperactive vertebrate sperm resembles that of some marine invertebrate sperm as they respond to chemoattractive factors from eggs (e.g., Miller 1985; Cosson 1990). Regardless of whether hyperactive motility possibly represents a form of chemotactic behavior in vertebrate sperm (Suarez et al. 1993), similar mechanisms could underlie this flagellar-beating pattern in marine invertebrates and vertebrates. It will be important for future work to measure the Ca^{2+} permeability of homo- and hetero-oligomeric sperm CNG channels and to examine the spatial pattern of Ca^{2+} entry into sperm via CNG channels.

4.5 Function of CNG Channels in Sperm

In many invertebrates, chemoattraction of sperm is strongly dependent on extracellular Ca^{2+} (for review, see e.g., Cosson 1990), and in sea urchin, the best studied species so far, on cyclic nucleotides as well (e.g., Garbers 1989; Cook et al. 1994). Recent studies also argue for chemoattraction of vertebrate sperm (e.g., Ralt et al. 1994); however, the molecular basis of this cellular process is unknown. Figure 4 illustrates several speculative scenarios underlying chemoattraction. Some of the mechanisms and components depicted in Fig. 4 have been identified in sea urchin sperm, whereas others have been discovered in mammalian sperm. No coherent and complete picture has emerged from any one signaling pathway.

In sea urchin, a membrane-bound guanylyl cyclase has been identified as receptor for a chemoattractive peptide (Shimomura et al. 1986); however, the underlying signaling pathway and the Ca^{2+} entry mechanism are still a matter of debate. In vertebrates, neither chemoattractive factors nor their receptors, let alone the internal messenger(s), have been identified. Recently, members of the family of putative olfactory receptors have been identified in mammalian sperm, leading to the hypothesis that these proteins may serve as receptors for chemotactic signals (Van-

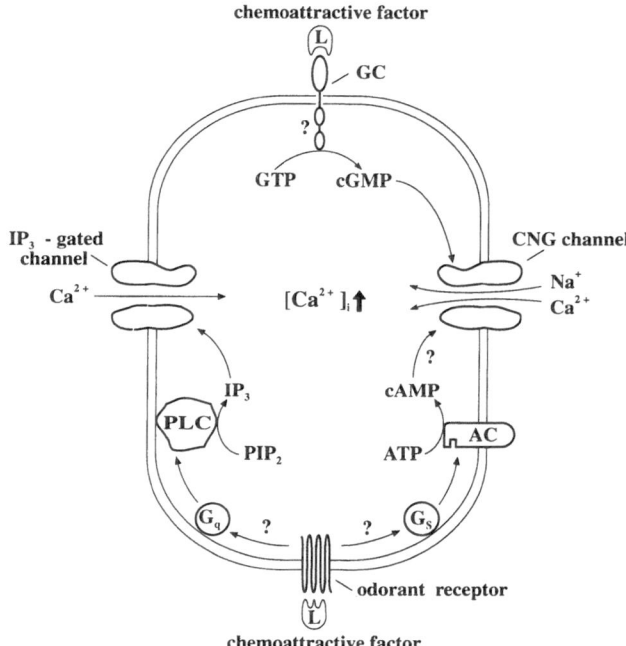

Fig. 4. Hypothetical signaling pathways of sperm chemoattraction. Binding of chemoattractive factors to membrane receptors causes a transient increase of $[Ca^{2+}]_i$. The change in $[Ca^{2+}]_i$ could lead to alteration in sperm swimming. The membrane receptors might belong either to the family of guanylyl cylases (*GC*) (as shown for invertebrate sperm) or to the family of G-protein-coupled receptors for odorants. By analogy to olfactory signal transduction, chemoattractive factors might use a signaling pathway involving cAMP and possibly also inositol 1,4,5-trisphosphate (IP₃) as intracellular messengers. Adenylyl cyclase (*AC*), phospholipase C (*PLC*); *L*, ligand

derhaeghen et al. 1993; Walensky et al. 1995). In analogy to olfactory signal transduction, these receptors might couple to a cAMP- or an IP₃-signaling pathway (for review, see e.g., Breer et al. 1994). This hypothesis relies either on CNG channels with high selectivity for cAMP or IP₃-gated channels as Ca^{2+} entry pathways. Experimental evidence for IP₃-gated channels in the plasma membrane of sperm does not exist. However, such channels reside in acrosomal membranes and are believed to mediate an IP_3-gated Ca^{2+} release from the acrosome (Walensky and Snyder 1995). This acrosomal Ca^{2+} release, as well as the Ca^{2+} influx into sperm via L-type voltage-activated Ca^{2+} channels, may trigger the acrosomal exocytosis by increasing $[Ca^{2+}]_i$ (Florman et al. 1992). Whether IP_3-gated channels or voltage-activated Ca^{2+} channels serve as Ca^{2+} entry mechanisms in sperm chemoattraction is unknown.

Vertebrate sperm express CNG channels. It is tempting to speculate that these channels serve as the Ca^{2+} entry pathway, regardless of whether cAMP or cGMP is the physiological ligand of the native channel. Binding of chemoattractive factors to membrane receptors of sperm might cause an increase in the concentration of cyclic nucleotides and thereby allow Ca^{2+} to enter the cell via CNG channels. The resulting change in $[Ca^{2+}]_i$ could lead to alteration of the direction of sperm swimming (cf. Shapiro 1987). Several lines of evidence support this hypothesis: (1) The behavioral response of sea urchin sperm induced by egg-derived peptides depends on external Ca^{2+} (Ward et al. 1985; Cook et al. 1994). (2) These peptides specifically bind to membrane receptors of sperm. Subsequently, the intracellular concentrations of cGMP, cAMP and Ca^{2+} are elevated (for reviews, see Garbers 1989; Ward and Kopf 1993). (3) Inhibition of a sperm cGMP-phosphodiesterase leads to prolongation of the increase in $[Ca^{2+}]_i$, suggesting that Ca^{2+} influx is coupled to the increase in cGMP (Schackmann and Chock 1986). (4) In sea urchin, putative receptors for chemoattractive peptides have been localized on the tail (Cardullo et al. 1994) as well as the putative odorant receptors in vertebrate sperm (Vanderhaeghen et al. 1993; Walensky et al. 1995). (5) The CNG channel in bovine sperm is localized on the tail as well. (6) The α-subunit of the sperm CNG channel is highly permeable to Ca^{2+} (Frings et al. 1995).

This hypothesis needs to be tested more directly, and it certainly is an important task for future work to identify the molecular mechanisms underlying sperm chemoattraction.

4.6 Summary

Recent studies suggest that vertebrate sperm may utilize signaling pathways similar to those of photoreceptors and OSNs. Bovine sperm express a CNG channel which is identical (at least with regard to the α-subunit) to that expressed in cone photoreceptors. This channel is highly permeable to Ca^{2+} ions. The targets for the CNG channel-mediated Ca^{2+} entry and their physiological function in sperm are still unclear. CNG channels may play a crucial role in regulating motility or chemoattraction of sperm.

Acknowledgments. I thank all my colleagues, whose ideas and experiments have contributed so much to this research. I am grateful to U.B. Kaupp for helpful comments and critical reading of the manuscript, A. Eckert for typing the manuscript, and the Deutsche Forschungsgemeinschaft for financial support (DFG We 1750/1–2, -1–3).

References

Biel M, Zong X, Distler M, Bosse E, Klugbauer N, Murakami M, Flockerzi V, Hofmann F (1994) Another member of the cyclic nucleotide-gated channel family, expressed in testis, kidney, and heart. Proc Natl Acad Sci USA 91:3505–3509

Bönigk W, Altenhofen W, Müller F, Dose A, Illing M, Molday RS, Kaupp UB (1993) Rod and cone photoreceptor cells express distinct genes for cGMP-gated channels. Neuron 10:865–877

Bradley J, Li J, Davidson N, Lester HA, Zinn K (1994) Heteromeric olfactory cyclic nucleotide-gated channels: a new subunit that confers increased sensitivity to cAMP. Proc Natl Acad Sci USA 91:8890–8894

Breer H, Raming K, Krieger J (1994) Signal recognition and transduction in olfactory neurons. Biochim Biophys Acta 1224:277–287

Cardullo RA, Herrick SB, Peterson MJ, Dangott LJ (1994) Speract receptors are localized on sea urchin sperm flagella using a fluorescent peptide analog. Dev Biol 162:600–607

Chen T-Y, Peng Y-W, Dhallan RS, Ahamed B, Reed RR, Yau K-W (1993) A new subunit of the cyclic nucleotide-gated cation channel in retinal rods. Nature 362:764–767

Cook SP, Brokaw CJ, Muller CH, Babcock DF (1994) Sperm chemotaxis: egg peptides control cytosolic calcium to regulate flagellar responses. Dev Biol 165:10–19

Cosson MP (1990) Sperm chemotaxis. In: Gagnon C (ed) Controls of sperm motility: biological and clinical aspects. CRC Press, Boca Raton, pp 103–135

del Pilar Gomez M, Nasi E (1995) Activation of light-dependent K^+ channels in ciliary invertebrate photoreceptors involves cGMP but not the IP_3/Ca^{2+} cascade. Neuron 15:607–618

Dhallan RS, Yau K-W, Schrader KA, Reed RR (1990) Primary structure and functional expression of a cyclic nucleotide-activated channel from olfactory neurons. Nature 347:184–187

Fesenko EE, Kolesnikov SS, Lyubarsky AL (1985) Induction by cyclic GMP of cationic conductance in plasma membrane of retinal rod outer segment. Nature 313:310–313

Florman HM, Corron ME, Kim TD-H, Babcock DF (1992) Activation of voltage-dependent calcium channels of mammalian sperm is required for zona pellucida-induced acrosomal exocytosis. Dev Biol 152:304–314

Foltz KR, Lennarz WJ (1993) The molecular basis of sea urchin gamete interactions at the egg plasma membrane. Dev Biol 158:46–61

Fraser LR, Monks NJ (1990) Cyclic nucleotides and mammalian sperm capacitation. J Reprod Fertil [Suppl] 42:9–21

Frings S, Seifert R, Godde M, Kaupp UB (1995) Profoundly different calcium permeation and blockage determine the specific function of distinct cyclic nucleotide-gated channels. Neuron 15:169–179

Garbers DL (1989) Molecular basis of fertilization. Annu Rev Biochem 58:719–742

Garbers DL, Kopf GS (1980) The regulation of spermatozoa by calcium and cyclic nucleotides. In: Greengard P, Robison GA (eds) Advances in cyclic nucleotide research, vol 13. Raven, New York, pp 251–306

Garbers DL, Lust WD, First NL, Lardy HA (1971) Effects of phosphodiesterase inhibitors and cyclic nucleotides on sperm respiration and motility. Biochemistry 10:1825–1831

Goulding EH, Ngai J, Kramer RH, Colicos S, Axel R, Siegelbaum SA, Chess A (1992) Molecular cloning and single-channel properties of the cyclic nucleotide-gated channel from catfish olfactory neurons. Neuron 8:45–58

Gray JP, Drummond GI, Luk DWT, Hardman JG, Sutherland EW (1976) Enzymes of cyclic nucleotide metabolism in invertebrate and vertebrate sperm. Arch Biochem Biophys 172:20–30

Hansbrough JR, Garbers DL (1981) Speract – purification and characterization of a peptide associated with eggs that activates spermatozoa. J Biol Chem 256:1447–1452

Haynes LW, Yau K-W (1985) Cyclic GMP-sensitive conductance in outer segment membrane of catfish cones. Nature 317:61–64

Henn DK, Baumann A, Kaupp UB (1995) Probing of the transmembrane topo-
    logy of cyclic nucleotide-gated channels by a gene fusion approach. Proc
    Natl Acad Sci USA 92:7425–7429
Hsu Y-T, Molday RS (1993) Modulation of the cGMP-gated channel of rod
    photoreceptor cells by calmodulin. Nature 361:76–79
Kaupp UB (1995) Family of cyclic nucleotide gated ion channels. Curr Opin
    Neurobiol 5:434–442
Kaupp UB, Niidome T, Tanabe T, Terada S, Bönigk W, Stühmer W, Cook NJ,
    Kangawa K, Matsuo H, Hirose T, Miyata T, Numa S (1989) Primary struc-
    ture and functional expression from complementary DNA of the rod
    photoreceptor cyclic GMP-gated channel. Nature 342:762–766
Koch K-W (1994) Calcium as modulator of phototransduction in vertebrate
    photoreceptor cells. Rev Physiol Biochem Pharmacol 125:149–192
Körschen HG, Illing M, Seifert R, Sesti F, Williams A, Gotzes S, Colville C,
    Müller F, Dosé A, Godde M, Molday L, Kaupp UB, Molday RS (1995) A
    240 K protein represents the complete β-subunit of cyclic nucleotide-gated
    channel from rod photoreceptors. Neuron 15:627–636
Liman ER, Buck LB (1994) A second subunit of the olfactory cyclic nucleo-
    tide-gated channel confers high sensitivity to cAMP. Neuron 13:611–621
Liu M, Chen T-Y, Ahamed B, Li J, Yau K-W (1994) Calcium-calmodulin
    modulation of the olfactory cyclic nucleotide-gated cation channel. Science
    266:1348–1354
Ludwig J, Margalit T, Eismann E, Lancet D, Kaupp UB (1990) Primary struc-
    ture of cAMP-gated channel from bovine olfactory epithelium. FEBS Lett
    270:24–29
Ludwig J, Terlau H, Wunder F, Brüggemann A, Pardo LA, Marquardt A,
    Stühmer W, Pongs O (1994) Functional expression of a rat homologue of
    the voltage gated ether á go-go potassium channel reveals differences in se-
    lectivity and activation kinetics between the Drosophila channel and its
    mammalian counterpart. EMBO J 13:4451–4458
Makler A, Stoller J, Reichler A, Blumenfeld Z, Yoffe N (1995) Inability of
    human sperm to change their orientation in response to external chemical
    stimuli. Fertil Steril 63:1077–1082
Miller RL (1985) Sperm chemo-orientation in the metazoa. In: Metz CB, Man-
    ory A (eds) Biology of fertilization, vol 2: biology of the sperm. Academic,
    New York, pp 275–337
Molday RS, Molday LL, Dose A, Clark-Lewis I, Illing M, Cook NJ, Eismann
    E, Kaupp UB (1991) The cGMP-gated channel of the rod photoreceptor
    cell characterization and orientation of the amino terminus. J Biol Chem
    266:21917–21922
Morisawa M (1994) Cell signaling mechanisms for sperm motility. Zool Sci
    11:647–662

Myles DG (1993) Molecular mechanisms of sperm-egg membrane binding and fusion in mammals. Dev Biol 158:35–45

Nakamura T, Gold GH (1987) A cyclic nucleotide-gated conductance in olfactory receptor cilia. Nature 325:442–444

Nakatani K, Yau K-W (1988) Calcium and magnesium fluxes across the plasma membrane of the toad rod outer segment. J Physiol (Lond) 395:695–729

Perry RJ, McNaughton PA (1991) Response properties of cones from the retina of the tiger salamander. J Physiol (Lond) 433:561–587

Picones A, Korenbrot JI (1995) Permeability and interaction of Ca^{2+} with cGMP-gated ion channels differ in retinal rod and cone photoreceptors. Biophys J 69:120–127

Ralt D, Goldenberg M, Fetterolf P, Thompson D, Dor J, Mashiach S, Garbers DL, Eisenbach M (1991) Sperm attraction to a follicular factor(s) correlates with human egg fertilizability. Proc Natl Acad Sci USA 88:2840–2844

Ralt D, Manor M, Cohen-Dayag A, Tur-Kaspa I, Ben-Shlomo I, Makler A, Yuli I, Dor J, Blumberg S, Mashiach S, Eisenbach M (1994) Chemotaxis and chemokinesis of human spermatozoa to follicular factors. Biol Reprod 50:774–785

Santos-Sacchi J, Gordon M (1980) Induction of the acrosome reaction in guinea pig spermatozoa by cGMP analogues. J Cell Biol 85:798–803

Schackmann RW, Chock PB (1986) Alteration of intracellular $[Ca^{2+}]$ in sea urchin sperm by the egg peptide speract. J Biol Chem 261:8719–8728

Shapiro BM (1987) The existential decision of a sperm. Cell 49:293–294

Shepherd GM (1994) Discrimination of molecular signals by the olfactory receptor neuron. Neuron 13:771–790

Shimomura H, Dangott LJ, Garbers DL (1986) Covalent coupling of a resact analogue to guanylate cyclase. J Biol Chem 261:15778–15782

Suarez SS, Varosi SM, Dai X (1993) Intracellular calcium increases with hyperactivation in intact, moving hamster sperm and oscillates with the flagellar beat cycle. Proc Natl Acad Sci USA 90:4660–4664

Tash JS (1990) Role of cAMP, calcium, and protein phosphorylation in sperm motility. In: Gagnon C (ed) Controls of sperm motility: biological and clinical aspects. CRC Press, Boca Raton, pp 229–240

Toowicharanont P, Shapiro BM (1988) Regional differentiation of the sea urchin sperm plasma membrane. J Biol Chem 263:6877–6883

Vanderhaeghen P, Schurmans S, Vassart G, Parmentier M (1993) Olfactory receptors are displayed on dog mature sperm cells. J Cell Biol 123:1441–1452

Walensky LD, Snyder SH (1995) Inositol 1,4,5-trisphosphate receptors selectively localized to the acrosomes of mammalian sperm. J Cell Biol 130:857–869

Walensky LD, Roskams AJ, Lefkowitz RJ, Snyder SH, Ronnett GV (1995) Odorant receptors and desensitization proteins colocalize in mammalian sperm. Mol Med 1:130–141

Ward CR, Kopf GS (1993) Molecular events mediating sperm activation. Dev Biol 158:9–34

Ward GE, Brokaw CJ, Garbers DL, Vacquier VD (1985) Chemotaxis of Arbacia punctulata spermatozoa to resact, a peptide from the egg jelly layer. J Cell Biol 101:2324–2329

Warmke JW, Ganetzky B (1994) A family of potassium channel genes related to eag in Drosophila and mammals. Proc Natl Acad Sci USA 91:3438–3442

Weyand I, Godde M, Frings S, Weiner J, Müller F, Altenhofen W, Hatt H, Kaupp UB (1994) Cloning and functional expression of a cyclic-nucleotide-gated channel from mammalian sperm. Nature 368:859–863

Wohlfart P, Haase W, Molday RS, Cook NJ (1992) Antibodies against synthetic peptides used to determine the topology and site of glycosylation of the cGMP-gated channel from bovine rod photoreceptors. J Biol Chem 267:644–648

Yau K-W (1994) Cyclic nucleotide-gated channels: an expanding new family of ion channels. Proc Natl Acad Sci USA 91:3481–3483

Zufall F, Firestein S, Shepherd GM (1994) Cyclic nucleotide-gated ion channels and sensory transduction in olfactory receptor neurons. Annu Rev Biophys Biomol Struct 23:577–607

5 CREM: A Transcriptional Master Switch Governing the cAMP Response in the Testis

L. Monaco, F. Nantel, N.S. Foulkes, and P. Sassone-Corsi

5.1	Introduction	70
5.2	Induction of Gene Expression by Activation of the cAMP Signaling Pathway	71
5.3	Transcriptional Activation	72
5.3.1	Phosphorylation	72
5.3.2	Interaction with Coactivator CBP	74
5.4	CREM Is an Early Response Gene	74
5.4.1	Kinetics of Induction	74
5.4.2	ICER: An Inducible Repressor and Its Autoregulation	76
5.4.3	Kinetics of Attenuation	78
5.5	CREM and Spermatogenesis	79
5.5.1	High Levels of the Activator in Germ Cells	79
5.5.2	A Regulator of Haploid Gene Expression	80
5.6	CREM Expression in Sertoli Cells	81
5.6.1	Induction of the Repressor ICER by FSH	81
5.6.2	ICER Involvement in the Long-Term Desensitization of the FSH Receptor	82
5.7	Homologous Recombination of the CREM Gene	83
5.7.1	Early Block of Spermiogenesis	83
5.7.2	Apoptosis of Germ Cells	85
5.7.3	Block of Postmeiotic Gene Expression	85
References		88

5.1 Introduction

The structural organization of most transcription factors is intrinsically modular, in most cases including a DNA-binding domain and an activation domain. It has been shown that these domains can be interchanged between different factors and still retain their functional properties. This modularity suggests that during evolution, the increasing complexity of gene expression may have resulted not only by duplication and divergence of existing genes, but also by a domain shuffling process to generate factors with novel properties (Harrison 1991). An important step forward in the study of transcription factors has been the discovery that many constitute final targets of specific signal transduction pathways. The two major signal transduction systems are those including cAMP and diacylglycerol (DAG) as second messengers (Nishizuka 1986). Each pathway is also characterized by a specific protein kinase (protein kinase A (PKA) and protein kinase C (PKC), respectively) and its ultimate target DNA control element [cAMP-responsive element (CRE) and TPA-responsive element (TRE), respectively]. Although initially characterized as distinct systems, accumulating evidence points towards extensive cross-talk between these pathways (Cambier et al. 1987; Yoshimasa et al. 1987; Masquilier and Sassone-Corsi 1992).

Intracellular levels of cAMP are regulated primarily by adenylyl cyclase. This enzyme is in turn modulated by various extracellular stimuli mediated by receptors and their interaction with G proteins (McKnight et al. 1988). cAMP binds cooperatively to two sites on the regulatory subunits of PKA, releasing the active catalytic subunits (Roesler et al. 1988; Lalli and Sassone-Corsi 1994). These are translocated from cytoplasmic and Golgi complex anchoring sites and phosphorylate a number of cytoplasmic and nuclear proteins on serines in the context X-Arg-Arg-X-*Ser*-X (Lalli and Sassone-Corsi 1994). In the nucleus, PKA-mediated phosphorylation ultimately influences the transcriptional regulation of various genes through distinct, cAMP-inducible promoter responsive sites (Ziff 1990; Borrelli et al. 1992).

5.2 Induction of Gene Expression by Activation of the cAMP Signaling Pathway

The consensus CRE is constituted by an 8-bp palindromic sequence (TGACGTCA) with a higher conservation in the 5' half of the palindrome than the 3' sequence. Several genes which are regulated by a variety of endocrine stimuli contain similar sequences in their promoter regions although at different positions (Sassone-Corsi 1988; Borrelli et al. 1992).

The first CRE-binding factor to be characterized was CREB (CRE-binding protein; Hoeffler et al. 1988) but subsequently at least ten additional CRE-binding factor cDNAs have been cloned (Lalli and Sassone-Corsi 1994). They were obtained by screening a variety of cDNA expression libraries, with CRE and ATF sites (Hai et al. 1989; Foulkes et al. 1991). These proteins belong to the bZip transcription factor class.

The different factors are able to heterodimerize with each other but only in certain combinations. A "dimerization code" exists which seems to be a property of the leucine zipper structure of each factor. Some ATF/CREB factors are able to heterodimerize with Fos and Jun, and this may change the specific affinity of binding to a CRE with respect to a Fos–Jun binding site (Hai and Curran 1991). This property resides in the similarity between the CRE (TGACGTCA) and TRE (TGACTCA) sequences (Sassone-Corsi et al. 1990; Masquilier and Sassone-Corsi 1992) and demonstrates the versatility of the transcriptional response to signal transduction pathways.

There are both activators and repressors of cAMP-responsive transcription. The CREM (CRE modulator) gene is unique because of its cell-specific expression and the large variety of isoforms with various functions (Mellström et al. 1993; Lalli and Sassone-Corsi 1994). Some alternatively spliced CREM isoforms act as antagonists of cAMP-induced transcription (Laoide et al. 1993). The inducible cAMP early repressor (ICER) product deserves special mention since it is generated from an alternative promoter of the CREM gene and is responsible for its early response inducibility which is unique among CRE-binding factors (see Sect. 5.4; Molina et al. 1993; Stehle et al. 1993).

5.3 Transcriptional Activation

5.3.1 Phosphorylation

The characterization of the transcriptional activators CREB and CREM (Gonzalez and Montminy 1989; Foulkes et al. 1992; Laoide et al. 1993) has helped to elucidate the molecular mechanisms involved in transcriptional activation. These factors contain a transcriptional activation domain which is divided into two independent regions (Fig. 1). The first, known as the phosphorylation box (P box), contains several consensus phosphorylation sites for various kinases, such as PKA, PKC, p34cdc2, glycogen synthase kinase-3 and casein kinases (CK) I and II (Gonzalez and Montminy 1989; Lee et al. 1990; de Groot et al. 1993a, b). The second region flanks the P box and is constituted by domains rich in glutamine residues (Lalli and Sassone-Corsi 1994).

Upon activation of the adenylyl cyclase pathway, a serine residue at position 133 of CREB and at position 117 of CREM is phosphorylated by PKA (Gonzalez and Montminy 1989; de Groot et al. 1993a). The major effect of phosphorylation is to convert CREB and CREM into powerful transcriptional activators. Within the P box, serine 133/117 is located in a region of about 50 amino acids containing an abundance of phosphorylatable serines and acidic residues (Fig. 1) which was shown to be essential for *trans*-activation by CREB and CREM (Lee et al. 1990; de Groot et al. 1993a).

Interestingly, increases in the levels of intracellular Ca^{2+} in PC12 cells caused by membrane depolarization have been shown to induce the phosphorylation of serine 133 in CREB and a concomitant activation of c-*fos* gene expression mediated by a CRE in the promoter (Sassone-Corsi et al. 1988; Sheng et al. 1990). Although Ca^{2+}/calmodulin-dependent protein kinase (CamK) was shown to be able to phosphorylate serine 133 in vitro (Dash et al. 1991), the in vivo significance remains unclear, since PKA also seems to be necessary for c-*fos* induction mediated by Ca^{2+} influx in PC12 cells (Ginty et al. 1991).

An important finding that reveals the complexity of the transcriptional response elicited by these factors concerns the mitogen-induced p70 S6 kinase (p70s6k), which phosphorylates and activates CREM (de Groot et al. 1994). This finding implicates p70s6k in the mitogenic response also at the nuclear level. Interestingly, since CREM and other

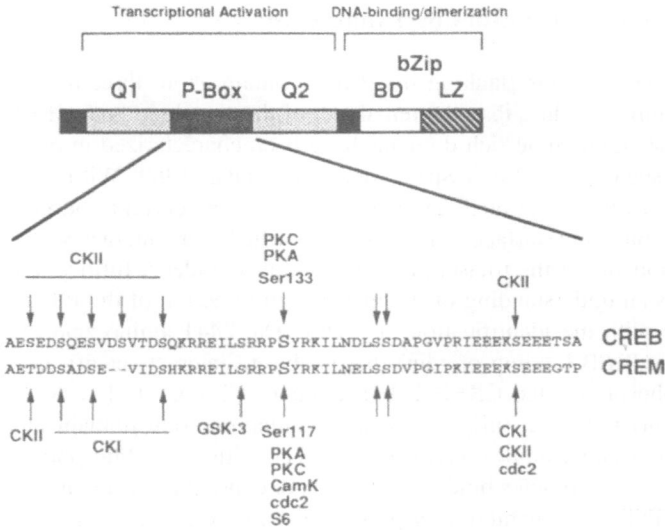

Fig. 1. Structure of a CRE-binding protein activator. The two glutamine-rich domains (*Q1* and *Q2*) and the bZip region (*BD* and *LZ*) are indicated in addition to the P box. This schematic representation is valid for the transcriptional activators cAMP-responsive element binding protein (*CREB*) and cAMP-responsive element modulator (*CREM*-τ). The detailed amino acid sequence of the CREM and CREB P box domains is shown. *Arrows* indicate the serine and threonine residues in CREB and CREM which have been demonstrated in vivo or in vitro to be phosphorylated by the protein kinases indicated. *PKC*, protein kinase C; *PKA*, protein kinase A; *CK*, casein kinase; *CamK*, Ca^{2+}/calmodulin-dependent protein kinase; *GSK-3*, glycogen synthase kinase

factors of the CREB/ATF family represent the final targets of the cAMP-pathway, these results show that they act as effectors of converging signaling systems and possibly as mediators of pathway cross-talk (de Groot et al. 1994).

5.3.2 Interaction with Coactivator CBP

The two domains flanking the P box contain about three-times more glutamine residues than the remainder of the protein in both CREB and CREM. Glutamine-rich domains have been characterized in other factors, such as AP-2 and Sp1 (Courey and Tjian 1989; Williams et al. 1988) as transcriptional activation domains. The current notion is that they constitute surfaces of the protein which can interact with other components of the transcriptional machinery. Indeed, further steps towards an understanding of the mechanism of action of the P box have come with the identification of a 265-kDa, 2441 amino acid protein, CBP (CREB-binding protein) that is able to interact specifically with the phosphorylated CREB P box domain (Chrivia et al. 1993). CBP contains two zinc finger domains, a glutamine-rich domain at its C terminus and a single consensus PKA recognition site. Phosphorylation of Ser-133 promotes binding to CBP and, consequently, the interaction with TFIIB, a general transcription factor involved in RNA polymerase II activity (Kwok et al. 1994). Thus, CBP may act as a link between CREB and the transcription preinitiation complex. This interaction may need some RNA polymerase II cofactors, such as TAF110. Finally, the adenoviral E1A oncoprotein-associated p300, which is thought to play a role in preventing the cell cycle G0/G1 transition, is structurally closely related to CBP (Arany et al. 1995). Both CBP and p300 appear to have intrinsic activating properties which are inhibited by the E1A protein (Arany et al. 1995). Thus, it is clear that studies of the transcriptional activation domain of CRE-binding bZip factors provide important insights into the function of transcription factors in general.

5.4 CREM Is an Early Response Gene

5.4.1 Kinetics of Induction

During studies of CREM expression within the neuroendocrine system, an unexpected new facet emerged; namely, the transcription of the CREM gene is inducible by cAMP (Molina et al. 1993). Furthermore, the kinetics of this induction are those of an early response gene (Verma and Sassone-Corsi 1987). This important finding further reinforces the

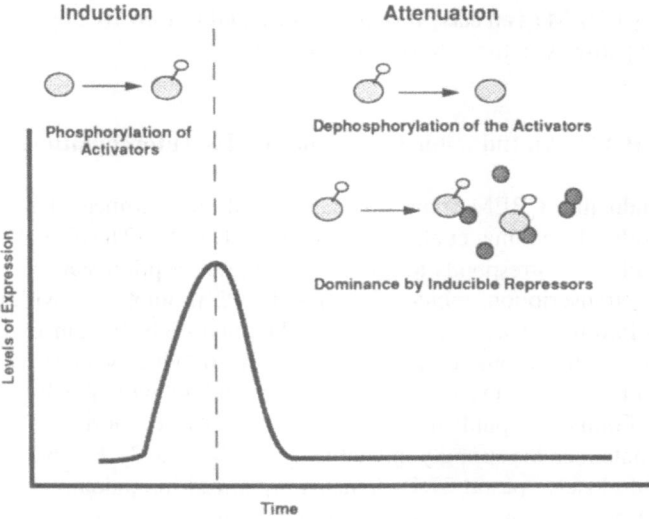

Fig. 2. Kinetics of cAMP-responsive element modulator (CREM) inducibility. After the induction phase, due to the phosphorylation of the activators (i.e., cAMP-responsive element binding protein, CREB), expression is attenuated by at least two mechanisms: (1) Dephosphorylation of the activators by some specific phosphatases and (2) negative autoregulation by the de novo synthesized ICER repressor on the P2 promoter (see also Fig. 3) (Molina et al. 1993; Sassone-Corsi 1994b)

notion that CREM products play a fulcral role in the nuclear response to cAMP, since the expression of no other CRE-binding factor has been shown to be cAMP-inducible to date.

The demonstration of cAMP inducibility first came from the finding that adrenergic signals direct CREM transcription in the pineal gland (Stehle et al. 1993). The inducibility phenomenon was then characterized in detail in the pituitary corticotroph cell line AtT20 (Molina et al. 1993; M. Lamas, unpublished). In unstimulated cells the level of CREM transcript is undetectable. However, upon treatment with forskolin (or cAMP analogs), within 30 min there is a rapid increase in CREM transcript levels which peak after 2 h and then progressively decline to basal levels by 5 h (Fig. 2). These characteristic kinetics

classify CREM as an early response gene and thus directly implicate the
cAMP pathway in the cell's early response.

5.4.2 ICER: An Inducible Repressor and Its Autoregulation

The inducible CREM transcript corresponds to a truncated product,
termed ICER (Molina et al. 1993; Stehle et al. 1993). The 5' end of the
ICER clones corresponds to an alternative transcription start site. The
start of transcription, which identifies the P2 promoter, is within the
10-kb intron which is 3' to the Q2 glutamine-rich domain exon. In
contrast to the promoter generating all the previously characterized
CREM isoforms (P1) and which is GC-rich and not inducible by cAMP
(N. S. Foulkes, unpublished), the P2 promoter has a normal A-T and
G-C content and is strongly inducible by cAMP (Fig. 3). It contains two
pairs of closely spaced CRE elements organized in tandem, where the
separation between each pair is only three nucleotides. These features
make P2 unique among cAMP-regulated promoters and are suggestive
of cooperative interactions among the factors binding to these sites.

The ICER open reading frame is constituted by the C-terminal segment of CREM. The predicted open reading frame encodes a small
protein of 120 amino acids with a predicted molecular mass of
13.4 kDa. This protein, compared with the previously described CREM
isoforms, essentially consists of only the DNA-binding domain, which
is constituted by the leucine zipper and basic region. The structure of
ICER is suggestive of its function and makes it one of the smallest
transcription factors ever described (Molina et al. 1993; Stehle et al.
1993).

The intact DNA-binding domain directs specific ICER binding to a
consensus CRE element. Importantly, ICER is able to heterodimerize
with the other CREM proteins and with CREB. ICER functions as a
powerful repressor of cAMP-induced transcription in transfection assays using an extensive range of reporter plasmids carrying individual
CRE elements or cAMP-inducible promoter fragments (Molina et al.
1993). Interestingly, ICER-mediated repression is obtained at substoi-
chiometric concentrations, similarly to the previously described CREM
antagonists (Laoide et al. 1993). ICER escapes from PKA-dependent
phosphorylation and thus constitutes a new category of CRE binding

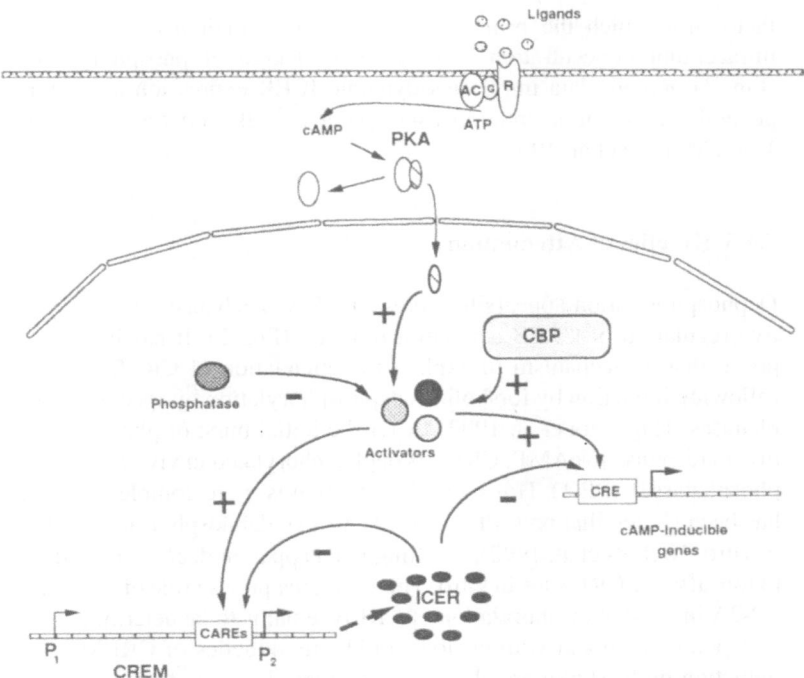

Fig. 3. The cAMP signal transduction pathway. Schematic representation of the route whereby ligands at the cell surface interact with membrane receptors (*R*) and result in altered gene expression. Ligand binding activates coupled G proteins (*G*) which in turn stimulates the activity of the membrane-associated adenylyl cyclase (*AC*). This converts ATP to cAMP which causes the dissociation of the inactive tetrameric protein kinase A (*PKA*) complex into the active catalytic subunits and the regulatory subunits. Catalytic subunits migrate into the nucleus where they phosphorylate and thereby activate transcriptional activators such as cAMP-responsive element binding protein (*CREB*), cAMP-responsive element modulator (*CREMτ*), and ATF-1. Attenuation of the activators may occur via a nuclear phosphatase (see also Fig. 2). Transcriptional induction appears to require interaction of the activators with *CBP*, a cofactor. These then interact with the CRE found in the promoters of cAMP-responsive genes to activate transcription. Phosphorylated factors activate also transcription from the CREM P2 promoter (*P2*) via the cAMP regulatory elements (*CARE*) and ultimately lead to a rapid increase in inducible cAMP early repressor (*ICER*) protein levels. ICER represses cAMP-induced transcription, including that from its own promoter. The subsequent fall in ICER protein levels eventually leads to a release of repression and permits a new cycle of transcriptional activation (see also Fig. 2). *P1*, CREM P1 promoter

factor, for which the principle determinant of their activity is their intracellular concentration and not their degree of phosphorylation (Fig. 3). Recent data implicates dynamic ICER expression as a more general feature of neuroendocrine systems (Lalli and Sassone-Corsi 1995; Monaco et al. 1995).

5.4.3 Kinetics of Attenuation

Dephosphorylation appears to represent a key mechanism in the negative regulation of CREB activation function (Fig. 2). It has been proposed that a mechanism to explain the attenuation of CREB activity following induction by forskolin is dephosphorylation by specific phosphatases (Hagiwara et al. 1992). After the initial burst of phosphorylation in response to cAMP, CREB is dephosphorylated in vivo by protein phosphatase-1 (PP-1). However, the situation is more complex since it has been shown that both PP-1 and PP-2A can dephosphorylate CREB in vitro (Nichols et al. 1992), resulting in an apparent decreased binding to low affinity CRE sites in vitro. Therefore, the precise role of PP-1 and PP-2A in the dephosphorylation of CREB remains to be determined.

Upon cotreatment with cycloheximide, the kinetics of CREM gene induction by forskolin are altered in that there is a significant delay in the postinduction decrease in the transcript; elevated levels persist for as long as 12 h. This implicates a de novo synthesized factor which might downregulate CREM transcription (Molina et al. 1993). This observation, combined with the presence of CRE elements in the P2 promoter, suggested that the transient nature of the inducibility could be due to ICER. Consistently, the CRE elements in the P2 promoter have been shown to bind to the ICER proteins. Detailed studies have demonstrated that the ICER promoter is indeed a target for ICER-negative regulation (Molina et al. 1993). Thus, there exists a negative autoregulatory mechanism controlling ICER expression (Figs. 2, 3). The CREM feedback loop predicts the presence of a refractory inducibility period in the gene's transcription (Sassone-Corsi 1994a).

5.5 CREM and Spermatogenesis

5.5.1 High Levels of the Activator in Germ Cells

CREM is a highly abundant transcript in adult testis while in prepubertal animals it is expressed at very low levels. Thus, in testis CREM is the subject of a developmental switch in expression (Foulkes et al. 1992; Delmas and Sassone-Corsi 1994). Further characterization revealed that the abundant CREM transcript encodes exclusively the activator form, while in prepubertal testis only the repressor forms were detected at low levels. Thus, the developmental switch of CREM expression also constitutes a reversal of function (Foulkes and Sassone-Corsi 1992).

Spermatogenesis is a process occurring in a precise and coordinated manner within the seminiferous tubules (Jégou et al. 1992). During this entire developmental process the germ cells are maintained in intimate contact with the somatic Sertoli cells. As the spermatogonia mature, they move from the periphery towards the lumen of the tubule until the mature spermatozoa are conducted from the lumen to the collecting ducts.

A remarkable aspect of the CREM developmental switch in germ cells is constituted by its exquisite hormonal regulation (Sassone-Corsi 1994b). The spermatogenic differentiation program is under the tight control of the hypothalamic–pituitary axis (Jégou et al. 1992). The regulation of CREM function in testis seems to be intricately linked to follicle-stimulating hormone (FSH) both at the level of the control of transcript processing and at the level of protein activity. For example, surgical removal of the pituitary gland leads to the loss of CREM expression in the rat adult testis (Foulkes et al. 1993). Furthermore, hypophysectomy in prepubertal animals prevents the switch in CREM expression at the pachytene spermatocyte stage, thus implicating the pituitary directly in both the maintenance and the switch to high levels of CREM expression. Injection of FSH leads to a rapid and significant induction of the CREM transcript. The hormonal induction of CREM by FSH is not transcriptional, consistent with the housekeeping nature of the P1 promoter. Instead, by a mechanism of alternative polyadenylation, AUUUA destabilizer elements present in the 3' untranslated region of the gene are excluded, dramatically increasing the stability of the CREM message. CREM is the first example of a gene whose expression is modulated by a pituitary hormone during spermatogenesis (Foulkes et al. 1993). The implication of these findings is that hormones can regulate gene expression at the level of RNA processing and stability. Importantly, the effect of FSH cannot be direct since germ cells do not have FSH receptors. Recent data suggest that another hormonal message originating from the Sertoli cells upon FSH stimulation mediates CREM activation in germ cells (L. Monaco, unpublished results).

5.5.2 A Regulator of Haploid Gene Expression

A first hint as to the role of CREM during spermatogenesis was indicated by its protein expression pattern. In the seminiferous epithelium, CREM transcripts accumulate in spermatocytes and spermatids, but CREM protein is detected only in haploid spermatids (Delmas et al. 1993). The absence of CREM protein in spermatocytes reflects a strict translational control and indicates multiple levels of regulation of gene expression in testis. It will be extremely important to analyze further the mechanism of this delay in translation and to define whether it is also hormonally regulated.

The expression of CREM activator protein in spermatids coincides with the transcriptional activation of several genes containing a CRE motif in their promoter region. These genes encode mainly structural proteins required for spermatozoon differentiation (transition protein, protamine, etc.), suggesting a role for CREM in the activation of genes required for the late phase of spermatid differentiation. This observation implies that the transcription of some key structural genes is directly linked to hormonal control and consequently to the level of cAMP present in seminiferous epithelium. To date at least three genes, RT7 (Delmas et al. 1993), transition protein-1 (Kistler et al. 1994), and calspermin (Sun et al. 1995), have been shown to be targets of CREM-mediated *trans*-activation in germ cells. A demonstration of the role of CREM in the expression of one of these genes, RT7, was shown using in vitro transcription experiments. A CREM-specific antibody blocks RT7 in vitro transcription with nuclear extracts from seminiferous tubules but not with extracts from liver (Delmas et al. 1993). In conclusion, CREM might participate in testis- and developmental-specific regulation of genes containing a CRE in their promoter region, by expressing the repressor isoforms before meiosis, and high levels of the activator after meiosis.

5.6 CREM Expression in Sertoli Cells

5.6.1 Induction of the Repressor ICER by FSH

The complex structure and function of the mammalian testis is maintained by cell–cell interactions as well as by endocrine signals originating from the hypothalamic–pituitary axis (Skinner 1991; Fritz 1978; Means et al. 1980). The gonadotropins FSH and LH (luteinizing hormone), released by the gonadotrophs of the pituitary gland, regulate spermatogenesis by directing the function of the somatic Sertoli and Leydig cells, respectively. LH and FSH interact with specific G protein-coupled membrane receptors and thereby stimulate adenylyl cyclase activity (Borrelli et al. 1992). On the basis of all the data which document the central role played by CREM during spermatogenesis and the involvement of gonadotropins in directing its expression (Delmas and Sassone-Corsi 1994), we have further characterized the role of these nuclear effectors. Treatment of primary cultures of Sertoli cells with FSH, forskolin, and dbcAMP results in a rapid and transient increase in the PKA-mediated phosphorylation of the activators CREB and CREMτ. Thus, upon pituitary hormonal stimulation there is a powerful and prolonged nuclear response to the activation of the adenylyl cyclase pathway (Monaco et al. 1995).

The induced phosphorylation of the activators results in a dramatic stimulation in the expression of the ICER repressor. The induction is detectable at 1 h, reaches a peak at 4 h, and then returns to basal levels by 24 h. In Sertoli cells ICER induction by FSH is retarded when compared to c-fos, being more similar to inhibin or other delayed genes (Hall et al. 1988; Hamil et al. 1994). Furthermore, cotreatment of the primary cells with FSH or forskolin together with the protein synthesis inhibitor cycloheximide leads to an extended ICER mRNA induction. Indeed, as observed in other systems (Greenberg et al. 1986; Molina et al. 1993), the presence of cycloheximide potentiates ICER induction. Interestingly, the kinetics of protein accumulation demonstrate persistent levels of ICER. There is a rapid increase in the protein levels at 4 h after treatment; however, elevated levels persist until 24 h and only start to significantly decline by 36 h (Monaco et al. 1995). This property distinguishes ICER from other early response genes where the hallmark of transient inducibility is common to both transcript and protein (Greenberg et al. 1986).

5.6.2 ICER Involvement in the Long-Term Desensitization of the FSH Receptor

In contrast to the CREMτ isoform, which is highly expressed in post-meiotic male germ cells and acts as transcriptional activator, ICER functions as a powerful repressor in Sertoli cells (Monaco et al. 1995). Interestingly, the function of ICER in Sertoli cells seems to be of major physiological importance since one of its targets is the FSH receptor gene (FSH-R). Specifically, it appears that ICER may be implicated in the downregulation of FSH-R expression, leading to the long-term desensitization phenomenon (Themmen et al. 1991). Consistently, no ICER induction is detected in gonadotropin-desensitized Sertoli cells. The stability of the ICER protein combined with the rapid and transient induction by FSH of ICER RNA are properties consistent with this scenario. ICER-mediated downregulation appears to involve a direct transcriptional repression of the FSH-R promoter activity. There is a functional CRE-like site at position −115 in the FSH-R promoter which is required for its expression in Sertoli cells (Heckert et al. 1992). Upon FSH stimulation, the intracellular levels of ICER increase dramatically. ICER binds efficiently to the CRE-like site in the FSH-R promoter, causing the transcriptional downregulation. In this manner, ICER completes a hormonal negative feedback loop, central to the regulation of Sertoli cell function. Indeed, the kinetics of ICER induction and the potentiation by cychloheximide is again consistent with the model for ICER-negative autoregulation. Thus, ICER appears to be a key determinant in the phenomenon of long-term desensitization of the receptor. Importantly, downregulation of FSH-R expression has also been correlated with a decreased stability of the transcript (Themmen et al. 1991). This observation, together with our results, suggests that more than one mechanism may be involved in long-term desensitization of this receptor.

These observations have many implications for the function of ICER in Sertoli cells and more generally in endocrine systems. Namely, it implies that ICER mediates a long-term downregulation of the cAMP transcriptional response following transient hormonal stimulation of the pathway. Thus, it is apparent that the stability of ICER protein may play a fundamental role in defining its function. Indeed, it is apparent that ICER may be involved in the long-term desensitization of other G protein-coupled receptors in other neuroendocrine tissues (Lalli and Sassone-Corsi 1995).

Recent molecular cloning studies reported the presence of several genes regulated positively or negatively by FSH in the Sertoli cells (Hall et al. 1988; Hamil et al. 1994; Hamil and Hall 1994). It is well known that the gonadotropin stimulates the expression of early genes, such as c-*fos* and *jun*B. Furthermore, these genes have been implicated in mediating the late response, i.e., the synthesis and secretion of several factors necessary for germ cell development. In this complex hormonal regulation of spermatogenesis, ICER induction could be involved in the mechanism to downregulate FSH activation of specific Sertoli cell genes. Our preliminary studies indicate that ICER may be responsible for the repression of FSH-induced expression of the c-*fos* and urokinase-type plasminogen activator genes in Sertoli cells (in preparation). All these data strengthen the important role played by the CREM family of transcription factors in the spermatogenic process.

5.7 Homologous Recombination of the CREM Gene

5.7.1 Early Block of Spermiogenesis

Spermatids are sculptured into the shape of mature spermatozoa in the process of spermiogenesis which involves extensive biochemical and morphological restructuring (Santen 1987). During male germ cell differentiation, dramatic changes in gene expression occur. Transcriptional activation of several genes has been described at very precise stages during differentiation (Propst et al. 1988; Wolgemuth and Watrin 1991). Genes that are transcribed specifically in male germ cells include those whose products are required for sperm structure and motility. For example, protamines and transition proteins are well known to be involved in the process of DNA condensation which is required for sperm head formation. These are candidate target genes for CREM transcriptional activation in postmeiotic germ cells.

To address the role of CREM in development and physiological processes we generated mutant mice with a gene disrupted by homologous recombination in mouse embryonic stem cells. We constructed a targeting vector containing a CREM genomic fragment in which a portion of the 3'-terminal exon encoding the DNA-binding domain was deleted and replaced by a PGK-neomycin cassette. The selection of the construct was dictated by the need to inactivate all the numerous CREM and ICER isoforms (Laoide et al. 1993; Stehle et al. 1993). Reduced fertility was observed in the breeding of the heterozygous mice. Comparison of the homozygous CREM-deficient mice with their normal littermates showed no macroscopic physical aberrations or reduction in body weight. Analysis of internal organs revealed no apparent changes in their structure as compared to wild-type mice. However, the testes of the CREM-deficient mice displayed a reduction of 20%–25% in their weight. Analysis of the seminal fluid of heterozygous mice compared to normal littermates demonstrated a 46% reduction in the overall number of spermatozoa, a 35% decrease in the ratio of motile spermatozoa, and a twofold increase in the number of spermatozoa with aberrant structures. Most of the aberrant spermatozoa were characterized by a kink and bubble-like structure midway along the tail. Strikingly, analysis of the seminal fluid from homozygous CREM-deficient mice revealed a complete absence of spermatozoa. This result demonstrates a dramatic impairement of spermatogenesis in the CREM-deficient mice. The homozygous males are sterile, demonstrating the necessity of a functional CREM transcription factor for male fertility. The homozygous female mice were fertile and displayed apparently normal ovary structure.

To determine the nature of the sperm deficiency in the CREM-deficient mice we perfomed a detailed anatomical analysis of the seminiferous epithelium. Consecutive spermatogenic cycles are classically depicted as waves of differentiating germ cells within each tubule (Parvinen 1982). In the mouse, each wave is divided into 12 stages, each representing a specific cellular association (Perey et al. 1961). Tubular segments containing postmeiotic germ cells which undergo spermiogenesis appear as dark sections under transillumination because of the higher DNA compaction of these haploid cells (Parvinen 1982).

Tubuli from CREM-deficient mice display a 20%–30% reduced diameter and completely lack the normal spermatogenic wave and the corresponding dark sections. Squash preparations (Parvinen and Hecht 1981) from consecutive segments of the seminiferous epithelium demonstrate that spermatogenesis in the CREM-deficient mice is interrupted at the stage of very early spermatids. Neither elongating spermatids nor spermatozoa are observed, while somatic Sertoli cells appear to be normal.

5.7.2 Apoptosis of Germ Cells

In stages VII–X we observe significant numbers of multinucleated giant cells, normally present at very low frequency in wild-type animals (Henriksen et al. 1995a). Interestingly, it has been previously shown that these cellular bodies correspond to apoptotic cells (Henriksen et al. 1995a). To confirm this observation, we have used in situ terminal transferase 3'-end labeling (Henriksen et al. 1995b) to reveal cells containing high levels of DNA-free ends, a diagnostic feature of apoptotic cells. The number of apoptotic cells in the CREM-deficient animals is 10- to 20-fold higher than in normal mice. Thus, these analyses indicate that the lack of CREM causes germ cells to cease differentiation and to undergo apoptosis. Histological analysis of the testis from 8-week-old CREM-deficient animals confirmed a reduced tubule diameter and revealed the corresponding absence of developing spermatids and spermatozoa. The somatic cell components of the testis and Sertoli and Leydig cells appeared normal. In addition, in tubules corresponding to stages VII–X the apoptotic cells were clearly visible (Fig. 4).

5.7.3 Block of Postmeiotic Gene Expression

Given the importance of the activation of specific postmeiotic genes in the process of spermiogenesis and the involvement of CREM in their regulation, we decided to compare the expression of a battery of genes in the CREM-deficient mice with that of the normal and heterozygous littermates. This analysis confirms the key role of CREM in the activa-

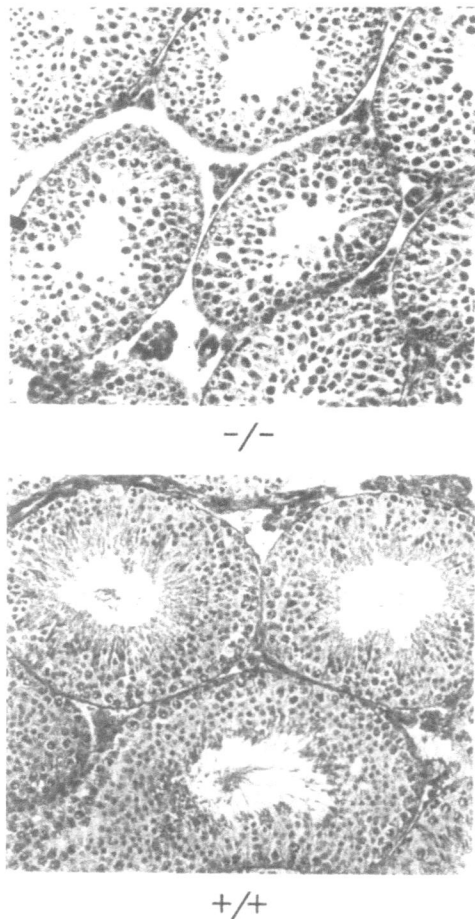

Fig. 4. cAMP-responsive element modulator (CREM) deficiency causes spermiogenesis arrest and male germ cell apoptosis. Testes from a 8-week-old homozygous mutant (-/-) and a wild type (+/+) mouse littermate. Histological
analysis of testis sections (magnification 200×). The tubules from the CREM-
deficient mice show impaired spermatogenesis and some multinucleated,
apoptotic cells

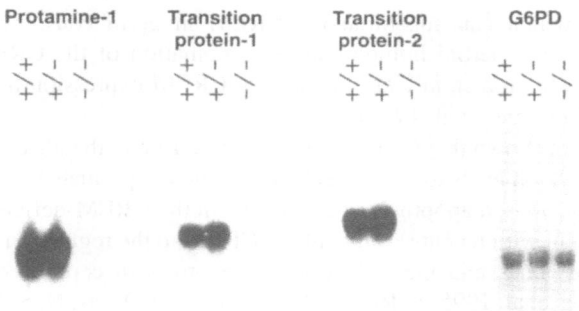

Fig. 5. Deregulation of postmeiotic gene expression in cAMP-responsive element modulator (CREM)-deficient mice. Analysis of mRNA expression of protamine 1, transition proteins 1 and 2, and G6PD by Northern blot analysis. Total testis RNA from wild type (+/+), heterozygote (+/-) and homozygous mutant (-/-) mice was used

tion of genes such as protamine 1 and 2 and transition proteins 1 and 2. The lack of expression of these genes may explain the impairment in the structuring of a mature spermatozoon in the CREM-deficient mice (Fig. 5). Moreover, the expression of genes such as calspermin (Sun et al. 1995), *Krox*–20 (Chevrier et al. 1988) and *Krox*–24 (Lemaire et al. 1988) is strongly reduced in both the heterozygous and homozygous mutant animals. In contrast, other genes normally expressed in premeiotic germ cells such as proacrosin-binding protein (Baba et al. 1994) and *Hoxa*–1 (Rubin and Nguyen-Huu 1991) were expressed at unchanged levels in the mutant mice.

It is important to note that CREB expression is unchanged with respect to normal littermates. CREB is the only other cAMP-responsive factor to be detected in male germ cells (Waeber et al. 1991; Ruppert et al. 1992). However, the germ cell-specific CREB isoforms are C terminally truncated, lacking dimerization and DNA-binding function, and their physiological role remains unclear. Furthermore, the expression of ATF-1, the only other member of the CREB/CREM subfamily of cAMP-responsive factors which are directly phosphorylated by PKA (Rehfuss et al. 1991), appears unchanged in various tissues. Also the levels of the coactivator CBP (Chrivia et al. 1993) and of ATF-2 (Hai et al. 1989) appear unchanged. Thus, apparently there is no redundant function which can substitute for CREM in germ cells. This is in contrast to the partial homologous recombination of the CREB gene which results in a significant increase of CREM expression in various tissues (Hummler et al. 1994).

We have shown that CREM plays a crucial role in the differentiation program which leads to the correct structuring of spermatozoa. In addition, the increased apoptosis of germ cells in the CREM-deficient mice is consistent with recent results linking CREM to the regulation of some cell cycle genes and the induction of apoptosis in certain cell types (Desdouets et al. 1995; S. Ruchaud, M. Lanotte, S. Vyas, N. S. Foulkes, P. Sassone-Corsi, in preparation). Spermatogenic arrest as exhibited in CREM-deficient mice is also a feature of many cases of infertility in human males (Chaganti and German 1979; Micic et al. 1992). Thus, these mice may constitute a tool for dissection of the altered physiological processes in human male infertility. Finally, the use of the CREM-deficient mice will help to understand the long-term desensitization phenomenon in both the Sertoli cells and other neuroendocrine systems.

References

Arany Z, Newsome D, Oldread E, Livingston DM, Eckner R (1995) A family of transcriptional adaptor proteins targeted by the E1A oncoprotein. Nature 374:81–84

Baba T, Niida Y, Michikawa Y, Kashiwabara SI, Kodaira K, Takenada M, Kohno N, Gerton G, Arai Y (1994) An acrosomal protein, sp32, in mammalian sperm is a binding protein specific for two proacrosins and an acrosin intermediate. J Biol Chem 269:10133–10140

Borrelli E, Montmayeur JP, Foulkes NS, Sassone-Corsi P (1992) Signal transduction and gene control: the cAMP pathway. Crit Rev Oncog 3:321–338

Cambier JC, Newell MK, Justement LB, McGuire JC, Leach KL, Chen ZZ (1987) Ia binding ligands and cAMP stimulate nuclear translocation of PKC in B lymphocytes. Nature 327:629–632

Chaganti RS, German J (1979) Human male fertility, probably genetically determined, due to defective meiosis and spermatogenic arrest. Am J Hum Genet 31:634–641

Chevrier P, Zerial M, Lemaire P, Almendral J, Bravo R, Charnay P (1988) A gene encoding a protein with zinc fingers is activated during Go/Gi transition in cultured cells. EMBO J 7:29–35

Chrivia, JC, Kwok RPS, Lamb N, Haniwawa M, Montminy MR, Goodman RH (1993) Phosphorylated CREB binds specifically to the nuclear protein CBP. Nature 365:855–859

Courey AJ, Tjian R (1989) Analysis of Sp1 in vivo reveals multiple transcriptional domains, including a novel glutamine activation motif. Cell 55:887–898

Dash PK, Karl KA, Colicos MA, Prywes R, Kandel ER (1991) cAMP response element-binding protein is activated by Ca^{2+}/calmodulin as well as cAMP-dependent protein kinase. Proc Natl Acad Sci USA 88:5061–5065

de Groot RP, den Hertog J, Vandenheede JR, Goris J, Sassone-Corsi P (1993a) Multiple and cooperative phosphorylation events regulate the CREM activator function. EMBO J 12:3903–3911

de Groot RP, Derua R, Goris J, Sassone-Corsi P (1993b) Phosphorylation and negative regulation of the transcriptional activator CREM by p34cdc2. Mol Endocrinol 7: 1495–1501

de Groot RP, Ballou LM, Sassone-Corsi P (1994) Positive regulation of the cAMP-responsive activator CREM by the p70 S6 kinase: an alternative route to mitogen-induced gene expression. Cell 79:81–91

Delmas V, Sassone-Corsi P (1994) The central role of CREM in the cAMP signalling pathway in testis. Mol Cell Endocrinol 100:121–124

Delmas V, van der Hoorn F, Mellström B, Jégou B, Sassone-Corsi P (1993) Induction of CREM activator proteins in spermatids: down-stream targets and implications for haploid germ cell differentiation. Mol Endocrinol 7: 1502–1514

Desdouets C, Matesic G, Molina CA, Foulkes NS, Sassone-Corsi P, Brechot C, Sobczak-Thepot J (1995) Cell cycle regulation of cyclin A gene expression by the cyclic AMP-responsive transcription factors CREB and CREM. Mol Cell Biol 15:3301–3309

Foulkes NS, Sassone-Corsi P (1992) More is better: activators and repressors from the same gene. Cell 68:411–414

Foulkes NS, Borrelli E, Sassone-Corsi P (1991) CREM gene: Use of alternative DNA binding domains generates multiple antagonists of cAMP-induced transcription. Cell 64:739–749

Foulkes NS, Mellstrom B, Benusiglio E, Sassone-Corsi P (1992) Developmental switch of CREM function during spermatogenesis: from antagonist to transcriptional activator. Nature 355:80–84

Foulkes NS, Schlotter F, Pévet P, Sassone-Corsi P (1993) Pituitary hormone FSH directs the CREM functional switch during spermatogenesis. Nature 362:264–267

Fritz IB (1978) Site of action of androgens and follicle-stimulating hormone on cells of the seminiferous tubule. In: Litwach G (ed) Biochemical actions of hormones. Academic, New York, pp 249–281

Ginty DD, Glowacka D, Bader DS, Hidaka H, Wagner JA (1991) Induction of immediate early genes by Ca^{2+} influx requires cAMP-dependent protein kinase in PC12 cells. J Biol Chem 266:17454–17458

Gonzalez GA, Montminy MR (1989) Cyclic AMP stimulates somatostatin gene transcription by phosphorylation of CREB at Ser 133. Cell 59:675–680

Greenberg ME, Hermanowski AL, Ziff EB (1986) Effect of protein synthesis inhibitors on growth factor activation of c-fos, c-myc, and actin gene transcription. Mol Cell Biol 6:1050–1057

Hagiwara M, Alberts A, Brindle P, Meinkoth J, Feramisco J, Deng T, Karin M, Shenolikar S, Montminy M (1992) Transcriptional attenuation following cAMP induction requires PP-1-mediated dephosphorylation of CREB. Cell 70:105–113

Hai T-Y, Curran T (1991) Cross-family dimerization of transcription factors Fos:Jun and ATF/CREB alters DNA binding specificity. Proc Natl Acad Sci USA 88: 3720–3724

Hai T-Y, Liu F, Coukos WJ, Green MR (1989) Transcription factor ATF cDNA clones: an extensive family of leucine zipper proteins able to selectively form DNA binding heterodimers. Genes Dev 3:2083–2090

Hall SH, Joseph DR, Conti M (1988) Follicle-stimulating hormone induces transient expression of the protooncogene c-fos in primary Sertoli cell cultures. Mol Endocrinol 2:55–61

Hamil KG, Hall SH (1994) Cloning of rat Sertoli cell follicle-stimulating hormone primary response complementary deoxyribonucleic acid: regulation of TSC-22 gene expression. Endocrinology 134:1205–1212

Hamil KG, Conti M, Shimasaki S, Hall SH (1994) Follicle-stimulating hormone regulation of AP1: inhibition of c-jun and stimulation of jun-B gene transcription in the rat Sertoli cell. Mol Cell Endocrinol 99:269–277

Harrison SC (1991) A structural taxonomy of DNA-binding domains. Nature 353:715–719

Heckert LL, Daley IJ, Griswold MD (1992) Structural organization of the follicle-stimulating hormone receptor gene. Mol Endocrinol 6: 70–80

Henriksen K, Hakovirta H, Parvinen M (1995a) In situ quantification of stage-specific apoptosis in the rat seminiferous epithelium: effects of short-term experimental cryptorchidism. Int J Androl (in press)

Henriksen K, Hakovirta H, Parvinen M (1995b) Testosterone inhibits and induces apoptosis in rat seminiferous tubules in a stage-specific manner: in situ quantification in squash preparations after administration of ethane dimethane sulfonate. Endocrinology 136:3285–3291

Hoeffler JP, Meyer TE, Yun Y, Jameson JL, Habener JF (1988) Cyclic AMP responsive DNA-binding protein: structure based on a cloned placental cDNA. Science 242:1430–1433

Hummler E, Cole TJ, Blendy JA, Ganss R, Aguzzi A, Schmid W, Beermann F, Schütz G (1994) Targeted mutation of the CREB gene: compensation within the CREB/ATF family of transcription factors. Proc Natl Acad Sci USA 91:5647–5651

Jégou B, Syed V, Sourdaine P, Byers S, Gérard N, Velez de la Calle J, Pineau C, Garnier DH, Bauché F (1992) The dialogue between late spermatids and Sertoli cells in vertebrates: a century of research. In: Nieschlag E, Habenicht U-F (eds) Spermatogenesis. Fertilization. Contraception. Molecular, cellular and endocrine events in male reproduction. Springer, Berlin Heidelberg New York, pp 56–95 (Ernst Schering Research Foundation Workshop, vol 4)

Kistler M, Sassone-Corsi P, Kistler SW (1994) Identification of a functional cAMP response element in the 5'-flanking region of the gene for transition protein 1 (TP1), a basic chromosomal protein of mammalian spermatids. Biol Reprod 51:1322–1329

Kwok RP, Lundblad J, Chrivia JC, Richards JP, Bachinger HP, Brennan RG, Roberts SG, Green MR, Goodman RH (1994) Nuclear protein CBP is a coactivator for the transcription factor CREB. Nature 370:223–226

Lalli E, Sassone-Corsi P (1994) Signal transduction and gene regulation: the nuclear response to cAMP. J Biol Chem 269:17359–17362

Lalli E, Sassone-Corsi P (1995) Long-term desensitization of the TSH receptor involves TSH-directed induction of CREM in the thyroid gland. Proc Natl Acad Sci USA 92:9633–9637

Laoide BM, Foulkes NF, Schlotter F, Sassone-Corsi P (1993) The functional versatility of CREM is determined by its modular structure. EMBO J 12:1179–1191

Lee CQ, Yun Y, Hoeffler JP, Habener JF (1990) Cyclic-AMP-responsive transcriptional activation involves interdependent phosphorylated subdomains. EMBO J 9:4455–4465

Lemaire P, Relevant O, Bravo R, Charnay P (1988) Two mouse genes encoding potential transcription factors with identical DNA-binding domains are activated by growth factors in cultured cells. Proc Natl Acad Sci USA 85:4691–4695

Masquilier D, Sassone-Corsi P (1992) Transcriptional cross-talk: nuclear factors CREM and CREB bind to AP-1 sites and inhibit activation by Jun. J Biol Chem 267:22460–22466

McKnight SG, Clegg CH, Uhler MD, Chrivia JC, Cadd GG, Correll LA, Otten AD (1988) Analysis of the cAMP-dependent protein kinase system using molecular genetic approaches. Rec Prog Horm Res 44:307–335

Means AR, Dedman JR, Tash JS, Tindall DJ, van Sickle M, Welsh MJ (1980) Regulation of the testis Sertoli cell by follicle-stimulating hormone. Annu Rev Physiol 42:59–70

Mellström B, Naranjo JR, Foulkes NS, Lafarga M, Sassone-Corsi P (1993) Transcriptional response to cAMP in brain: specific distribution and induction of CREM antagonists. Neuron 10:655–665

Micic M, Nikolis J, Micic S (1992) Clinical and meiotic studies in an infertile man with Y; 13 translocation. Hum Reprod 7:1118–1120

Molina CA, Foulkes NS, Lalli E, Sassone-Corsi, P (1993) Inducibility and negative autoregulation of CREM: an alternative promoter directs the expression of ICER, an early response repressor. Cell 75:875–886

Monaco L, Foulkes NS, Sassone-Corsi P (1995) Pituitary follicle- stimulating hormone (FSH) induces CREM gene expression in Sertoli cells: involvement in long-term desensitization of the FSH receptor. Proc Natl Acad Sci USA 92:10673–10677

Nichols M, Weih F, Schmid W, DeVack C, Kowenz-Leutz E, Luckow B, Boshart M, Schütz G (1992) Phosphorylation of CREB affects its binding to high and low affinity sites: implications for cAMP induced gene transcription. EMBO J 11:3337–3346

Nishizuka Y (1986) Studies and perspectives of protein kinase C. Science 233:305–312

Parvinen M (1982) Regulation of the seminiferous epithelium. Endocr Rev 3:404–417

Parvinen M, Hecht NB (1981) Identification of living spermatogenic cells of the mouse by transillumination-phase contrast microscopic technique for "in situ" analyses of DNA polymerase activities. Histochemistry 71:567–579

Perey B, Clermont Y, Leblond CP (1961) The wave of the seminiferous epithelium. Am J Anat 108:47–77

Propst F, Rosenberg MP, Vande Woude GF (1988) Proto-oncogene expression in germ cell development. Trends Genet 4:183–187

Rehfuss RP, Walton KM, Loriaux MM, Goodman RH (1991) The cAMP-rgulated enhancer-binding protein ATF-1 activations transcription in response to cAMP-dependent protein kinase A. J Biol Chem 266:18431–18434

Roesler WJ, Vanderbark GR, Hanson RW (1988) Cyclic AMP and the induction of eukaryotic gene expression. J Biol Chem 263:9063–9066

Rubin MR, Nguyen-Huu MC (1991) Murine embryonic spinal cord and adult testis Hox-1.4 cDNAs are identical 3' to the homeobox. DNA Seq 1:329–334

Ruppert S, Cole TJ, Boshart M, Schmid E, Schütz G (1992) Multiple mRNA isoforms of the transcription activator protein CREB: generation by alternative splicing and specific expression in primary spermatocytes. EMBO J 11:1503–1512

Santen RJ (1987) The testis. In: Felig P, Baxter JD, Broadus AE, Frohman LA (eds) Endocrinology and metabolism. McGraw-Hill, New York, pp 821–905

Sassone-Corsi P (1988) Cyclic AMP induction of early adenovirus promoters involves sequences required for E1A-transactivation. Proc Natl Acad Sci USA 85:7192–7196

Sassone-Corsi P (1994a) Rhythmic transcription and autoregulatory loops: winding up the biological clock. Cell 78:361–364

Sassone-Corsi P (1994b) The nuclear response to cAMP during spermatogenesis: the key role of transcription factor CREM. In: Verhoeven G, Habenicht UF (eds) Molecular and cellular endocrinology of the testis. Springer, Berlin Heidelberg New York, pp 219–252 (Ernst Schering Research Foundation Workshop, Suppl 1)

Sassone-Corsi P, Visvader J, Ferland L, Mellon PL, Verma IM (1988) Induction of proto-oncogene fos transcription through the adenylate cyclase pathway: characterization of a cAMP-responsive element. Genes Dev 2:1529–1538

Sassone-Corsi P, Ransone LJ, Verma IM (1990) Cross-talk in signal transduction: TPA-inducible factor Jun/AP-1 activates cAMP responsive enhancer elements. Oncogene 5:427–431

Sheng M, McFadden G, Greenberg ME (1990) Membrane depolarization and calcium induce c-fos transcription via phosphorylation of transcription factor CREB. Neuron 4:571–582

Skinner MK (1991) Cell-cell interactions in the testis. Endocr Rev 12:45–77

Stehle JH, Foulkes NS, Molina CA, Simonneaux V, Pévet P, Sassone-Corsi P (1993) Adrenergic signals direct rhythmic expression of transcriptional repressor CREM in the pineal gland. Nature 365:314–320

Sun Z, Sassone-Corsi P, Means A (1995) Calspermin gene transcription is regulated by two cyclic AMP response elements contained in an alternative promoter in the calmodulin kinase IV gene. Mol Cell Biol 15:561–571

Themmen APN, Blok LJ, Post M, Baarends WM, Hoogerbrugge JW, Parmentier M, Vassart G, Grootegoed JA (1991) Follitropin receptor down-regulation involves a cAMP-dependent post-transcriptional decrease of receptor mRNA expression. Mol Cell Endocrinol 78:R7–R13

Verma IM, Sassone-Corsi P (1987) Proto-oncogene fos: complex but versatile regulation. Cell 51:513–514

Waeber G, Meyer TE, LeSieur M, Hermann HL, Gérard N, Habener JF (1991) Developmental stage-specific expression of cyclic adenosine 3',5'-monophosphate response element-binding protein CREB during spermatogenesis involves alternative exon splicing. Mol Endocrinol 5:1418–1430

Williams T, Admon A, Luscher B, Tjian R (1988) Cloning and expression of AP-2, a cell-type-specific transcription factor that activates inducible enhancer elements. Genes Dev 2:1557–1569

Wolgemuth DJ, Watrin F (1991) List of cloned mouse genes with unique expression pattern during spermatogenesis. Mammalian Genome 1:283–288

Yoshimasa T, Sibley DR, Bouvier M, Lefkowitz RJ, Caron MG (1987) Cross-talk between cellular signalling pathways suggested by phorbol ester adenylate cyclase phosphorylation. Nature 327:67–70

Ziff EB (1990) Transcription factors: a new family gathers at the cAMP response site. Trends Genet 6:69–72

6 Targeted Disruption
of the Protein Kinase A System in Mice

G.S. McKnight, R.L. Idzerda, E.R. Kandel, E.P.Brandon,
M. Zhuo, M. Qi, R. Bourtchouladze, Y. Huang, K.A. Burton,
B.S. Skålhegg, D.E. Cummings, L. Varshavsky, J.V. Planas,
K. Motamed, K.A. Gerhold, P.S. Amieux, C.R. Guthrie,
K.M. Millett, M. Belyamani, and T. Su

6.1	Introduction	96
6.1.1	Expression of R and C Isoforms	97
6.1.2	Holoenzyme Formation	98
6.1.3	Anchoring of PKA in Subcellular Compartments	98
6.1.4	PKA Regulates Gene Expression	99
6.1.5	PKA, Synaptic Modulation, and Learning	101
6.2	Gene Targeting Overview	102
6.2.1	Embryonic Stem Cell Lines and Targeting Vectors	103
6.2.2	Germline Mutations in PKA Subunits	104
6.2.3	Compensatory Changes in R and C Isoforms	105
6.3	Synaptic Plasticity: Defects in PKA Knockout Mice	105
6.3.1	LTP in the Schaffer Collateral Pathway	107
6.3.2	LTD in the Schaffer Collateral Pathway	109
6.3.3	LTP in the Mossy Fiber Pathway	112
6.3.4	Analysis of Behavior in PKA Mutant Mice	114
6.4	RIIβ Knockout Mice Are Genetically Lean	116
6.5	Concluding Remarks	117
References		118

6.1 Introduction

The holoenzyme of cAMP-dependent protein kinase (PKA) is composed of two regulatory (R) and two catalytic (C) subunits and forms the
major mediator of cAMP action in animal cells. Additional responses to
cAMP are also elicited by the cyclic nucleotide-gated ion channels such
as those expressed in the olfactory epithelium and recently found in heart,
kidney, testis, and brain (Biel et al. 1994). Four R subunit genes (RIα,
RIβ, RIIα, and RIIβ) have been cloned in mouse and are highly conserved in all mammals, whereas only two C subunit genes (Cα and Cβ)
have been reported in mouse (McKnight 1991) and a third Cγ subunit has
been found only in humans (Beebe et al. 1990). We have discovered a
processed pseudogene (no introns) that is apparently derived from Cα
and since the pseudogene is located on the mouse X chromosome, we
have named it Cx . We find no transcripts from the Cx pseudogene and
the sequence has mutated such that it would not give rise to a functional
C subunit (Cummings et al. 1994). The human Cγ subunit is also most
closely related to Cα, and although it is transcribed, no protein has yet
been detected in vivo. Like Cx, the Cγ gene is intronless (T. Jahnsen,
personal communication), suggesting that Cγ and Cx both evolved from
a retroposon derived from the Cα gene early in the mammalian lineage
and may have retained functionality only in humans.

We have recently found that there are at least three splice variants
derived from the Cβ gene and refer to these as Cβ1, Cβ2, and Cβ3. The
published Cβ sequence for mouse (Uhler et al. 1986) corresponds to
Cβ1 and this subunit is expressed in most mouse tissues, although it
usually represents 30% or less of the total C subunit. The Cβ2 and Cβ3
variants are truncated at the amino terminus and Cβ2 is missing the
amino-terminal glycine required for myristylation. Both Cβ2 and Cβ3
subunits are expected to produce active C subunits capable of interacting with R subunit as well as the heat stable inhibitor PKI. We have not
explored the tissue specific expression of Cβ2/3 in detail but they are
abundantly expressed in brain and appear to be absent from heart and
kidney. An alternatively spliced form of bovine Cβ mRNA has been
reported (Wiemann et al. 1991) that changes the amino terminus and is
missing the myristylation site present on both Cα and Cβ1. This bovine
splice variant does not appear to correspond to either of the Cβ2/3 splice
variants we have discovered in mice. The C subunits are also modified

by phosphorylation but these phosphates appear to be constitutive and, in the case of Thr197, required for full activity (Orellana and McKnight 1992). The RII subunits can be modified by both autophosphorylation, which reduces the affinity for C subunit (Rosen and Erlichman 1975), and by phosphorylation by other kinases, including casein kinase II, glycogen synthase kinase (GSK)-3, and cdc2 (Keryer et al. 1993). Possible regulatory roles for these phosphorylations remain unclear.

6.1.1 Expression of R and C Isoforms

The expression of the various R and C isoforms has been extensively studied at both the mRNA and protein level. The RIα, RIIα, and Cα subunits show the broadest distribution and are present, although in varying amounts, in nearly all tissues – including brain. The RIβ subunit is the most tissue specific of the mouse subunits, with expression concentrated primarily in neurons, although mRNA has been reported in testis, adrenal, spleen, and pituitary. The RIIβ gene is expressed in brain, fat, and bone marrow, and is regulated by follicle-stimulating hormone (FSH) in Sertoli cells in the testis (Øyen et al. 1988) and granulosa cells in the ovary (Kurten et al. 1992). In addition, RIIβ is developmentally expressed in embryonic liver during erythrogenesis, but is turned off in adult liver (Cadd and McKnight 1989). The Cβ gene is preferentially expressed in brain but shows substantial levels of mRNA in nearly all other tissues. With a newly developed peptide antibody against Cβ we have detected the protein in heart, liver, spleen, testis, and most other tissues in addition to brain.

Messenger RNA for all six isoforms of R and C are expressed in mouse brain but the localized expression differs greatly. Of particular note is the high level of expression of RIβ in CA1-CA3 pyramidal cells of the hippocampus, the concentrated expression of RIIβ in the dentate granule cells and striatum, and the preferential expression of Cβ in the dentate granule cells. In addition, all three β subunits are highly expressed in cortex. RIIα mRNA is very highly expressed in the medial habenula but is also found in a variety of other sites, including the hippocampus and cortex. Expression of RIα and Cα appears to be rather ubiquitous over all brain regions and at least part of this expression is in glial cells (Cadd and McKnight 1989).

6.1.2 Holoenzyme Formation

The formation of holoenzyme depends on dimerization of R subunits which occurs at the amino terminus and is likely to be predominantly a homodimerization reaction rather than promiscuous heterodimerization between various R isoforms. However, RIα/RIβ heterodimers have been reported (Taskén et al. 1993) and we have suggestive evidence that RIIα and RIIβ can interact as well (Otten et al. 1991). The amino-terminal region is the most diverse in terms of sequence and, in addition to promoting dimerization, this region is also involved in anchoring as discussed below. It appears that there is no specificity in terms of R dimer interactions with C subunits and we would expect to find every possible combination in cells based on in vitro association properties and results from cell culture. We have noted a rather remarkable preference for RII-C holoenzyme in cells that also express RI. This preferential association may result from either the subcellular location of the RII protein or a higher affinity binding with C subunit under in vivo conditions (Otten and McKnight 1989). The ability of cAMP to dissociate holoenzyme and release active C subunit differs between the various R and C subunits and may constitute a biochemical feature that confers specific functional properties to the cell. The RIβ-containing holoenzyme is more sensitive to cAMP than the RIα holoenzyme (Cadd et al. 1990) and recent evidence demonstrates that Cβ1 forms a more sensitive holoenzyme in combination with the RIIα subunit (M. Uhler, personal communication).

6.1.3 Anchoring of PKA in Subcellular Compartments

One of the intriguing aspects of the PKA system is the evidence demonstrating that the holoenzyme is directed to specific subcellular sites by interaction with specific anchoring proteins (AKAPs) (Bregman et al. 1989; Luo et al. 1990; Scott and McCartney 1994). It is estimated that some cell types express as many as 10–15 different AKAPs that bind RII-containing holoenzyme with nanomolar affinities. This targeting of PKA may provide a mechanism to increase the specificity of substrate selection in response to localized accumulation of cAMP and it is clear that many of the AKAPs are themselves substrates for PKA phosphorylation. Subcellular anchoring may also reflect the kinetic requirements of systems that depend on rapid modulation such as voltage-gated ion channels (Hell et al. 1994; Li et al. 1993) and glutamate and GABA receptors (Moss et al. 1992; Raymond et al. 1993a, b). There is recent evidence demonstrating a functional role of AKAPs in the rapid modulation of voltage-gated Ca^{2+} channels (Johnson et al. 1994) and AMPA receptors (Rosenmund et al. 1994). Whereas the RII subunits both bind avidly to AKAPs, the RI subunits are generally thought to remain cytoplasmic, although an interesting example of membrane localization exists for RIα in T cells (Skålhegg et al. 1994).

The hypothesis that AKAPs play an important role in regulatory phosphorylation gained recent support with the exciting discovery that AKAP79 (the human homologue of mouse AKAP150) binds the calcium/calmodulin (Ca^{2+}/CaM)-regulated phosphatase, calcineurin, as well as RII (Coghlan et al. 1995). Anchoring of a kinase/phosphatase complex that can be sequentially activated (the kinase by cAMP, the phosphatase by Ca^{2+}) could allow rapid modulation of nearby ion channels or receptors. More than 20 AKAPs have been cloned to date but many more have been detected by overlay blots with labeled RII as the probe.

6.1.4 PKA Regulates Gene Expression

Cyclic AMP has been shown to be one of the principal regulators of gene induction and cAMP response elements (CREs) are found in many gene promoters. These CREs bind an array of transcription factors of the CREB/ATF family, some of which are directly activated by PKA phosphorylation and some acting in an inhibitory fashion. The binding of phospho-CREB to a CRE leads to interactions with the coactivator CBP (CREB-binding protein) that is then thought to communicate with the basal transcription complex and RNA polymerase (Ferreri et al. 1994; . Chrivia et al. 1993). When cAMP is elevated by hormones or neurotransmitters, PKA dissociates and the C subunit has been shown to migrate to the nucleus where CREB and other members of this family are concentrated (Hagiwara et al. 1993). PKA has also been shown to be essential for the basal transcriptional activity of several genes and the activation level of PKA may be a determinant of differentiation pathways. For example, we have demonstrated that the expression of adrenal cell-specific genes such as P450scc (the rate-limiting enzyme in steroid biosynthesis) is shut off if PKA activity is inhibited (Clegg et al. 1992). In a more recent study we have demonstrated that expression of CFTR (the cystic fibrosis chloride channel) requires basal PKA activity (McDonald et al. 1995).

Several groups have used a genetic approach to study the differentiation of hepatocytes, and a tissue-specific extinguisher (TSE-1) that modulates expression of a subset of hepatocyte genes was characterized. Rather unexpectedly, TSE-1 turned out to be the RIα regulatory subunit of PKA . When expressed in hepatocytes, it inhibits expression of the genes coding for tyrosine aminotransferase (TAT), phosphoenolpyruvate carboxykinase (PEPCK), and glucose-6-phosphatase (Boshart et al. 1991; Jones et al. 1991). These gene products are important in gluconeogenesis and are normally induced at birth although premature stimulation of the fetus with glucagon can induce expression prenatally. These developmental changes in gene expression are normally accompanied by a decrease in RIα gene expression at birth that we suggest could lead to an elevation in the basal PKA activity, inducing gene expression and inhibiting replication. After partial hepatectomy, the liver has the extraordinary ability to regenerate, and this process is accompanied by a substantial induction of RIα mRNA and protein and a decline in basal PKA activity. Since cAMP is known to inhibit hepatocyte replication (Vintermyr et al. 1993), the induction of RIα may be important in lowering the basal activity of PKA to allow the program of cell division and regeneration to occur.

Recently a novel role of PKA in *Drosophila* limb patterning has been discovered by analysis of PKA mutants that appear to act downstream of the hedgehog signal in development (Lepage et al. 1995; Li et al. 1995; Jiang and Struhl 1995; Pan and Rubin 1995). The implication from the *Drosophila* work is that PKA is involved in transducing the hedgehog signal and directing localized expression of wnt (wingless) and dpp (decapentaplegic) genes during development. Mice with disruptions in murine wnt genes show a variety of developmental abnormalities (McMahon and Bradley 1990; Takada et al. 1994), indicating that function is conserved for the wnt pathway in mammals. If decreased C subunit activity causes inappropriate expression of dpp and wnt, as reported, then the RIα mutant mice might be expected to have increased C activity and inhibition of wnt gene expression.

6.1.5 PKA, Synaptic Modulation, and Learning

The role of cAMP and the cAMP-regulated kinases in behavior and synaptic transmission has been under intense scrutiny over the past few years. *Drosophila* learning mutants have been isolated from genetic screens and some of the mutated genes have been characterized. The *dunce* gene codes for a low K_m phosphodiesterase (Chen et al. 1986) and *rutabaga* codes for a Ca^{2+}-sensitive adenylyl cyclase (Livingston 1985). Mutations in the C subunit or expression of dominant inhibitors of PKA behind a heat shock promoter also lead to defects in *Drosophila* learning (Skoulakis et al. 1993). Studies using the marine snail *Aplysia* have demonstrated a role for cAMP and PKA in simple forms of learning that involve both short-term modifications (ion channel phosphorylation) and long-term effects on gene induction and synaptic remodeling (Schacher et al. 1993).

In mammals, electrophysiologists have focused considerable attention on two forms of use-dependent synaptic changes that are thought to be likely candidates for the underlying mechanism of learning. Long-term potentiation (LTP) is an enhancement of synaptic transmission that is input specific and generally requires coactivation of both pre- and postsynaptic elements of the synapse during high-frequency stimulation. The most attractive features of LTP as a model of memory are its long duration (several weeks in vivo), synaptic specificity, and correlation with gene-inductive events (Frey et al. 1993). An opposing change in synaptic strength occurs after low-frequency stimulation, resulting in long-term depression (LTD) (Bear and Malenka 1994). It is quite interesting that a stimulus that produces LTD can also erase LTP at specific synapses. Although both LTP and LTD can be demonstrated in hippocampus, cortex, and cerebellum, it is the hippocampus that has enjoyed the most attention because lesions in either the rodent or human hippocampus lead to defects in certain forms of spatial learning. Studies involving stimulators and inhibitors of second messenger pathways as well as analysis of knockout mice have implicated the cAMP pathway as well as the Ca^{2+} second messenger system.

The initial phase of LTP in the Schaffer collateral/CA1 pathway is *N*-methyl-d-asparate (NMDA) receptor dependent and does not require cAMP (Bear and Malenka 1994). However, the late phase of LTP at this synapse is dependent on both gene induction and cAMP (Frey et al.

1993) and is diminished in the CREB knockout mice (Bourtchuladze et al. 1994). In contrast, LTP in the mossy fiber/CA3 pathway is NMDA receptor independent and can be initiated directly by cAMP acting presynaptically. LTP at this synapse is thought to be the result of a Ca^{2+}/CaM-mediated activation of adenylyl cyclase followed by a cAMP-dependent increase in glutamate release from the mossy fiber terminals (Weisskopf et al. 1994). The late phase of LTP at the CA3 synapse is also dependent on gene induction and protein synthesis (Huang et al. 1994). Clearly both Ca^{2+} and cAMP are interacting to produce the synaptic changes seen in the hippocampus, and cAMP-mediated changes in gene expression are implicated in learning and behavior.

6.2 Gene Targeting Overview

The technology for producing targeted disruptions and mutations in genes first became available in the late 1980s and has already led to an explosive increase in the available mouse mutants. When we compiled a summary of the published gene knockouts at the end of 1994 (Brandon et al. 1995b), there were about 270 unique gene disruptions – and the number is likely to double in 1995. Although at first it seemed as if many null mutations did not give any phenotype, further study has uncovered defects in all but 5% of the 270 reported by the end of 1994. It is also interesting to note that only about 25% of the null mutants are embryonic or neonatal lethals, indicating that most genes do serve specific functions but are not essential for life. This is comforting from an evolutionary standpoint since most of the genes disrupted are highly conserved among all mammalian species and many are more broadly conserved across the animal kingdom.

As with any new technology, it has taken time for laboratories to fully appreciate how best to take advantage of it and also to come to grips with some of the limitations inherent in all genetic studies. One consideration has been the potential for compensatory changes in the expression of other proteins when a single gene product is eliminated. We suggest that compensatory changes are likely to occur in all gene knockouts and that in nearly every case one is studying a novel organism that is attempting to compensate for the function of a normal component of the cellular machinery. The same situation occurs in all genetic mutants whether they be mice, *Drosophila*, zebra fish, or yeast. By examining both the compensatory changes in other biological components and the functional deficits that arise from the inability to compensate fully, we can begin to understand the physiological role played by individual proteins. Studies in the mouse are further complicated when the null mutation is in a protein that is expressed in several tissues and intricate hormonal, metabolic, or behavioral changes occur. The PKA system is complex, involving regulatory and catalytic isoforms that interact with each other, subunit isoforms that are expressed in more than one tissue, and the expression of multiple isoforms within a given cell. The kinase holoenzyme is just one link in a complex signaling system that involves receptors, G proteins, cyclases, phosphodiesterases, and phosphatases. Given the potential for homeostatic controls within this system, it is not unexpected that mice carrying a null mutation in a PKA isoform will exhibit many compensatory alterations.

6.2.1 Embryonic Stem Cell Lines and Targeting Vectors

Embryonic stem (ES) cell lines are derived from the pluripotent cells of the inner cell mass in 3.5-day mouse blastocysts. They must be manipulated in culture by electroporation, drug selection, and screening for homologous recombination. The ES cells must then be reinjected into recipient blastocysts to produce chimeric mice. In order to obtain mutant mice, the ES cells must maintain their ability to contribute to the germline throughout their clonal expansion in cell culture and exposure to drugs and cryopreservation. Not surprisingly, many of the mutated cell lines are capable of producing chimerism in the recipient mouse but have not retained germline competence and do not give rise to knockout mice. In order to improve the frequency of obtaining germline-competent cells we have derived four ES cell lines from the 129Sv/J mouse and demonstrated that each has the ability to contribute to the germline (Brandon et al. 1995a). These ES cell lines (REK1-4) have been used to produce mutations in each of the six PKA subunit isoforms in mice.

Targeting vectors have generally been constructed from clones isolated from 129 genomic libraries although we have also used BALB/c genomic DNA with success and with high frequencies of homologous recombination. Our strategies have varied somewhat with each subunit, but typically we have attempted to remove the transcriptional start site of the gene and the initiation codon of the protein. The targeting vectors have all been of the replacement type in which the exogenous DNA integrates by homologous recombination, leaving the gene interrupted by the neomycin resistance gene.

6.2.2 Germline Mutations in PKA Subunits

We have now obtained germline mutations in each of the PKA subunits and are beginning to study the physiological and biochemical abnormalities associated with these mutations. Mice that have null mutations in RIβ, RIIβ, RIIα, and Cβ1 are apparently healthy and fertile and are beginning to provide interesting clues about compensatory mechanisms and physiological roles. The Cβ1 null mutants continue to produce Cβ2/3 as described earlier and efforts are underway to produce a knockout of all of the Cβ isoforms. Surprisingly, the Cα null mutant mice appear relatively normal at birth although they show severe growth retardation and usually die within the first 6 weeks of life. Only the RIα gene disruption gives rise to embryonic lethality and further studies are needed to determine the timing of this developmental block. In keeping with the topic of this conference, we are very interested in the potential changes in spermatogenesis that might arise in these knockout mice. The fact that the mice remain fertile does not preclude more subtle defects in testicular function. We are particularly interested in examining sperm motility in RIIα mutant mice since RIIα is normally a major PKA subunit associated with the flagellum in mature sperm and cAMP is thought to participate in the regulation of motility.

Our initial studies on the RIβ and Cβ1 null mutants focused on electrophysiology and behavior since both of these subunits are expressed most highly in the brain. Studies on the RIIβ mice have initially focused on adipose tissue and metabolic regulation although RIIβ is also expressed at high levels in brain.

6.2.3 Compensatory Changes in R and C Isoforms

One of the initial studies that is essential for each knockout is an evaluation of changes in other R or C subunits and the net effect on basal and cAMP-stimulated PKA activity. Disruption of the RIβ subunit does not change the total activity of brain PKA but we do see an increase in the RIα subunit that may roughly substitute for the lost RIβ. What effect might this have at a biochemical level? We have shown previously that holoenzymes assembled from RIβ and either Cα or Cβ1 display an increased sensitivity to activation by cAMP compared with RIα. A cell that has compensated for the lost RIβ by increasing levels of RIα might now be expected to require a higher threshold of cAMP accumulation to achieve PKA activation. This reduced sensitivity to activation could interfere with sensitive synaptic modulation in neurons where RIβ is specifically expressed.

Disruption of RIIβ leads to a profound change in PKA in both white and brown adipose tissue where the principal regulatory subunit is normally RIIβ. We find a large increase in RIα and a small decrease in total C protein and activity. In adipocytes from RIIβ mutant mice the PKA has switched from a type II to a type I holoenzyme. This may disturb the normal localization of PKA since it appears that RII but not RI can interact specifically with AKAPs. We have not detected any changes in other subunits in the Cβ1 mutants but this C subunit is generally expressed at a much lower level than Cα and would not be expected to contribute more than 10%–20% of the total C activity.

6.3 Synaptic Plasticity: Defects in PKA Knockout Mice

One of the most fascinating functions of the signal transduction systems is the modulation of synaptic plasticity in the brain. Changes in synaptic strength can be measured both in vitro and in vivo after electrical stimulation and these changes can be synapse specific and long lasting. It is not difficult to see why this phenomenon of LTP might seem like a ready mechanism to underlie learning and memory and intensive effort has been devoted to both understand the mechanism at a biochemical level and demonstrate its role in learning. The rat was the focus of most electrophysiological and behavioral studies done prior to the advent of

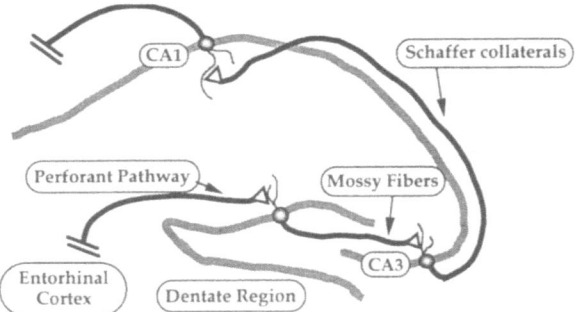

Fig. 1. Hippocampal pathways. The perforant pathway leading from the entorhinal cortex to the dentate granule cells, the mossy fiber pathway from the granule cells to the CA3 pyramidal cells, and the Schaffer collateral pathway from CA3 to CA1 pyramidal cells are shown

gene knockouts. Now, however, it is more often knockout mice that are swimming around in water mazes and being subjected to electrophysiological scrutiny. At an electrophysiological level, the hippocampal trisynaptic pathway has been intensely studied both because of the relative ease in recording from this discrete region and because lesions within the hippocampal pathway cause profound losses in spatial memory. As shown in Fig. 1, the input into the hippocampus arrives via the perforant pathway from the entorhinal cortex and projects to the granule cells of the dentate gyrus. The granule cells in turn project their axons via the mossy fiber pathway to the CA3 pyramidal cells. Finally, the pyramidal cells of the CA3 region project by means of the Schaffer collateral pathway to the CA1 pyramidal cells. In addition to this network of connections, additional pathways exist within the hippocampus, including connections from the entorhinal cortex directly to the CA1 pyramidal cells.

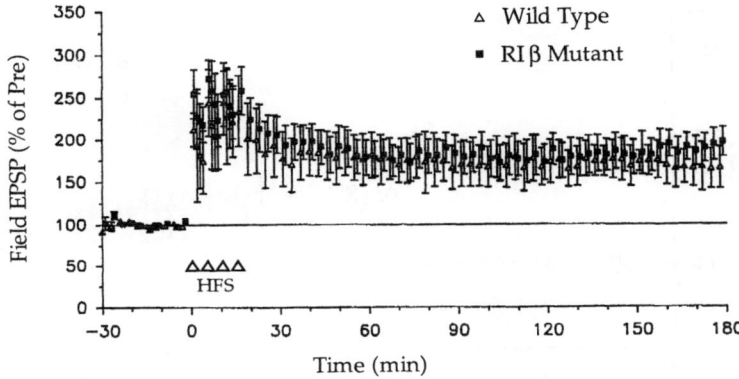

Fig. 2. Schaffer collateral long-term potentiation (LTP) in RIβ knockout mice. Tetanic stimulation to produce LTP was 100 Hz for 1 s, delivered four times with an intertrain interval of 4 min. All experiments were done blind to genotype with slices from six to nine mice in each group. Adapted from Brandon et al. (1995c). *HFS*, high-frequency stimulation; *EPSP*, excitatory postsynaptic potential

6.3.1 LTP in the Schaffer Collateral Pathway

We have examined the ability of RIβ and Cβ1 mutant mice to sustain LTP in the Schaffer collateral pathway after high-frequency stimulation in a hippocampal slice preparation. The RIβ mutants were indistinguishable from wild types (Fig. 2) and were capable of late-phase LTP extending beyond the 3-h experiment. The Cβ mutants responded normally to a single high-frequency stimulus with transient potentiation indicating no difference in the early phase of LTP (Fig. 3a). However, after a series of four high-frequency stimuli, wild-type slices displayed LTP that lasted for the 3-h duration of the experiment, whereas the Cβ mutant slices were unable to maintain the potentiation and displayed nearly a 70% loss in late-phase LTP (Fig. 3b). Both RIβ and Cβ1 mutant mice displayed normal synaptic transmission and normal facilitation after a paired pulse stimulation.

The loss of LTP in the Cβ1 mutants is quite interesting and at face value agrees well with the observations that the late phase of LTP in this pathway is cAMP dependent, with PKA and CREB transcriptional

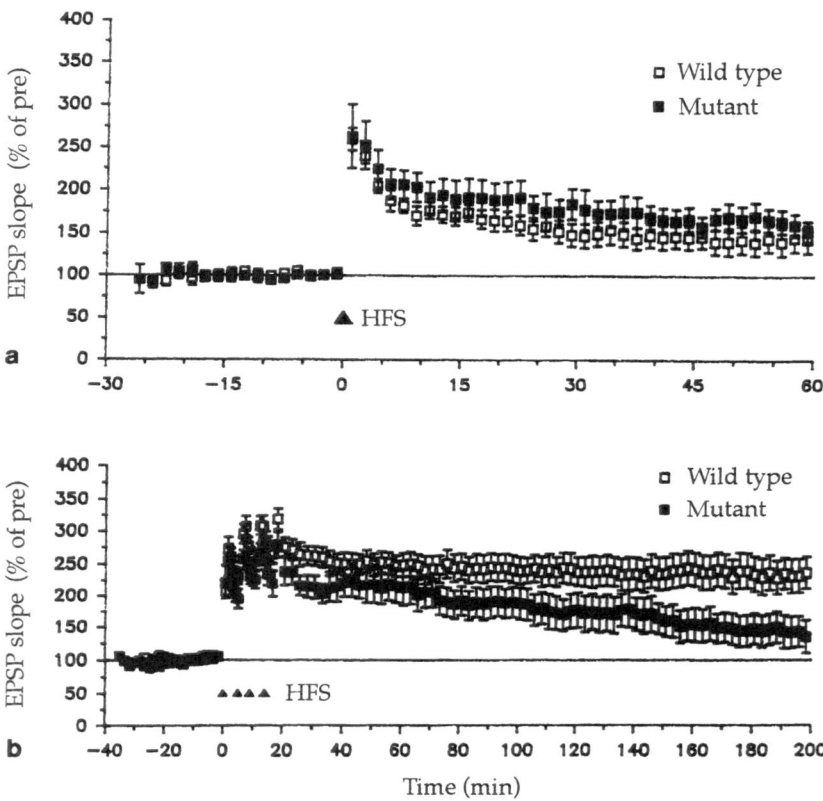

Fig. 3a,b. Schaffer collateral long-term potentiation (LTP) in Cβ1 knockout mice. **a** The early phase of LTP induced by a one-train high frequency stimulation (*HFS*). **b** Late-phase LTP after four trains of HFS. Adapted from Qi et al. (1996). *EPSP*, excitatory postsynaptic potential

activation likely being involved. However, this may be a simplistic interpretation since Cβ1 is likely to be a small proportion of the total C subunit in the CA3 and CA1 neurons. An additional possibility is that Cβ associates into a holoenzyme which differs in biochemical properties or subcellular localization from its Cα counterpart. For example, it has recently been discovered that when Cβ1 is complexed with the RIIα subunit, the resulting holoenzyme shows an increased sensitivity to activation by cAMP (E. Baude and M. Uhler, personal communication). The subcellular localization of Cβ1 in the hippocampus has not yet been explored.

6.3.2 LTD in the Schaffer Collateral Pathway

Both RIβ and Cβ mutant mice have lost the ability to undergo LTD in the Schaffer collateral pathway (Qi et al. 1996; Brandon et al. 1995c). A low-frequency stimulus (1 Hz for 15 min) applied to the Schaffer collateral–CA1 pyramidal cell synapse of wild-type mice resulted in a depression of the field excitatory postsynaptic potential (EPSP) that lasted at least 35 min. When RIβ mutant mice were tested using the same paradigm, the ability to evoke LTD was nearly completely lost, as shown in Fig. 4a. A related electrophysiological phenomenon, depotentiation or erasure, is also affected in the RIβ knockouts. As shown in Fig. 4b, after LTP induction in the Schaffer collateral pathway, a low-frequency stimulus will erase or depotentiate the synapse in wild-type mice but is ineffective in RIβ knockout mice. The same electrophysiological measurements were made on the Cβ knockout mice and both LTD and depotentiation were defective in these mice as well (Fig. 5).

It is interesting to compare these results with the effects of pharmacological inhibition of PKA in the slice using KT5720. This drug effectively prevents the appearance of LTD in wild-type slices, suggesting that the biochemical effects of the RIβ and Cβ1 knockouts are mediated by a diminished ability to phosphorylate specific substrates (Brandon et al. 1995c).

In order to understand the mechanistic events which are influenced by PKA during LTD induction we must first understand in more detail the biochemical mechanisms underlying LTD itself. One model to explain LTD has been proposed by Lisman (Lisman 1989) and further updated by Malenka (Malenka 1994). This model suggests that low-frequency stimulation leads to a modest rise in calcium that may couple preferentially to phosphatase activation during LTD induction, leading to the decreased level of synaptic transmission. Our experiments demonstrate that cAMP and the PKA signaling system must also be incorporated into a model for LTD. This is not surprising since the two

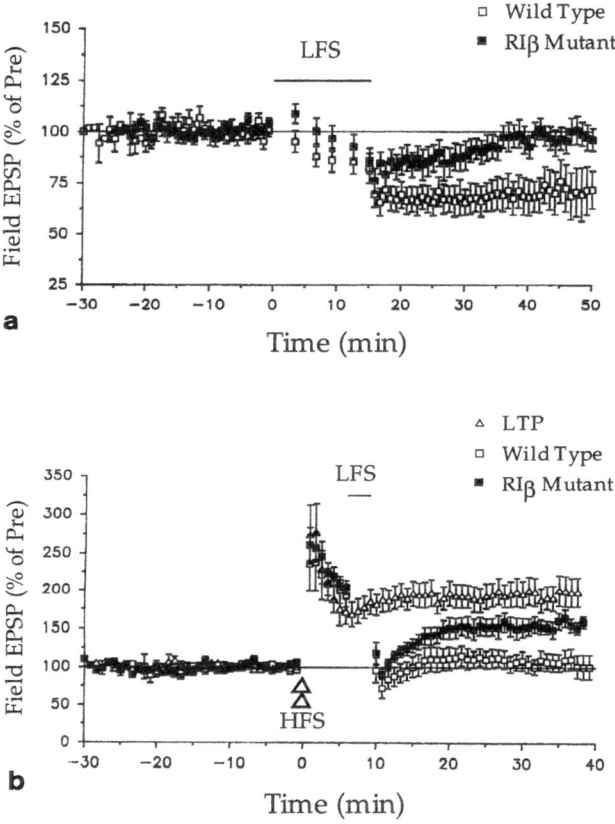

Fig. 4a,b. Synaptic long-term depression (LTD) at the Schaffer collateral–CA1 pyramidal cell synapse in hippocampal slices from RIβ knockout mice. **a** LTD was produced by a low-frequency stimulation (*LFS*) delivered for 15 min at 1 Hz. **b** The high-frequency stimulus (*HFS*) to produce long-term potentiation (*LTP*) was 100 Hz for 1 s delivered twice with an intertrain interval of 20 s. The LFS was delivered at 5 Hz for 3 min to produce depotentiation. Measurements from wild-type slices in which LTP was evoked without subsequent depotentiation are shown as *open triangles*. Adapted from Brandon et al. (1995c). *EPSP*, excitatory postsynaptic potential

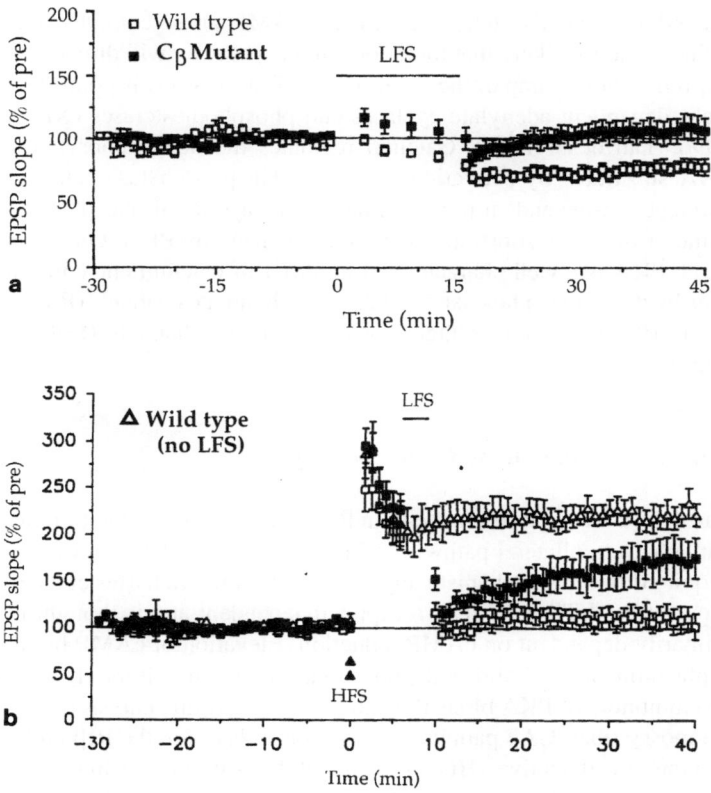

Fig. 5a,b. Long-term depression (LTD) and depotentiation in Cβ1 knockout mice. The same protocol described in Fig. 4 was applied to hippocampal slices from the Cβ1 knockout mice. Adapted from Qi et al. (1996). *EPSP*, excitatory postsynaptic potential; *LFS*, low-frequency stimulation; *HFS*, high-frequency stimulation

second messenger systems, calcium and cAMP, are so completely inter-twined that it is likely that mutations in one pathway will directly affect the other. For example, the level of cAMP in neurons is controlled by CaM-dependent adenylate cyclases and phosphodiesterases (Xia et al. 1996; Yan et al. 1994). Calcium regulates the dephosphorylation of PKA substrates by activation of the protein phosphatase calcineurin, and calcium-dependent protein kinases are capable of phosphorylating some of the same substrates that are recognized by PKA. On the other hand, PKA is a well-characterized modifier of calcium entry into neu-rons by direct phosphorylation of AMPA glutamate channels (Raymond et al. 1993a, b) and voltage-sensitive calcium channels (Hell et al. 1993).

6.3.3 LTP in the Mossy Fiber Pathway

The defects in synaptic plasticity in RIβ and Cβ1 mice are not limited to the Schaffer collateral pathway. LTP in the mossy fiber–CA3 pathway is quite different mechanistically from LTP in the Schaffer collaterals. Mossy fiber LTP is NMDA receptor independent and is thought to be primarily dependent on cAMP induction. Elevation of cAMP by direct application of forskolin and phosphodiesterase inhibitors elicits LTP and inhibitors of PKA block this induction. A careful analysis of LTP in the mossy fiber–CA3 pathway demonstrates that both the RIβ and Cβ1 mutants are defective (Huang et al. 1995). Although a low level of mossy fiber LTP remains in the RIβ mutants, we could detect no evidence for LTP in Cβ1 mutants in response to two trains of high-fre-quency stimulation (Fig. 6). However, if the slices were challenged with forskolin, which elicits a robust LTP in wild-type mice, both RIβ and Cβ1 mutants responded with LTP that was indistinguishable from wild type (Fig. 7). This suggests that the defect depends on the strength of the initiating signal; a weaker stimulation mediated through electrical stimulation may not reach threshold in the mutants, whereas complete activation of PKA in response to forskolin is capable of overcoming the defect. This makes sense since we have not completely eliminated PKA from the neurons but rather have caused a more subtle shift in the isoforms expressed by selective gene knockout. A daunting task is now to discover what the RIβ and Cβ1 isoforms are doing in neurons. Which

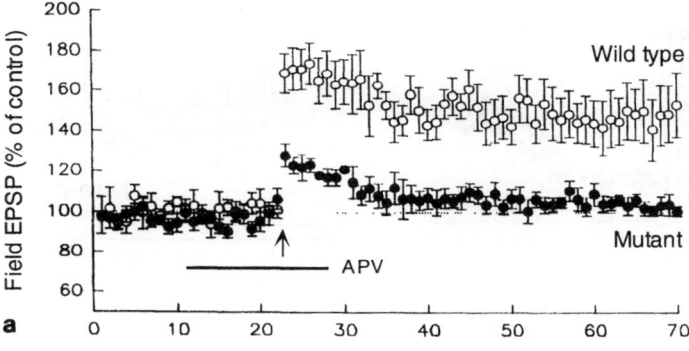

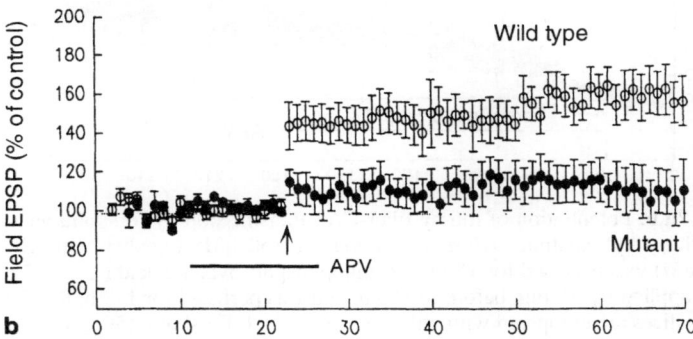

Fig. 6a,b. Mossy fiber long-term potentiation (LTP) in Cβ1 and RIβ knockout mice. Two trains of tetanus (100 Hz, 1 s, 0.1-ms pulse duration in 10-s intervals) induced robust LTP in the presence of aminophosphosovaleric acid (*APV*) in wild-type mice. **a** Cβ1 knockout mice are compared with wild-type controls. **b** RIβ knockout versus wild type. Adapted from Huang et al. (1995). *EPSP*, excitatory postsynaptic potential

substrates are they targeting that cannot be efficiently phosphorylated by the other (Cα- and RIα-containing) PKA isoforms?

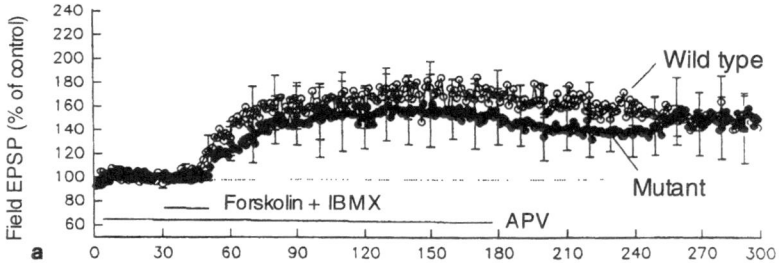

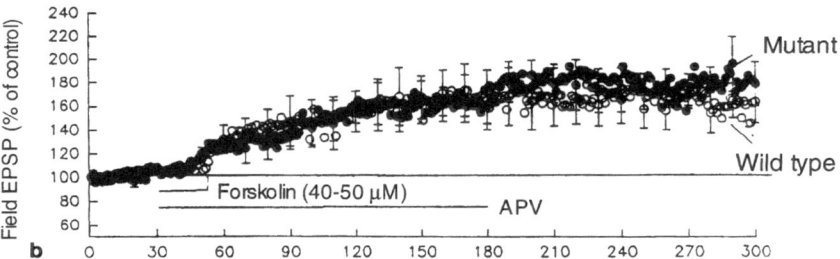

Fig. 7a,b. Potentiation of mossy fiber-CA3 transmission by forskolin and iso-butyl methyl xanthine (*IBMX*). **a** Forskolin (50 μ*M*) together with IBMX (50 μ*M*) was perfused for 15 min. Aminophosphosovaleric acid (*APV*; 25 μ*M*) was applied for 10 min before forskolin and was perfused for 1–2 h. RIβ knockout slices are compared with wild-type controls. **b** Forskolin (50 μ*M*) was applied as in part **a** in the absence of IBMX and long-term potentiation was measured in both Cβ1 knockout and wild-type slices. Adapted from Huang et al. (1995). *EPSP*, excitatory postsynaptic potential

6.3.4 Analysis of Behavior in PKA Mutant Mice

Targeted disruptions of the PKA isoforms produce mice with specific electrophysiological defects and these mice can then be tested in a battery of behavioral studies to determine whether there is any correlation between the two parameters. Since most of our electrophysiological measurements were done in hippocampus, we have begun by examining spatial and contextual learning and memory tasks that are thought to rely heavily on hippocampal processes. RIβ and Cβ1 mutant mice have been tested in the Barnes maze and Morris water maze. In these tasks the mice develop a spatial representation of the environment surrounding the maze and use this in their search strategy to find a goal (hole or platform) that allows them to escape from an unpleasant situation (buzzer and lights or swimming). In addition, mice were tested in behavioral tasks involving context or cued conditioning. In these tasks, the mice learn to fear a new environment or react to a conditioned cue because of its temporal association with an aversive unconditioned stimulus (foot shock). In all of these tests and in open field observation we were unable to detect differences between wild-type and either RIβ or Cβ1 mutant mice (Huang et al. 1995). Although disappointing in terms of linking behavior with electrophysiological phenomena, this negative result is in some ways more informative than one in which the animals exhibit defects. We can conclude from these studies that the ability to sustain potentiation in the mossy fiber pathway and the ability to undergo depression in the Schaffer collateral pathway are not essential for mice to perform within normal parameters in the most frequently used spatial memory tasks. Several caveats must be considered. First, we have only measured LTP and LTD under in vitro slice conditions and in response to high- or low-frequency electrical stimulation. We have shown that the mossy fiber pathway in mutant mice can still undergo potentiation in response to forskolin, a powerful activator of cyclases, and it is possible that LTP may still occur in vivo in response to different stimulation. Second, we must keep in mind that these mutant animals have developed from conception with this mutation and that alternative neuronal pathways may have been stimulated to take over some of the normal functions in defective synapses. Finally, the behavioral tests may not be sensitive enough or may not be testing the correct function that would correlate with hippocampal plasticity. Unfortunately we cannot give these mice a battery of cognitive tests as one can a graduate student. It is quite likely that a Morris water maze for humans would not distinguish between a Norwegian mountaineer guide and a shopper who loses his/her car in the parking lot. Clearly, more refinement is needed in all of these measurements.

6.4 RIIβ Knockout Mice Are Genetically Lean

We have disrupted the RIIβ gene and begun studies on these mutant mice focusing on both neuronal and adipocyte functions. Homozygotic mutant mice appear quite healthy and show no gross changes in behavior. They are fertile, which was somewhat surprising since the RIIβ protein is expressed in both Sertoli (testis) and granulosa (ovary) cells where it is strongly induced by FSH. However, when we examined fat tissue from these animals it was apparent that the loss of RIIβ had a dramatic effect on adipocyte function. The RIIβ knockout mice had a 60% reduction in white fat compared to age-matched controls. The number of fat cells in the knockout mice was the same as controls but the histology of knockout fat in adult mice displayed a characteristic depletion of triglyceride stores similar to that seen in mice which have been fasted. When we separated type I and II kinases on an high-performance liquid chromatography (HPLC) DEAE-ion exchange column, we found that nearly all of the PKA activity in wild type fat is in the form of a type II (RIIβ) holoenzyme whereas the knockout fat has undergone a dramatic compensatory change in kinases and now contains a high level of type I (RIα) kinase. Total PKA activity was decreased by about 50% and there was a corresponding decrease in C subunit as shown by Western blot analysis of adipocyte protein from wild-type and knockout mice. However, we observe a large (three- to fivefold) increase in RIα protein in the RIIβ mutant fat, indicating the presence of a compensatory mechanism similar to that seen in brain from RIβ knockout mice. Recent studies indicate a critical change in brown adipose tissue (BAT) in RIIβ mutant mice. BAT facilitates non-shivering thermogenesis during cold acclimation by the induction of uncoupling protein (UCP). UCP is a proton translocator which uncouples mitochondrial respiration from oxidative phosphorylation so that energy derived from oxidation of fatty acids is dissipated as heat, rather than stored as ATP. BAT from RIIβ mutant mice has an increase in basal PKA activity accompanied by an induction of UCP mRNA and protein. The increased expression of uncoupling protein leads to an elevation in body temperature by 0.8 °C and an increased O_2 consumption (Cummings et al. 1996). These results suggest that brown fat may be a key regulator of total body fat in agreement with another mouse genetic experiment in which brown fat was eliminated in mice with a toxic transgene giving rise to obesity (Lowell et al. 1993). The RIIβ mice provide a novel genetic model in which to study the regulation of obesity.

6.5 Concluding Remarks

The techniques of targeted gene disruption in mice allow us to manipulate the genome of a mammalian organism in ways that would have seemed impossible to most biologists just 10 years ago. In response to this success, many molecular biologists are now attempting to address issues of physiological function and even behavior, and this has necessitated a tremendous recruitment of experienced physiologists, behavioral neuroscientists, biophysicists, and anatomists to the study of the rapidly increasing number of mutant lines of mice. Insights into a gene product's overall role in the organism are within reach in contrast to the more limited view based on cell culture experiments that we were previously left with.

The family of six genes that code for the subunits of PKA are in many ways ideal for targeted genetic experiments. The proteins are very well characterized biochemically and structurally and we think the complete set has been isolated although other splice variants and perhaps completely unique genes might have escaped our notice as yet. In terms of function, PKA plays a central role in signal transduction mechanisms and many specific substrates have been identified, so there is no lack of physiological questions that can be pursued in virtually every tissue. Nevertheless when your Southern blot or polymerase chain reaction finally tells you that you are looking at a mouse that has lost the ability to make RIIα and yet seems unperturbed, there is a strong sensation that much remains to be learned. The detective work that one hopes will eventually lead to some understanding of why the RIIα gene is a highly conserved member of this gene family is just beginning. RIIα is abundantly expressed in skeletal muscle and in cardiac tissues. Why is this mouse able to hang upside down from his cage with his heart obviously beating? RIIα is highly induced late in spermatid development and the protein binds tightly to mitochondria in the midpiece and the fibrous sheath in the distal portion of the flagellum, yet the RIIα knockout mouse has successfully fathered several litters of pups. We clearly have a lot to learn about the essential functions of the PKA system and, hopefully, the available mutant PKA mouse lines will provide a good starting point for these studies.

References

Bear MF, Malenka RC (1994) Synaptic plasticity: LTP and LTD. Curr Opin Neurobiol 4:389–399

Beebe SJ, Øyen O, Sandberg M, Frøysa A, Hansson V, Jahnsen T (1990) Molecular cloning of a tissue-specific protein kinase (Cγ) from human testis – representing a third isoform for the catalytic subunit of cAMP-dependent protein kinase. Mol Endocrinol 4:465–475

Biel M, Zong X, Distler M, Bosse E, Klugbauer N, Murakami M, Flockerzi V, Hofmann F (1994) Another member of the cyclic nucleotide-gated channel family, expressed in testis, kidney, and heart. Proc Natl Acad Sci USA 91:3505–3509

Boshart M, Weih F, Nichols M, Schutz G (1991) The tissue-specific extinguisher locus TSE1 encodes a regulatory subunit of cAMP-dependent protein kinase. Cell 66:849–859

Bourtchuladze R, Frenguelli B, Blendy J, Cioffi D, Schutz G, Silva AJ (1994) Deficient long-term memory in mice with a targeted mutation of the cAMP-responsive element-binding protein. Cell 79:59–68

Brandon EP, Gerhold KA, Qi M, McKnight GS, Idzerda RL (1995a) Derivation of novel embryonic stem cell lines and targeting of cyclic AMP-dependent protein kinase genes. Rec Prog Horm Res 50:403–408

Brandon EP, Idzerda RL, McKnight GS (1995b) Targeting the mouse genome: a compendium of knockouts. Curr Biol 5:625–634

Brandon EP, Zhuo M, Huang Y-Y, Qi M, Gerhold KA, Burton KA, Kandel ER, McKnight GS, Idzerda RL (1995c) Hippocampal long-term depression and depotentiation are defective in mice carrying a targeted disruption of the gene encoding the RIβ subunit of cAMP-dependent protein kinase. Proc Natl Acad Sci USA 92:8851–8855

Bregman DB, Bhattacharyya N, Rubin CS (1989) High affinity binding protein for the regulatory subunit of cAMP-dependent protein kinase II-B. Cloning, characterization, and expression of cDNAs for rat brain P150. J Biol Chem 264:4648–4656

Cadd G, McKnight GS (1989) Distinct patterns of cAMP-dependent protein kinase gene expression in mouse brain. Neuron 3:71–79

Cadd GG, Uhler MD, McKnight GS (1990) Holoenzymes of cAMP-dependent protein kinase containing the neural form of type I regulatory subunit have an increased sensitivity to cyclic nucleotides. J Biol Chem 265:19502–19506

Chen CN, Denome S, Davis RL (1986) Molecular analysis of cDNA clones and the corresponding genomic coding sequences of the Drosophila dunce+ gene, the structural gene for cAMP phosphodiesterase. Proc Natl Acad Sci USA 83:9313–9317

Chrivia JC, Kwok RP, Lamb N, Hagiwara M, Montminy MR, Goodman RH (1993) Phosphorylated CREB binds specifically to the nuclear protein CBP. Nature 365:855–859

Clegg CH, Abrahamsen MS, Degen JL, Morris DR, McKnight GS (1992) Cyclic AMP-dependent protein kinase controls basal gene activity and steroidogenesis in Y1 adrenal tumor cells. Biochemistry 31:3720–3726

Coghlan VM, Perrino BA, Howard M, Langeberg LK, Hicks JB, Gallatin WM, Scott JD (1995) Association of protein kinase A and protein phosphatase 2B with a common anchoring protein. Science 267:108–111

Cummings DE, Edelhoff S, Disteche CM, McKnight GS (1994) Cloning of a mouse protein kinase A catalytic subunit pseudogene and chromosomal mapping of C subunit isoforms. Mammalian Genome 5:701–706

Cummings DE, Brandon EP, Planas JV, Motamed K, Idzerda RL, McKnight GS (1996) Genetically lean mice derived by targeted disruption of the RIIβ subunit of protein kinase A (manuscript submitted)

Ferreri K, Gill G, Montminy M (1994) The cAMP-regulated transcription factor CREB interacts with a component of the TFIID complex. Proc Natl Acad Sci USA 91:1210–1213

Frey U, Huang YY, Kandel ER (1993) Effects of cAMP simulate a late stage of LTP in hippocampal CA1 neurons. Science 260:1661–1664

Hagiwara M, Brindle P, Harootunian A, Armstrong R, Rivier J, Vale W, Tsien R, Montminy MR (1993) Coupling of hormonal stimulation and transcription via the cyclic AMP-responsive factor CREB is rate limited by nuclear entry of protein kinase A. Mol Cell Biol 13:4852–4859

Hell JW, Yokoyama CT, Wong ST, Warner C, Snutch TP, Catterall WA (1993) Differential phosphorylation of two size forms of the neuronal class C L-type calcium channel α_1 subunit. J Biol Chem 268:19451–19457

Hell JW, Appleyard SM, Yokoyama CT, Warner C, Catterall WA (1994) Differential phosphorylation of two size forms of the N-type calcium channel α_1 subunit which have different COOH termini. J Biol Chem 269:7390–7396

Huang YY, Li XC, Kandel ER (1994) cAMP contributes to mossy fiber LTP by initiating both a covalently mediated early phase and macromolecular synthesis-dependent late phase. Cell 79:69–79

Huang YY, Kandel ER, Varshavsky L, Brandon EP, Qi M, Idzerda RL, McKnight GS, Bourtchouladze R (1995) A genetic test of the effects of mutations in PKA on mossy fiber LTP and its relation to spatial and contextual learning. Cell 83:1211–1222

Jiang J, Struhl G (1995) Protein kinase A and hedgehog signaling in Drosophila limb development. Cell 80:563–572

Johnson BD, Scheuer T, Catterall WA (1994) Voltage-dependent potentiation of L-type Ca^{2+} channels in skeletal muscle cells requires anchored cAMP-dependent protein kinase. Proc Natl Acad Sci U S A 91:11492–11496

Jones KW, Shapero MH, Chevrette M, Fournier RE (1991) Subtractive hybridization cloning of a tissue-specific extinguisher: TSE1 encodes a regulatory subunit of protein kinase A. Cell 66:861–872

Keryer G, Luo Z, Cavadore JC, Erlichman J, Bornens M (1993) Phosphorylation of the regulatory subunit of type IIβ cAMP-dependent protein kinase by cyclin B/p34cdc2 kinase impairs its binding to microtubule-associated protein 2. Proc Natl Acad Sci USA 90:5418–5422

Kurten RC, Levy LØ, Shey J, Durica JM, Richards JS (1992) Identification and characterization of the GC-rich and cyclic adenosine 3',5'-monophosphate (cAMP)-inducible promoter of the type IIβ cAMP-dependent protein kinase regulatory subunit gene. Mol Endocrinol 6:536–550

Lepage T, Cohen SM, Diaz-Benjumea FJ, Parkhurst SM (1995) Signal transduction by cAMP-dependent protein kinase A in Drosophila limb patterning. Nature 373:711–715

Li M, West JW, Numann R, Murphy BJ, Scheuer T, Catterall WA (1993) Convergent regulation of sodium channels by protein kinase C and cAMP-dependent protein kinase. Science 261:1439–1442

Li W, Ohlmeyer JT, Lane ME, Kalderon D (1995) Function of protein kinase A in hedgehog signal transduction and Drosophila imaginal disc development. Cell 80:553–562

Lisman J (1989) A mechanism for the Hebb and the anti-Hebb processes underlying learning and memory. Proc Natl Acad Sci USA 86:9574–9578

Livingston MS (1985) Genetic dissection of Drosophila adenylate cyclase. Proc Natl Acad Sci USA 82:5992–5996

Lowell BB, S-Susulie V, Hamann A, Lawitts JA, Himms HJ, Boyer BB, Kozak LP, Flier JS (1993) Development of obesity in transgenic mice after genetic ablation of brown adipose tissue. Nature 366:740–742

Luo Z, Shafit ZB, Erlichman J (1990) Identification of the MAP2- and P75-binding domain in the regulatory subunit (RIIβ) of type II cAMP-dependent protein kinase. Cloning and expression of the cDNA for bovine brain RIIβ. J Biol Chem 265:21804–21810

Malenka RC (1994) Synaptic plasticity in the hippocampus: LTP and LTD. Cell 78:535–538

McDonald RA, Matthews RP, Idzerda RL, McKnight GS (1995) Basal expression of the cystic fibrosis transmembrane conductance regulator gene is dependent on protein kinase A activity. Proc Natl Acad Sci USA 92:7560–7564

McKnight GS (1991) Cyclic AMP second messenger systems. Curr Opin Cell Biol 3:213–217

McMahon AP, Bradley A (1990) The Wnt-1 (int-1) proto-oncogene is required for development of a large region of the mouse brain. Cell 62:1073–1085

Moss SJ, Smart TG, Blackstone CD, Huganir RL (1992) Functional modulation of GABAA receptors by cAMP-dependent protein phosphorylation. Science 257:661–665

Orellana SA, McKnight GS (1992) Mutations in the catalytic subunit of cAMP-dependent protein kinase result in unregulated biological activity. Proc Natl Acad Sci USA 89:4726–4730

Otten AD, McKnight GS (1989) Overexpression of the type II regulatory subunit of the cAMP-dependent protein kinase eliminates the type I holoenzyme in mouse cells. J Biol Chem 264:20255–20260

Otten AD, Parenteau LA, Døskeland S, McKnight GS (1991) Hormonal activation of gene transcription ins ras-transformed NIH3T3 cells overexpressing RIIα and RIIβ subunits of cAMP-dependent protein kinase. J Biol Chem 266:23074–23082

Øyen O, Eskild W, Beebe SJ, Hansson V, Jahnsen T (1988) Biphasic response to 3',5'-cyclic adenosine monophosphate (cAMP) at the messenger ribonucleic acid level for a regulatory subunit of cAMP-dependent protein kinase. Mol Endocrinol 2:1070–1076

Pan D, Rubin GM (1995) cAMP-dependent protein kinase and hedgehog act antagonistically in regulating decapentaplegic transcription in Drosophila imaginal discs. Cell 80:543–552

Qi M, Zhuo M, Skålhegg BS, Brandon EP, Kandel ER, McKnight GS, Idzerda RL (1996) Impaired hippocampal plasticity in PKA-Cβ1 mutant mice. Proc Natl Acad Sci USA (in press)

Raymond LA, Blackstone CD, Huganir RL (1993a) Phosphorylation and modulation of recombinant GluR6 glutamate receptors by cAMP-dependent protein kinase. Nature 361:637–641

Raymond LA, Blackstone CD, Huganir RL (1993b) Phosphorylation of amino acid neurotransmitter receptors in synaptic plasticity. Trends Neurosci 16:147–153

Rosen OM, Erlichman J (1975) Reversible autophosphorylation of a cyclic 3':5'-AMP-dependent protein kinase from bovine cardiac muscle. J Biol Chem 250:7788–7794

Rosenmund C, Carr DW, Bergeson SE, Nilaver G, Scott JD, Westbrook GL (1994) Anchoring of protein kinase A is required for modulation of AMPA/kainate receptors on hippocampal neurons. Nature 368:853–856

Schacher S, Kandel ER, Montarolo P (1993) cAMP and arachidonic acid simulate long-term structural and functional changes produced by neurotransmitters in Aplysia sensory neurons. Neuron 10:1079–1088

Scott JD, McCartney S (1994) Localization of A-kinase through anchoring proteins. Mol Endocrinol 8:5–11

Skålhegg BS, Taskén K, Hansson V, Huitfeldt HS, Jahnsen T, Lea T (1994) Location of cAMP-dependent protein kinase type I with the TCR-CD3 complex. Science 263:84–87

Skoulakis EM, Kalderon D, Davis RL (1993) Preferential expression in mushroom bodies of the catalytic subunit of protein kinase A and its role in learning and memory. Neuron 11:197–208

Takada S, Stark KL, Shea MJ, Vassileva G, McMahon JA, McMahon AP (1994) Wnt-3a regulates somite and tailbud formation in the mouse embryo. Genes Dev 8:174–189

Taskén K, Skålhegg BS, Solberg R, Andersson KB, Taylor SS, Lea T, Blomhoff HK, Jahnsen T, Hansson V (1993) Novel isozymes of cAMP-dependent protein kinase exist in human cells due to formation of RIα-RIβ heterodimeric complexes. J Biol Chem 268:21276–21283

Uhler MD, Chrivia JC, McKnight GS (1986) Evidence for a second isoform of the catalytic subunit of cAMP-dependent protein kinase [published erratum appears in J Biol Chem (1987) 262:5431]. J Biol Chem 261:15360–15363

Vintermyr OK, Bøe R, Bruland T, Houge G, Døskeland SO (1993) Elevated cAMP gives short-term inhibition and long-term stimulation of hepatocyte DNA replication: roles of the cAMP-dependent protein kinase subunits. J Cell Physiol 156:160–170

Weisskopf MG, Castillo PE, Zalutsky RA, Nicoll RA (1994) Mediation of hippocampal mossy fiber long-term potentiation by cyclic AMP. Science 265:1878–1882

Wiemann S, Kinzel V, Pyerin W (1991) Isoform Cβ2, an unusual form of the bovine catalytic subunit of cAMP-dependent protein kinase. J Biol Chem 266:5140–5146

Xia Z, Choi E-J, Blazynski C, Storm DR (1996) Do the calmodulin stimulated adenylyl cyclases play a role in neuroplasticity? Behav Brain Sci 18:429–440

Yan C, Bentley JK, Sonnenburg WK, Beavo JA (1994) Differential expression of the 61 kDa and 63 kDa calmodulin-dependent phosphodiesterases in the mouse brain. J Neurosci 14:973–984

7 Posttranscriptional Regulation of Postmeiotic Gene Expression

N.B. Hecht

7.1   Introduction 123
7.2   Many Messenger RNAs in Postmeiotic Male Germ Cells
        Undergo Deadenylation upon Translation 124
7.3   Testicular Poly(A) Binding Proteins 126
7.4   p48/52, Sequence-Independent RNA-Binding Proteins
        that also Bind to Specific Germ Cell Promoter Sequences 127
7.5   Subcellular Localization of Messenger RNAs in the Testis 128
7.6   TB-RBP, a Regulator of Translation and Cellular Localization
        of mRNAs 130
7.7   Superoxide Dismutase 1 Utilizes an Alternative Promoter
        Which Produces a Novel Postmeiotic mRNA
        Whose Translation Is Regulated by an RNA-Binding Protein ... 134
7.8   Conclusions 135
References 136

7.1 Introduction

In eukaryotic cells the expression of a gene is regulated at many different levels. In the nucleus, changes in chromatin structure and DNA methylation control the temporal and spatial transcription of genes. Although the time of transcription is frequently the primary regulator of gene expression in many tissues, including the testis, the actual time of synthesis of many proteins in male germ cells is often dependent upon posttranscriptional mRNA processing events. Posttranscriptional regulation is especially important towards the end of spermatogenesis because, in contrast to virtually every other eukaryotic cell type, nuclear transcription ceases during mid-spermiogenesis in male germ cells. This necessitates that mRNA storage and translational activation play prominent roles in the expression of a large number of spermatid and spermatozoal proteins that are synthesized in late stages of germ cell maturation. Many of the structural and isoprotein molecules of the spermatozoon are under this type of posttranscriptional control (reviewed in Eddy and O'Brien 1994; Erickson 1993; Handel 1987; Hecht 1993, 1995; Willison and Ashworth 1987; Wolgemuth et al. 1993).

After eukaryotic mRNAs are transcribed, they undergo a number of important modifications and movements essential for their physiological functioning. These include removal of introns by splicing, polyadenylation, transport from the nucleus to the cytoplasm, stabilization in the cytoplasm, and often movement to specific cytoplasmic locations before they are translated. Although little is known about the molecular mechanisms that regulate the splicing, transport, and stabilization of postmeiotic male germ cell mRNAs, the mechanisms regulating polyadenylation, translation, and mRNA localization during mammalian spermiogenesis are beginning to be deciphered.

In this chapter I limit my discussion to several posttranscriptional events novel to postmeiotic male germ cells. It is not my intent to present here an exhaustive review of posttranscriptional regulation in the testis and an apology is offered in advance to those whose research has not been discussed. Instead I plan to focus primarily on recent data presented at the 9th European Testis Workshop. Emphasis will be placed on several testicular RNA-binding proteins that modulate aspects of posttranscriptional regulation, especially translation in mammalian male germ cells.

7.2 Many Messenger RNAs in Postmeiotic Male Germ Cells Undergo Deadenylation upon Translation

Polyadenylation of mRNAs is often associated with the activation of stored mRNAs in the eggs of many species ranging from clams to mammals (Jackson and Standart 1990). In the testis, similar increases in poly(A) tail length have been seen in mRNAs encoding proteins such as lactate dehydrogenase C and cytochrome c_s, genes that are expressed during meiosis (Alcivar et al. 1991; Hake et al. 1990). However, the opposite appears to occur when stored mRNAs of postmeiotic male germ cells are activated. Many, if not all, of the temporally and translationally regulated mRNAs that are first transcribed during spermiogenesis undergo a poly(A) shortening upon activation for translation. For instance, the translationally repressed forms of the mRNAs encoding transition proteins 1 and 2, protamines 1 and 2 and a mitochondrial capsule selenoprotein are long and homogeneous, i.e., they contain poly(A) tails of about 130 A's, whereas the polysomal forms of these mRNAs become shorter and more heterogeneous as a result of partial deadenylation (Kleene 1989). These five mRNAs are testis specific and are first transcribed in round spermatids. After transcription, their introns are removed and they are stored as mature and apparently functional mRNAs (as determined in cell-free translation assays after RNA deproteinization) in the cytoplasm of spermatids until they are translated days later as spermatogenesis proceeds. It is not known what role, if any, the partial deadenylation plays in the activation of these mRNAs. This changeover from storage to translation of mRNAs occurs over a 7-day interval in the mouse with the activation of transition proteins 1 and 2 occurring several days before that of the protamines 1 and 2.

Although the function(s) of poly(A) shortening in mRNA metabolism remains a mystery, it appears to be characteristic of postmeiotic mRNAs and is not restricted to only stored and testis-specific mRNAs. The partial deadenylation also is seen with the polysomal form of the mRNA encoding γ enteric actin (Gu et al. 1996). γ enteric actin is a gene widely expressed in numerous somatic tissues, especially the smooth muscle cells of the intestine and interstitial blood vessels. It is also expressed in the germ cells of the testis and is found in the cytoplasm of developing spermatids (Oko et al. 1991). Posttranscriptional processing of the γ enteric actin mRNA in spermatids appears specific to this actin isoprotein since the ubiquitously expressed cytoplasmic β and γ actin mRNAs do not undergo similar deadenylations in the germ cells of the mouse testis. This suggests that the restricted temporal expression of an mRNA may influence the deadenylation process or specific *cis*-acting elements in mRNAs may be essential for the polyadenylation/deadenylation. In fact, the 3' untranslated region of the mouse γ enteric actin does share several conserved sequence elements that are also present in

other mRNAs that undergo deadenylation, such as the transition protein
1 and protamine mRNAs.

7.3 Testicular Poly(A) Binding Proteins

Although an extensive literature exists for the role of polyadenylation in
eukaryotic cells, the metabolic effects resulting from changes in poly(A)
tail length are unclear. One possible outcome from the alterations in
poly(A) tail lengths may be differential protein binding to the 3' untranslated regions of mRNAs. Among the proteins that bind to the poly(A) tail
is a widely expressed poly(A) binding protein (PABP) of about 70 kDa
(reviewed in Sachs 1993; Sachs and Wahle 1993). Sequence compari-
sons of cDNAs encoding PABP from yeast, human, mouse, *Xenopus*,
and *Drosophila* have revealed that the highly conserved protein contains
four RNA-binding domains near its amino terminus which facilitate its
preferential binding to groups of about 25 adenines. This protein–RNA
interaction is believed to stabilize the mRNAs, enhance their translation
by regulating interactions between the poly(A) tail and the 60S ribosomal
subunit, and also facilitate the shortening of the poly(A) tail in association with a poly(A)-specific nuclease.

To gain insight into the expression of PABP during spermiogenesis
and to determine whether the polyadenylated mRNAs of stored and
activated postmeiotic mRNAs differentially recognize PABP, the cellular and subcellular distributions of both PABP and its mRNA have been
examined (Gu et al. 1995a). PABP mRNA levels change greatly during
spermatogenesis, since the primary PABP mRNA, a 3.9-kb mRNA, is
developmentally regulated in the rodent testis. A low level of PABP
mRNA is detected in premeiotic testicular cells, while higher levels of
PABP mRNA are present in meiotic cells, early postmeiotic cells, and
adult testis. Although the highest levels of the 3.9-kb PABP mRNA are
found in round spermatids, little, if any, PABP mRNA is found in
elongating spermatids. Moreover, the PABP mRNA may be itself under
translational control, since less than 10% of the total PABP mRNA in
testicular extracts is polysome associated. Recently, in an "in vitro"
study, PABP binding to the A-rich sequence in the 5' untranslated
region (UTR) of PABP mRNA has been shown to repress translation in
a cell-free system (de Melo Neto et al. 1995).

At the protein level, PABP shows a widespread distribution in the mammalian testis with its highest level in round spermatids, the cell type especially enriched with stored mRNAs (Gu et al. 1995a). PABP levels increase during meiosis and, in the rat, attain their maximal level in the cytoplasm of steps 7–8 spermatids just before nuclear condensation and elongation. PABP levels remain high until steps 14–15 spermatids, suggesting that PABP is a stable protein, since these are the cell types that contain little, if any, PABP mRNA.

The subcellular distribution of PABP varies greatly among species. Sea urchin embryos contain large amounts of free PABP (Drawbridge et al. 1990), whereas most of the PABP in *Xenopus* embryos in bound to mRNAs (Zelus et al. 1989). Perhaps because of the large amount of stored mRNAs in postmeiotic male germ cells [round spermatids are estimated to contain nearly 11 ng of poly(A)$^+$ RNA/mg of total RNA (Kleene et al. 1983)], the mammalian testis contains very little free PABP. Immunoprecipitation studies have revealed that PABP is bound to both the stored and translated forms of the postmeiotic mRNAs encoding protamines 1 and 2, suggesting that, as assayed by immunoprecipitation, the 70-kDa PABP does not recognize differences in the poly(A) length of these mRNAs. Since the 70-kDa PABP is only one of a large family of PABPs (Belostotsky and Meagher 1993), any differential specificity of binding of PABP to the longer and shorter poly(A) tails may reside either with another PABP protein or in association with other testicular proteins. At least one other testicular PABP has been identified by cloning its cDNA from a testis cDNA library (Wang et al. 1992), and Northern blot analyses of testicular extracts suggest the presence of multiple PABP mRNAs, supporting the likelihood that additional testicular PABPs exist (Kleene et al. 1984; Gu et al. 1995a).

7.4 p48/52, Sequence-Independent RNA-Binding Proteins that also Bind to Specific Germ Cell Promoter Sequences

In the immature oocytes of *Xenopus*, a group of polypeptides (mRNPs 1–4) have been shown to constitute the majority of the protein associated with poly(A) mRNAs, whereas in late-stage oocytes only mRNPs 3 and 4 are detected (Darnbourgh and Ford 1981). The abundant mRNPs 3 and 4 in oocytes have apparent molecular masses of 54 and

56 kDa, respectively, and bind to a wide range of mRNAs. The p54/p56 proteins accumulate during oogenesis and are most abundant in the developmental stages when large amounts of maternal mRNAs are stored as stable nontranslated mRNAs (Richter and Evers 1984; Tafuri and Wolffe 1993; Murray et al. 1991, 1992). The p54/56 are isolated from 15S particles that contain several other mRNA-binding polypeptides including a protein kinase (Murray et al. 1991). Perhaps this kinase activity is involved in the phosphorylation of p54/56 (Cummings et al. 1989), which "in vitro" studies indicate is necessary for p54/56 to function as translational repressors (Kick et al. 1987). Recently, p54 and p56 were cloned (Murray et al. 1992), demonstrating that they represent two similar proteins. More importantly, sequence analysis of p56 showed it was identical to FRG Y2, a *Xenopus* germ cell-specific transcription factor (Tafuri and Wolffe 1990, 1992; Wolffe et al. 1992). The identity of FRGY2 and p54/56 has also been confirmed at the protein level by direct molecular mass determination (Deschamps et al. 1992).

Mammalian homologues of p54/56 have recently been identified in mouse testis (Kwon and Hecht 1993a). The mouse testis proteins, estimated by sodium dodecyl sulfate polyacrylamide gel electrophoresis (SDS-PAGE) to be about 48 and 52 kDa, form RNA–protein complexes with all tested RNA transcripts, suggesting that they also are sequence-independent RNA-binding proteins. The expression of the 48/52-kDa mouse proteins is developmentally regulated in the testis with maximal levels of the two proteins being found in round spermatids and is only found in oocytes in the ovary. The 48/52-kDa proteins are detected solely in the nonpolysomal fractions of postmitochondrial extracts from testis and are not detected in extracts of brain, liver, kidney, or prepuberal testes from 12-day-old mice. This indicates that as with the *Xenopus* p54/56, p48/52 are germ-cell specific in the mouse. It is likely that p48/52 facilitate storage of "paternal" mRNAs by forming sequence-independent mRNA–protein structural complexes.

As demonstrated with the *Xenopus* homologues of p48/52 (Tafuri and Wolffe 1993), p48/52 also bind DNA. In *Xenopus* FRG Y2 serves as a transcription factor by binding to a 12 nucleotide DNA sequence, CTGATTGGCCAA, that is present in many *Xenopus* germ cell-specific promoters. Since nine of the 12 nucleotides recognized by the *Xenopus* FRG Y2/p54/56 proteins are also present in many mammalian male germ cell promoters, including protamine 1 and 2, transition protein 2, phosphoglycerate kinase 2, the alternative promoter for cytochrome c_s, and cytochrome c_t, we have investigated whether the mouse homologues of *Xenopus* p54/p56 may also play a role in regulating transcription in the testis for genes such as the protamines (Nikolajczyk et al. 1995). Western blot analyses with both anti-p54/p56 and anti-FRG Y2 antibodies have confirmed that, in addition to being abundant in the cytoplasm, the mouse homologue of p54/p56 is also a nuclear protein and is present in mouse testis nuclear extracts that are transcriptionally active. Moreover, both the *Xenopus* p54/p56 and mouse testis homologues bind to a sequence in the conserved promoter element recognized by FRG Y2/p54/56 in the mouse protamine 2 gene. The interactions between the mouse testis p48/52 and its conserved transcriptional binding site in protamine 2 suggests that a coupled mechanism involving both transcription and translation is involved in the regulation of haploid gene expression in the testis (Ranjan et al. 1993).

7.5 Subcellular Localization of Messenger RNAs in the Testis

In mammals such as the mouse, transcription terminates 7–10 days before spermiogenesis is completed (Kierszenbaum and Tres 1978). As a result, many of the proteins of the elongating spermatid and spermatozoon must be synthesized under translational control.

To determine whether the inactivation/activation of stored transcripts during spermiogenesis could be mediated by subcellular or organellar compartmentalization of mRNAs, light and electron microscopy were used to localize by in situ hybridization in rat testis the subcellular sites of the stored and translating mRNAs encoding transition protein 1 and protamine 1 (Morales et al. 1991). During early spermiogenesis, only nuclear transcripts of transition protein 1 and protamine 1 are seen. After step 7, at about the time transcription ceases, transition protein 1 and protamine 1 mRNAs are only detected in the cytoplasm. In round spermatids (where transition protein 1 and protamine mRNAs are stored) and in elongated spermatids (where transition protein 1 and protamine 1 mRNAs are translated), no specific localization to any membrane-bound organelles such as the endoplasmic reticulum or mitochondria or to non-membrane-bound structures such as the chromatoid body is seen. Moreover, no changes in mRNA distribution are seen during translation of these mRNAs in elongated spermatids. These data suggest that the translational arrest and activation of the transition protein 1 and protamine 1 mRNAs are not primarily controlled by a compartmentalized storage of mRNAs in the cytoplasm or by movement into and out of specific organelles in the cytoplasm of spermatids.

Since it is possible that transition protein 1 and protamine 1 are atypical testicular postmeiotic mRNAs, the detection of mRNA localization in the testis was extended by repeating the in situ hybridizations at both light and electron microscope levels with a $[^3H]$-polyuridylic acid probe, thereby allowing examination of the cellular sites of all poly(A)$^+$ mRNAs of the testis (Morales and Hecht 1994). In both germ cells and somatic cells of the testis, poly(A)$^+$ RNA is mostly seen dispersed in the cytoplasm or in association with the endoplasmic reticulum. Poly(A)$^+$ RNAs are only occasionally found associated with mitochondria, lysosomes, lipid inclusions, or axonemes. No compartmentalization of poly(A)$^+$ RNA is detected in the cytoplasm of round or elongated spermatids, and, in most sections examined, the chromatoid body did not contain any significant amounts of poly(A)$^+$ RNA either. These data suggest that there is no distinct compartmentalization of the general population of male germ cell mRNAs in specific structures (such as the chromatoid body) or subcellular sites. From this approach, however, it is not possible to determine whether mRNA distribution and localization is influenced by the cytoskeleton (see below).

7.6 TB-RBP, a Regulator of Translation and Cellular Localization of mRNAs

Protein binding to the 3' untranslated region of mRNAs has been shown to play a prominent role in many cellular regulatory events, including mRNA stability (reviewed in Beelman and Parker 1995), translational control (reviewed in Curtis et al. 1995; Spirin 1994), and subcellular localization (reviewed in St. Johnston 1995). Braun et al. (1989) have demonstrated in transgenic mice that the 3' untranslated region of the protamine 1 mRNA attached to a human growth hormone reporter gene confers the necessary information to translate the transgene mRNA at the identical time that the endogenous protamine mRNAs are translated. When the 3' untranslated region of human growth hormone replaces the 3' untranslated region of the protamine 1, no delay in translation is seen – demonstrating the importance of this region of the mRNA for its temporal expression during spermiogenesis.

To define the mechanisms that control the expression of the protamine mRNAs, we have first identified *cis*-acting elements present in the 3' untranslated region of protamine mRNAs that are recognized by testicular cytoplasmic factors (Kwon and Hecht 1991, 1993b). Using gel retardation assays, two sequence elements (the Y and H elements) that form specific RNA–protein complexes were identified in the 3' untranslated regions of protamine 1 and 2 and transition protein 1 mRNAs. The protein binding sites of the two complexes are located between nucleotides +537 and +572 in the protamine 2 mRNA and to similar sites in the mRNAs of protamine 1 and transition protein 1. These sequence elements are highly conserved among many other postmeiotic translationally regulated mRNAs of the mammalian testis. UV-crosslinking studies reveal that a protein, hereafter called testis-brain RNA-binding protein (TB-RBP), specifically binds to the conserved sequences. These findings suggest that specific protein binding to highly conserved sequences present in the 3' untranslated regions of a group of translationally regulated testicular ("paternal") mRNAs is involved in their posttranscriptional regulation.

Since many proteins can bind to RNA, it is important to functionally demonstrate that protein binding to conserved *cis*-acting sequences can influence translation. To this end, three mRNAs containing a human growth hormone reporter gene and either the 3' untranslated region of human growth hormone, the 3' untranslated region of protamine 2, or a 46-nucleotide sequence containing the conserved Y and H elements of the 3' untranslated region of protamine 2 were synthesized. Translation of the fusion mRNAs was markedly repressed in reticulocyte lysates supplemented with a mouse testis extract enriched for TB-RBP when the mRNAs contained the 3' untranslated region of protamine 2 or the Y and H elements of protamine 2, but no decrease in translation was seen when the fusion mRNAs contained the 3' untranslated region of human growth hormone. Moreover, consistent with its role as a reversible translational repressor, TB-RBP is predominantly detected in round spermatids, requires phosphorylation for RNA binding and does not bind when dephosphorylated, and is detected solely in the ribonucleo-protein fractions of a testicular postmitochondrial extract. These data suggest that when TB-RBP is phosphorylated, it represses translation of mRNAs such as the protamine mRNAs by binding to the highly con-served Y and H elements in round spermatids. When protamine needs to be synthesized in elongating spermatids, TB-RBP detaches from the mRNAs, likely as a result of dephosphorylation.

Using RNA gel-retardation assays with cytoplasmic extracts pre-pared from six different mouse tissues, we recently found that, in addi-tion to testis, a TB-RBP-like protein is abundant in mammalian brain extracts (Han et al. 1995a). By many criteria, including electrophoretic mobilities of RNA–protein complexes, pH and salt requirements for RNA–protein complex formation, numerous chromatographic proper-ties, molecular size determinations of TB-RBP following UV-crosslink-ing, and peptide mapping of the crosslinked protein, we conclude that the TB-RBP of brain and testis are identical. Moreover, as seen in the testis, TB-RBP is solely found in the nonpolysomal fractions of brain postmitochondrial extracts.

Since the "paternal" mRNAs that are recognized by TB-RBP are testis specific, it was initially surprising to us that TB-RBP should be abundant in brain extracts. However, a search of the Genbank database with the conserved cis-acting elements that TB-RBP recognizes quickly identified many brain mRNAs, such as tau or myelin basic protein whose mRNAs contain similar sequences (Ainger et al. 1993; Litman et al. 1993). Gel shift and UV crosslinking studies with subclones of the 3' untranslated regions of mRNAs encoding tau and myelin basic protein reveal RNA–protein complexes and crosslinked proteins of molecular weights that are identical to those obtained bound to the Y and H elements of testicular mRNAs (Han et al. 1995a). TB-RBP from testis and brain also interchangeably bind with specificity to the similar, conserved sequences in the 3' untranslated regions of brain or testis mRNAs. Many of the brain mRNAs that contain the conserved Y or H elements share one property: They are transported along microtubules and thereby moved by an as yet to be defined mechanism to specific locations along the processes of the brain cells to the sites where they are translated (Wilhelm and Vale 1993).

Consistent with a role in mRNA transport and localization for TB-RBP, recent studies have indicated that TB-RBP from brain or testis bind specific mRNAs to microtubules in vitro (Han et al. 1995b). When TB-RBP is added to microtubules that are reassembled from either crude brain extracts or from purified tubulin, most of the TB-RBP is bound to microtubules. The association of TB-RBP with the microtubules requires the assembly of microtubules and is diminished by colcemid, low temperature, and high levels of salt and requires GTP. In the presence of TB-RBP, transcripts from the 3' untranslated regions of protamine 2, tau, and myelin basic protein, three mRNAs that contain one or both of the conserved sequence elements are linked to microtubules, whereas transcripts that lack the conserved sequences are not. We propose that TB-RBP serves as an attachment protein for the microtubule association of transported mRNAs. Considering its ability to arrest translation in vitro, we speculate that TB-RBP serves an important role in the storage and transportation of mRNAs to specific intracellular sites where they are translated. Whether TB-RBP also facilitates subcellular localization in male germ cells remains to be established.

RNA-binding proteins appear to play other important roles in spermatogenesis. Chromosomal deletion of a human RNA-binding protein encoded on the Y chromosome (Ma et al. 1993) or deletion of a *Drosophila* RNA-binding protein (Karsch-Mizrachi and Haynes 1993) both result in azoospermia without additional phenotypic changes. Several other testicular RNA-binding proteins have recently been characterized by Braun and colleagues (Fajardo et al. 1994; Schumacher et al. 1995a, b). Two proteins of 53 and 55 kDa that form RNA–protein complexes have been demonstrated to bind to specific 22 and 20 nucleotide sequences present in the 3' untranslated regions of protamine 1 and 2 mRNAs (Fajardo et al. 1994). A third RNA-binding protein, a 71-kDa protein, that is expressed at high levels in the testis, ovary, and brain has been localized to cytoplasmic microtubules (Schumacher et al. 1995a). A fourth RNA-binding protein of 72 kDa appears to be associated with the nuclear scaffold and may be involved in nuclear posttranscriptional processes (Schumacher et al. 1995b). Clearly, continued analysis of the functions that RNA-binding proteins play in regulating gene expression in the testis will be both challenging and rewarding.

7.7 Superoxide Dismutase 1 Utilizes an Alternative Promoter Which Produces a Novel Postmeiotic mRNA Whose Translation Is Regulated by an RNA-Binding Protein

Superoxide dismutase 1 (copper-zinc superoxide dismutase) is an important enzyme in a pathway that inactivates free radicals in cells. Overexpression of superoxide dismutase 1 leads to clinical symptoms similar to Down's syndrome (Avraham et al. 1988), whereas reduced levels of superoxide dismutase 1 are also highly deleterious (Deng et al. 1993; Rosen et al. 1993). In mammals, although superoxidase dismutase 1 is encoded by a single-copy gene (Levanon et al. 1985), multiple superoxide dismutase 1 transcripts have been found. Two superoxide dismutase 1 mRNAs that differ by about 200 nucleotides have been detected in human tissue culture cells (Lieman-Hurwiz et al. 1982). These mRNAs are identical in their 5' untranslated and coding regions, but differ in their 3' untranslated regions (Sherman et al. 1984). Although only one mRNA of about 0.70 kb has been detected in the somatic tissues of rat and mouse (Benedetto et al. 1991), in rat testes two transcripts of 0.77 and 0.94 kb have been reported (Jow et al. 1993).

Since spermatozoa are highly sensitive to free radical damage, we have started to analyze the expression and regulation of superoxide dismutase 1 as part of a group of genes that protect germ cells from reactive oxygen (Gu et al. 1995b). In mouse testis, multiple superoxide dismutase 1 mRNAs of about 0.73, 0.80, and 0.93 kb are detected. The 0.73-kb mRNA is present in somatic cells and in early stages of differentiating male germ cells. The 0.80-kb and 0.93-kb mRNAs are only found in postmeiotic germ cells. From RNase H and Northern blot analyses, it has been demonstrated that the three superoxide dismutase 1 mRNAs are derived from two transcripts: one, a ubiquitously expressed transcript and, the second, a postmeiotic transcript. The transcripts differ by 114 nucleotides. The additional sequence in the longer postmeiotic superoxide dismutase 1 mRNA is solely in the 5' untranslated region and originates from an alternative upstream promoter contiguous with the somatic superoxide dismutase 1 promoter. Polysomal gradient analysis of the superoxide dismutase 1 mRNAs in mouse testis reveals that over 90% of the 0.93-kb superoxide dismutase 1 mRNA is nonpolysomal, while the 0.80- and 0.73-kb superoxide dismutase 1 mRNAs are primarily polysomal. A more rapidly migrating form of the 0.93-kb superoxide dismutase 1 mRNA, resulting from partial deadenylation, is found on polysomes.

In cell-free assays the 0.93-kb superoxide dismutase 1 mRNA is translated only slightly less efficiently than the 0.73-kb superoxide dismutase 1 mRNA, suggesting that a *trans*-acting factor may be involved in the translational repression "in vivo" of the postmeiotic superoxide dismutase 1 mRNA. Recently, a 65-kDa protein that binds to the extended 5' untranslated region and suppresses its translation "in vitro" was purified and characterized (W. Gu and N. B. Hecht, unpublished results). This specific testicular RNA–protein interaction appears to be necessary to fine-tune protein synthesis, in this case controlling the level of superoxide dismutase 1 produced in maturing male germ cells, thereby preventing a cellular imbalance of this crucial enzyme that inactivates reactive oxygen species.

7.8 Conclusions

The study of male germ cells offers wonderful opportunities to understand the molecular mechanisms regulating gene expression in differentiating cells. In addition to utilizing traditional, i.e., the general regulatory mechanisms of all cell types, novel regulatory possibilities are especially prominent during spermiogenesis, a time in which massive morphological change occurs despite a "nuclear shutdown" culminating in the apparently quiescent spermatozoon. As our knowledge of the mechanisms regulating posttranscriptional gene expression in postmeiotic germ cells grows, we can predict that many new surprises and important regulatory processes will be discovered.

References

Ainger K, Avossa D, Morgan F, Hill SJ, Barry C, Barbarese E, Carson JH (1993) Transport and localization of exogenous myelin basic protein mRNA microinjected into oligodendrocytes. J Cell Biol 123:431–441

Alcivar AA, Trasler JM, Hake LE, Salchi-Ashtiana K, Goldberg E, Hecht NB (1990) DNA methylation and expression of the genes coding for lactate dehydrogenases A and C during rodent spermatogenesis. Biol Reprod 44:527–535

Avraham KB, Schickler M, Sapoznicov D, Yarom R, Groner Y (1988) Down's syndrome: abnormal neuromuscular junctions in the tongues of transgenic mice with elevated levels of human Cu/Zn superoxide dismutase. Cell 54:823–829

Beelman C, Parker R (1995) Degradation of mRNA in eukaryotes. Cell 81:179–183

Belostotsky DA, Meagher RB (1993) Differential organ-specific expression of three poly(A) binding protein genes from Arabidopsis thaliana. Proc Natl Acad Sci USA 90:6686–6690

Benedetto MT, Anzai Y, Gordon JW (1991) Isolation and analysis of the mouse genomic sequence encoding Cu^{2+}-Zn^{2+} superoxide dismutase. Gene 99:191–195

Braun RE, Peschon JJ, Behringer RR, Brinster RL, Palmiter RD (1989) Protamine 3'-untranslated sequences regulate temporal translational control and subcellular localization of growth hormone in spermatids of transgenic mice. Genes Dev 3:793–802

Cummings A, Barrett P, Sommerville J (1989) Multiple modifications in the phosphoproteins bound to stored messenger RNA in Xenopus oocytes. Biochim Biophys Acta 1014:319–326

Curtis D, Lehmann R, Zamore PD (1995) Translational regulation in development. Cell 81:171–178

Darnbourgh CH, Ford PJ (1981) Identification in Xenopus laevis of a class of oocyte-specific proteins bound to messenger RNA. Eur J Biochem 113:415–426

de Melo Neto O, Standart N, Martins de Sa C (1995) Autoregulation of poly(A)-binding protein synthesis in vitro. Nucleic Acids Res 23:2198–2205

Deng H-X, Hentati A, Tainer JA, Iqbal Z, Cayabyab A, Hung WY, Getzoff ED, Hu P, Herzfeldt B, Roos RP, Warner C, Deng G, Soriano E, Smyth C, Parge HE, Ahmed A, Roses AD, Hollewell RA, Pericak-Vouce MA, Siddique T (1993) Amyotrophic lateral sclerosis and structural defects in Cu, Zn superoxide dismutase. Science 261:1047–1050

Deschamps S, Viel A, Garrigos M, Denis H, Le Maire M (1992) mRNP4, a major mRNA-binding protein of Xenopus oocytes is identical to transcription factor FRG Y2. J Biol Chem 267:15799–13802

Drawbridge J, Grainger JL, Winkler MM (1990) Identification and characterization of poly (A) binding protein from the sea urchin: a quantitative analysis. Mol Cell Biol 10:3994–4006

Eddy EM, O'Brien DA (1994) The spermatozoon. In: Knobil E, Neil JD (eds) The physiology of reproduction, 2nd edn. Raven, New York, pp 29–68

Erickson RP (1993) Molecular genetics of mammalian spermatogenesis. In: Gwatkin R (ed) Genes in mammalian reproduction. Wiley-Liss, New York, pp 1–26

Fajardo MA, Butner KA, Lee K, Braun RE (1994) Germ cell-specific proteins interact with the 3' untranslated regions of Prm-1 and Prm-2 mRNA. Dev Biol 166:643–653

Gu W, Kwon Y, Hermo L, Oko R, Hecht NB (1995a) Poly (A) binding protein is bound to both stored and polysomal mRNAs in the mammalian testis. Mol Reprod Dev 40:273–285

Gu W, Morales C, Hecht NB (1995b) In male mouse germ cells Cu-Zn superoxide dismutase utilizes alternative promoters which produce multiple transcripts with different translation potential. J Biol Chem 270:236–243

Gu W, Kwon YK, Hecht NB (1996) Poly (A) shortening accompanies translation of the mRNA encoding γ enteric acid but not the cytoplasmic β and γ actin mRNAs in post-meiotic male germ cells. Mol Reprod Dev (in press)

Hake LE, Alcivar AA, Hecht NB (1990) Changes in mRNA length accompany translational regulation of the somatic and testis-specific cytochrome c genes during spermatogenesis in the mouse. Development 110:249–257

Han J, Gu W, Hecht NB (1995a) TB-RBP, a testicular translational regulatory RNA-binding protein that is abundant in the brain and binds to the 3'UTR of transported brain mRNA. Biol Reprod 53:707–717

Han JR, Yiu GKC, Hecht NB (1995b) Testis brain-RNA binding protein (TB-RBP) is a microtubule associated protein that attaches translationally repressed and transported mRNAs to microtubules. Proc Natl Acad Sci USA 92:9550–9554

Handel MA (1987) Genetic control of spermatogenesis in mice. In: Hennig W (ed) Results and problems in cell differentiation, spermatogenesis: genetic aspects, vol 15. Springer, Berlin Heidelberg New York, pp 1–62

Hecht NB (1993) Gene expression during male germ cell development. In: Ewing L, Desjardins C (eds) Cell and molecular biology of the testis. Oxford University Press, New York, pp 400–432

Hecht NB (1995) The making of a spermatozoon: a molecular perspective. Dev Gen 16:95–103

Jackson RJ, Standart N (1990) Do the poly (A) tail and 3' untranslated region control mRNA translation? Cell 62:15–24

Jow WW, Schlegel PN, Cichon Z, Philips D, Goldstein M, Bardin CW (1993) Identification and localization of copper-zinc superoxide dismutase gene expression in rat testicular development. J Androl 14:439–447

Karsch-Mizrachi I, Haynes SR (1993) The RB97D gene encodes a potential RNA-binding protein required for spermatogenesis in Drosophila. Nucleic Acids Res 21:2229–2235

Kick D, Barrett P, Cummings A, Sommerville J (1987) Phosphorylation of a 60 kDa polypeptide from Xenopus oocytes blocks messenger RNA translation. Nucleic Acids Res. 15:4099–4109

Kierszenbaum AL, Tres LL (1978) RNA transcription and chromatin structure during meiotic and post-meiotic stages of spermatogenesis. Fed Proc 37:2512–2516

Kleene KC (1989) Poly (A) shortening accompanies the activation of translation of five mRNAs during spermatogenesis in the mouse. Development 106:367–373

Kleene KC, Distel RJ, Hecht NB (1983) cDNA clones encoding poly (A) RNAs which first appear at detectable levels in haploid phases of spermatogenesis in the mouse. Dev. Biol. 98:455–464

Kleene KC, Distel RJ, Hecht NB (1984) Translational regulation and coordinate deadenylation of a haploid mRNA during spermiogenesis in the mouse. Dev Biol 105:71–79

Kwon YK, Hecht NB (1991) Cytoplasmic protein binding to highly conserved sequences in the 3' untranslated region of mouse protamine 2 mRNA, a translationally regulated gene of male germ cells. Proc Natl Acad Sci USA 88:3584–3588

Kwon YK, Hecht NB (1993a) Proteins homologous to the Xenopus germ cell-specific RNA-binding proteins p54/56 are temporally expressed in mouse male germ Cells. Dev Biol 158:90–100

Kwon YK, Hecht NB (1993b) Binding of a phosphoprotein to the 3' untranslated region of the mouse protamine 2 mRNA temporally represses its translation. Mol Cell Biol 13:6547–6557

Levanon D, Lieman-Hurwitz J, Dafni N, Wigderson M, Sherman L, Bernstein Y, Laver-Rudich Z, Danciger E, Stein O, Groner Y (1985) Architecture and anatomy of the chromosomal locus in human chromosome 21 encoding the Cu/Zn superoxide dismutase. EMBO J 4:77–84

Lieman-Hurwitz J, Dafni N, Lavie V, Groner Y (1982) Human cytoplasmic superoxide dismutase cDNA clone: a probe for studying the molecular biology of Down syndrome. Proc Natl Acad Sci USA 79:2808–2811

Litman P, Barg J, Rindzoonki L, Ginzburg I (1993) Subcellular localization of tau mRNA in differentiating cell culture: implications for neuronal polarity. Neuron 10:627–638

Ma K, Inglis JD, Sharkey A, Bickmore WA, Hill RE, Prosner EJ, Speed RM, Thomson EJ, Jobling M, Taylor K, Wolfe J, Cooke HJ, Hargreave TB, Chandley AC (1993) A Y chromosome gene family with RNA-binding protein homology: candidates for the azoospermia factor AZF controlling human spermatogenesis. Cell 75:1287–1295

Morales CR, Kwon YK, Hecht NB (1991) Cytoplasmic localization during storage and translation of the mRNAs of transition protein 1 and protamine 1, two translationally regulated transcripts of the mammalian testis. J Cell Sci 100:119–131

Morales CR, Hecht NB (1994) Poly (A)$^+$ RNAs are enriched in spermatocyte nuclei but not in chromatoid bodies in the rat testis. Biol Reprod 50:309–319

Murray MT, Krohne G, Franke WW (1991) Different forms of soluble cytoplasmic mRNA binding proteins and particles in Xenopus laevis oocytes and embryos. J Cell Biol 112:1–11

Murray MT, Schiller DL, Franke WW (1992) Sequence analysis of cytoplasmic mRNA-binding proteins of Xenopus oocytes identifies a family of RNA-binding proteins. Proc Natl Acad Sci USA 89:11–15

Nikolajczyk BS, Murray MT, Hecht NB (1995) A mouse homologue to the Xenopus germ-cell specific RNA/DNA-binding proteins p54/p56 interacts with the protamine 2 promoter. Biol Reprod 52:524–530

Oko R, Hermo L, Hecht NB (1991) Distribution of actin isoforms within cells of the seminiferous epithelium of the rat testis: evidence for a muscle form of actin in spermatids. Anat Record 231:63–81

Ranjan M, Tafuri SR, Wolffe AP (1993) Masking mRNA from translation in somatic cells. Genes Dev 7:1725–1736

Richter JD, Evers DC (1984) A monoclonal antibody to an oocyte-specific poly(A) RNA-binding protein. J Biol Chem 258:4864–4869

Rosen DR, Siddique T, David P, Figlewicz DA, Sapp P, Hentati A, Donaldson D, Goto JP, Deng H-X, Rahmani Z, Krizus A, McKenna-Yasek D, Cayabyab A, Gaston SM, Berger R, Tanzi RE, Halperin JJ, Herzfeldt B, Van der Bergh R, Hong WY, Bird T, Deng G, Mulder DW, Smyth C, Laing NG, Gusella JS, Horvitz HR, Brown Jr RH (1993) Mutations in Cu/Zn superoxide dismutase are associated with familial amyotrophic lateral sclerosis. Nature 362:59–62

Sachs AB (1993) Messenger RNA degradation in eukaryotes. Cell 74:41314–41421

Sachs A, Wahle E (1993) Poly (A) tail metabolism and function in eucaryotes. J Biol Chem 268:22955–22958

Schumacher JM, Lee K, Edelhoff S, Braun RE (1995a) Spnr, a murine RNA-binding protein that is localized to cytoplasmic microtubules. J Cell Biol 129:1023–1032

Schumacher JM, Lee K, Edelhoff S, Braun RE (1995b) Distribution of Tenr, an RNA-binding protein, in a lattice-like network within the spermatid nucleus in the mouse. Biol Reprod 52:1274–1283

Sherman L, Levanon D, Lieman-Hurwitz J, Dafni N, Groner Y (1984) Human Cu/Zn superoxide dismutase gene: molecular characterization of its two mRNA species. Nucleic Acids Res 12:9349–9365

Spirin AS (1994) Storage of messenger RNA in eukaryotes: envelopment with protein, translational barrier at 5' side, or conformational masking by 3' side? Mol Reprod Dev 38:107–117

St Johnson D (1995) The intracellular localization of messengers RNAs. Cell 81:161–170

Tafuri SR, Wolffe AP (1990) Xenopus Y-box transcription factors: molecular cloning, functional analysis, and developmental regulation. Proc Natl Acad Sci USA 87:9028–9032

Tafuri SR, Wolffe AP (1992) DNA binding multimerization and transcription stimulation by the Xenopus Y box proteins in vitro. New Biol 4:349–359

Tafuri SR, Wolffe AP (1993) Dual roles for transcription and translation factors in the RNA storage particles of Xenopus oocytes. Trends Cell Biol 3:94–98

Wang M-Y, Cutler M, Karimpour L, Kleene DC (1992) Nucleotide sequence of a mouse testis poly (A) binding protein cDNA. Nucleic Acids Res 20:3519

Wilhelm JE, Vale RD (1993) RNA on the move: the mRNA localization pathway. J Cell Biol 123:269–274

Willison K, Ashworth A (1987) Mammalian spermatogenic gene expression. Trends Genet 3:351–355

Wolffe AP, Tafuri S, Ranjan M, Familari M (1992) The Y-box factors: a family of nucleic acid binding proteins conserved from Escherichia coli to man. New Biol 4:290–298

Wolgemuth DJ, Gruppi C, Vambutas V, Wadewitz AG (1993) Patterns of expression and potential functions of cellular oncogenes and heat shock protein genes during germ cell development. In: Ewing L, Desjardins C (eds) Cell and molecular biology of the testis. Oxford University Press, New York, pp 433–451

Zelus BD, Giebelhaus DH, Eib DW, Kenner KA, Moon RT (1989) Expression of the poly (A) binding protein during development of Xenopus laevis. Mol Cell Biol 9:2756–2760

8 Isolation and Culture of Immature Rat Type A Spermatogonial Stem Cells

G. Dirami, N. Ravindranath, M.C. Jia, and M. Dym

8.1	Introduction	142
8.2	Materials and Methods	143
8.2.1	Isolation of Rat Type A Spermatogonia	143
8.2.2	Purification of Spermatogonia by Differential Plating	144
8.2.3	Morphological and Immunocytochemical Characterization of Rat Type A Spermatogonia	144
8.2.4	Sertoli Cell Preparation and Culture	145
8.2.5	Cell Viability Assay	146
8.2.6	Analysis of DNA Fragmentation by Flow Cytometry	146
8.2.7	Analysis of DNA Fragmentation by Agarose Gel Electrophoresis	147
8.2.8	Statistical Analysis of Data	147
8.3	Results	148
8.3.1	Characterization of Purified Rat Spermatogonia	148
8.3.2	Survivability of Isolated Spermatogonia in DMEM/F12 Medium	149
8.3.3	Spermatogonial Stem Cells Undergo an Apoptotic Form of Cell Death	150
8.3.4	Soluble Form of KL Enhances the Survival of Type A Spermatogonial Stem Cells in Culture	153
8.3.5	Effects of Sertoli Cell-Conditioned Media on the Viability of Spermatogonia in Culture	154
8.3.6	Effect of FBS and HS on the Viability of Spermatogonial Stem Cells	155
8.3.7	HS and SCCM Maintain the Viability of Isolated Spermatogonial Stem Cells in Culture	156
8.4	Discussion	157
8.5	Summary	161
References		162

8.1 Introduction

Spermatogenesis is a complex process of cellular renewal and differentiation that begins with the divisions of the type A spermatogonial stem cells and ends as late spermatids are released into the seminiferous tubule lumen as spermatozoa (Dym 1983). In vivo spermatogonial stem cells can be directed to one of three fates: (1) renew themselves into other stem cells; (2) differentiate into type B spermatogonia and eventually spermatocytes and more mature germ cells; or (3) degenerate. Despite abundant studies on the morphology and kinetics of spermatogonial cell renewal and differentiation (Clermont 1966, 1969; Dym and Clermont 1970; Huckins 1971; Oakberg 1971), very little is known about the regulation of spermatogonial cell proliferation or degeneration in mammals. Attempts to study spermatogonial proliferation in organ cultures have been made by several investigators (Martinovitch 1937, 1939; Steinberger et al. 1964; Ghatnekar et al. 1974; Aizawa and Nishimune 1979; Curtis 1981; Boitani et al. 1993). In all these studies, differentiation stopped at the pachytene spermatocyte stage. Similarly, spermatogonial proliferation and differentiation up to pachytene spermatocytes have been observed in cocultures of spermatogenic cells with Sertoli cells in serum-free defined medium supplemented with hormone and growth factors (Tres and Kierszenbaum 1983; Hadley et al. 1985). However, differentiation beyond pachytene spermatocytes into young spermatids was observed in seminiferous tubule segments cultured for 4–6 days (Parvinen et al. 1983). Thus, it is likely that cellular interactions are important for spermatogonial proliferation and differentiation. However, the Sertoli cell factors which are responsible for regulating this process are not known. It has been observed that up to 75% of spermatogonia undergo spontaneous degeneration before maturation (Abe 1987; Huckins 1978). Although the withdrawal of gonadotropins by hypophysectomy or immunoneutralization enhances the degeneration of germ cells (Raj and Dym 1976; Russell and Clermont 1977), other factors promoting degeneration of germ cells in intact animals have not been identified. In order to examine the regulation of spermatogonial renewal, differentiation, and degeneration under controlled culture conditions, it is important to develop an in vitro model system. In this direction, we have isolated rat type A spermatogonial cells from 9-day-old rats (Dym et al. 1995) and purified them to greater than 95%

purity by sedimentation velocity at unit gravity followed by differential plating in fetal bovine serum (FBS)-supplemented medium. The present study was undertaken to standardize culture conditions which would allow the type A spermatogonia to survive for longer periods of time.

8.2 Materials and Methods

8.2.1 Isolation of Rat Type A Spermatogonia

Male Sprague-Dawley rats, 9 days of age, were purchased from the Charles River Breeding Laboratories (Wilmington, MA, USA). The testes were excised and decapsulated. Seminiferous epithelial cells were enzyme dispersed and separated by the method we described in 1977 (Bellvé et al. 1977) with minor modifications more recently (Dym et al. 1995). Briefly, the decapsulated testes were suspended in a 1:1 mixture of Dulbecco's modified Eagle's medium and Ham F12 medium (DMEM/F12) containing collagenase (1.5 mg/ml) and DNAse (1 μg/ml), and incubated at 34°C for 15 min in a shaking water bath operated at 100 cycles/min. After two washes in DMEM/F12 medium, seminiferous cord fragments, mostly devoid of interstitial cells, were incubated in DMEM/F12 medium containing collagenase (1.5 mg/ml), hyaluronidase (1.5 mg/ml), trypsin (0.5 mg/ml), and DNAse (1 μg /ml) for 20–30 min using the conditions described above. The dispersed cells were washed twice with medium and filtered through 80 μm and 40 μm nylon mesh (Tetco Inc., Briarcliff Manor, NY, USA), successively. The cells of the dissociated epithelium were then separated by sedimentation velocity at unit gravity at 4°C, with use of a 2%–4% bovine serum albumin (BSA) gradient in DMEM/F12 medium. The cells were bottom-loaded into an SP-120 chamber in a volume of 30 ml, and a BSA gradient was generated using 275 ml each of 2% and 4% BSA. The cells were allowed to sediment for a standard period of 2.5 h, and then 35 fractions of 15 ml were collected at 90-s intervals. The cells in each fraction were examined under a phase contrast microscope, and fractions containing cells of similar size and morphology were pooled and spun down by low-speed centrifugation and then resuspended in DMEM/F12 medium.

8.2.2 Purification of Spermatogonia by Differential Plating

The enriched spermatogonial fractions collected from the STAPUT apparatus were pooled and subjected to differential plating to eliminate the contaminating cells (myoid and Sertoli cells) which constitute about 10%–15% of the cell population. The pooled cells were incubated in DMEM/F12 containing 5% FBS for 4 h at 34°C. The spermatogonial cells which remained in suspension were collected and washed in DMEM/F12 before plating. The purity of the cell preparation was determined prior to and after differential plating.

8.2.3 Morphological and Immunocytochemical Characterization of Rat Type A Spermatogonia

Phase Contrast Microscopy. The cells recovered after differential plating were examined by phase contrast microscopy for an approximation of their size and to identify their morphological attributes.

Immunocytochemical Localization of c-kit Receptor. The isolated spermatogonial cells were centrifuged at $90 \times g$ for 5 min onto glass slides in a Cytospin centrifuge (Shandon L'upshaw, Pittsburgh, PA, USA). The cells were fixed and permeabilized with ice-cold methanol for 3 min and then washed three times with PBS. Streptavidin-biotin peroxidase immunostaining was carried out with Histostain-SP kits (Zymed Laboratories, Burlingame, CA, USA) according to the manufacturer's instructions and as described by our group (Dym et al. 1995). Briefly, endogenous peroxidase activity was blocked by a 45-s treatment with periodic acid solution, and endogenous biotin was blocked by using the avidin blocking solutions, followed by blocking of nonspecific antibody binding with 10% nonimmune goat serum. The cells were then incubated at 37°C for 1 h in a moist chamber with normal rabbit serum (1:500) or with rabbit anti-mouse *c-kit* receptor antibody (1:500) raised against the whole protein (gift from Dr. Peter Besmer, Sloan-Kettering Memorial Cancer Institute, New York, NY, USA). The cells were immunostained with, successively, biotinylated goat anti-rabbit antibodies (10 min), streptavidin-peroxidase (5 min), and substrate-chromogen mixture (10–15 min). The cells were counterstained for 3 min with hematoxylin and then examined with a Zeiss Axiophot light microscope fitted with Planapo objectives. A positive reaction is characterized by the deposition of a reddish-brown reaction product at the site of the antibody–antigen reaction.

8.2.4 Sertoli Cell Preparation and Culture

Sertoli cells were isolated from 9-day-old Sprague-Dawley rats (Charles River Breeding Laboratories, Inc., Wilmington, MA, USA) by sequential enzymatic digestion as described previously (Hadley et al. 1985) with some modifications (Dirami et al. 1995). Briefly, the testes were decapsulated, minced, and then digested with collagenase (150 units/ml) and DNAse (5 μg/ml) for 10 min at 34°C in a shaking water bath (100 cycles/min) to remove Leydig cells and other interstitial cells. The seminiferous tubule fragments were washed three times with DMEM (Gibco Laboratories Inc., Grand Island, NY, USA) and subjected to a second digestion with collagenase (500 units/ml), hyaluronidase (1.5 mg/ml), and DNAse (5 μg/ml) for 20–30 min to remove the peritubular myoid cell layer. The seminiferous cord fragments, which are now much smaller in size, were washed twice with DMEM and subjected to a third digestion with collagenase, hyaluronidase, and DNAse to obtain smaller Sertoli cell aggregates of 5–10 cells.

Sertoli cell aggregates were cultured either in DMEM/F12 alone or in DMEM/F12 supplemented with FSH (100 ng/ml), testosterone (30 ng/ml), retinoic acid (100 ng/ml), vitamin E (200 ng/ml), insulin (5 μg/ml), transferrin (5 μg/ml), selenium (5 ng/ml), and 1 mM sodium pyruvate (serum-free defined medium, SFDM). The conditioned media from cells cultured in DMEM/F12 alone (SCCM$_A$), and the cells cultured in DMEM/F12 supplemented with hormones and growth factors (SCCM$_B$) were collected at 24-h intervals for 3 days, centrifuged, and dialyzed/concentrated using Centriprep-10 microconcentrators (10 000 MW cut off) (Amicon). Total protein concentration was determined as previously described (Bradford 1976).

8.2.5 Cell Viability Assay

Cell viability was determined with the MTT colorimetric assay as described recently (Dirami et al. 1995). The principle of the assay is that MTT (3-[4.5-dimethylthiazol-2-yl]-2,5-diphenyltetrazolium bromide), a nontoxic pale yellow substrate, is taken up by living cells to yield a dark blue formazan product. The process requires active mitochondria, thus dead cells will not form formazan. The formazan that is formed is read spectrophotometrically at 570-nm absorbance and is directly proportional to the number of viable cells. A calibration curve relating absorbance to cell number was determined for freshly isolated spermatogonial cells. For this assay, cells were seeded at a density of 10^5 cells/well ($n=8$) in 96-well plates. The cells were cultured in DMEM/F12 in the presence or absence of 10% horse serum (HS) for various lengths of time, or in DMEM/F12 supplemented with 100 ng/ml rat kit ligand (KL) (gift from Dr. J.L. Tilly, The Johns Hopkins University, MD), 10 µl of the concentrated SFDM, 10 µl (10 µg total protein) of concentrated Sertoli cell conditioned medium (SCCM), or 10% FBS for 24 h at 34°C. After the indicated time of incubation, 10 µl of labeling reagent (MTT) was added and the cells were further incubated for an additional 4 h at 34°C. Cells were solubilized by incubating in 100 µl of a solubilization solution (10% SDS in 0.01 M HCl) overnight at 37°C. The absorbance at 570 nm was determined in a microtiter plate reader (Bio-Rad, Hercules, CA, USA). The results were expressed as a percentage of viable cells at time zero.

8.2.6 Analysis of DNA Fragmentation by Flow Cytometry

Quantitation of cells with degraded DNA was performed as we described previously (Dirami et al. 1995). Briefly, the spermatogonial stem cells (5×10^6 cells), obtained immediately after differential plating or cultured for 24 h in DMEM/F12, were washed in cold PBS. After a brief centrifugation, the pellet was resuspended in 1 ml 95% ethanol at 4°C by gentle pipetting and then stored at −20°C until analysis. Prior to flow cytometry, the cells were washed in cold PBS and incubated in fresh PBS at 37°C for 20 min. After centrifugation, the pelleted cells were resuspended in 1–2 ml propidium iodide (Sigma Chemical Co, St.

Louis, MO, USA) solution (PBS containing 0.1% triton X-100, 0.1 mM EDTA, 50 µg/ml propidium iodide). Samples were stored in the dark at room temperature and flow cytometrically analyzed within 24 h using a Becton-Dickinson Flow Cytometer (Lombardi Cancer Research Center, Georgetown University, Washington, DC, USA).

8.2.7 Analysis of DNA Fragmentation by Agarose Gel Electrophoresis

Low-molecular-weight genomic DNA was isolated as previously described (Dirami et al. 1995). Briefly, DNA was isolated from spermatogonial stem cells (5×10^6 cells) obtained immediately after differential plating or after culture in DMEM/F12 for 24 h. The cells were pelleted and resuspended in a lysis buffer containing 10 mM Tris-HCl (pH 7.4), 10 mM EDTA, and 0.5% Triton X-100 (Sigma) and kept on ice for 10 min. The low-molecular-weight genomic DNA was extracted twice with phenol:chloroform/isoamyl alcohol (24:1) and the aqueous phase was separated by centrifugation for 15 min at 15 000 rpm. The DNA was precipitated by addition of two volumes of ice-cold ethanol, and the samples were stored at –20°C overnight. The precipitated DNA was pelleted at 15 000 rpm for 30 min and washed successively with 100% and 75% ice-cold ethanol. The pellets were dried, dissolved in 10 µl Tris/EDTA buffer (10 mM Tris-HCl, 0.2 mM EDTA, pH 7.5), then loaded on a 1.8% agarose gel. Electrophoretic separation of DNA was performed at 40 V for 6 h, and the DNA was visualized by staining with ethidium bromide. For sizing of DNA bands, 5 µg of a standard preparation (100-bp ladder from Gibco BRL) were run along with the samples.

8.2.8 Statistical Analysis of the Data

All the experiments were performed at least three times with replicate samples. Significance between controls and experimental samples was established by one-way analysis of variance. The difference was considered significant when p was less than 0.05.

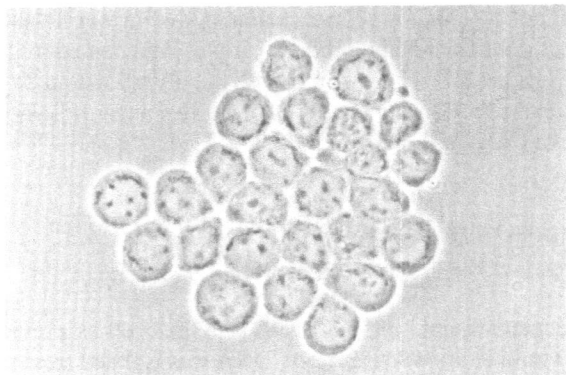

Fig. 1. Phase contrast micrograph of freshly isolated type A spermatogonia after differential plating. The type A spermatogonia are spherical in shape and contain organelles located generally in the perinuclear region. The large nuclei posses several prominent nucleoli. (×675)

8.3 Results

8.3.1 Characterization of Purified Rat Spermatogonia

Figure 1 represents a phase contrast micrograph of freshly isolated type A spermatogonia from 9-day-old rats after differential plating. The spermatogonial cells appeared to be approximately 20–25 μm in diameter and had large spherical nuclei containing several prominent nucleoli. The cytoplasm was characterized by organelles located mostly in the perinuclear region. Generally, the type A spermatogonia looked almost identical to their in vivo counterparts present in 9-day-old rat testes (Dym et al. 1995).

Using the *c-kit* receptor as a marker for the type A spermatogonia, the purity of the spermatogonial preparation before and after differential plating was established. The purity of the preparation before differential plating was in the range of 80%–85%. After removal of myoid and Sertoli cell contaminants, the percentage of spermatogonia in the final preparation ranged between 95% and 100%. In these preparations, a number of unstained cells were present in the spermatogonial prepara-

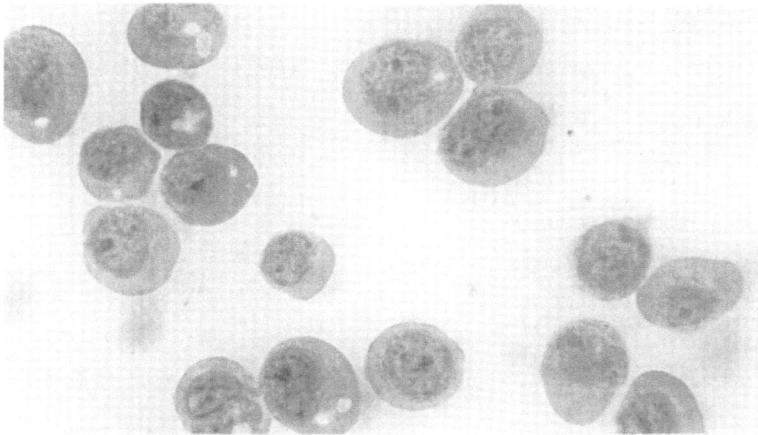

Fig. 2. Immunostaining of isolated type A spermatogonia for the *c-kit* receptor after differential plating.Spermatogonial cells were cytocentrifuged onto glass slides, fixed in cold methanol, and immunostained with the *c-kit* receptor antibody. In this preparation, all the spermatogonia stained for the c-kit receptor. (×1200)

tion prior to differential plating (results not shown), whereas very few unstained cells (<2%) were observed after differential plating (Fig. 2).

8.3.2 Survivability of Isolated Spermatogonia in DMEM/F12 Medium

Purified spermatogonia were cultured in plain DMEM/F12 medium for up to 96 h at 34°C, and the viability was monitored at 24-h intervals (Fig. 3). The spermatogonial cells showed a progressive decline in viability. By 24 h, more than 50% of cells were nonviable. Less than 20% of the cells were viable at the end of 96 h.

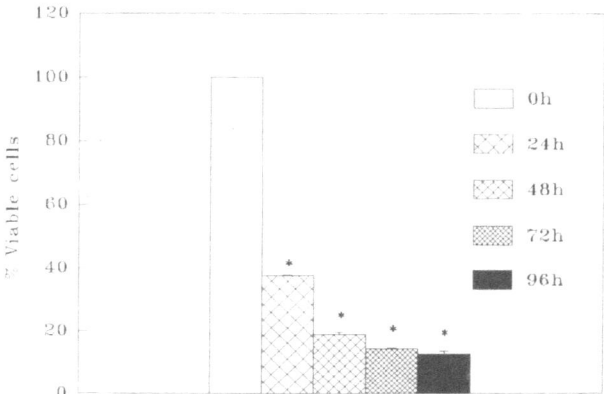

Fig. 3. Viability of type A spermatogonial stem cells cultured in Dulbecco's modified Eagle's and Ham F12 (DMEM/F12) medium.Isolated type A spermatogonial cells were seeded at a density of 10^5 cells/well in 96-well plates, and cultured for 24, 48, 72, and 96 h in DMEM/F12 medium at 34°C. Spermatogonia exhibited a significant decrease in cell viability with time (*$p<0.05$), and less than 20% viable cells were present by 96 h

8.3.3 Spermatogonial Stem Cells Undergo an Apoptotic Form of Cell Death

Flow cytograms of the spermatogonial cells obtained immediately after differential plating and after culture for 24 h in DMEM/F12 medium is depicted in Fig. 4. The freshly isolated cells (after differential plating for 4 h) exhibited a prominent diploid peak at channel 100 and a very small broad apoptotic peak (Fig. 4a). The peak between channels 150 and 200 represents cell clumps. The majority of the cells cultured for 24 h exhibited a reduction in DNA content, and the pool of these cells is represented by a hypodiploid peak at channel 50. A small peak representing normal diploid cells is seen at channel 100 (Fig. 4b).

To further assess whether the reduction in cellular DNA depicted by flow cytometric analysis is due to internucleosomal breakdown and generation of small fragments of DNA, low-molecular-weight DNA extracted from the spermatogonial stem cells immediately after differential plating and after culture for 24 h in DMEM/F12 was subjected

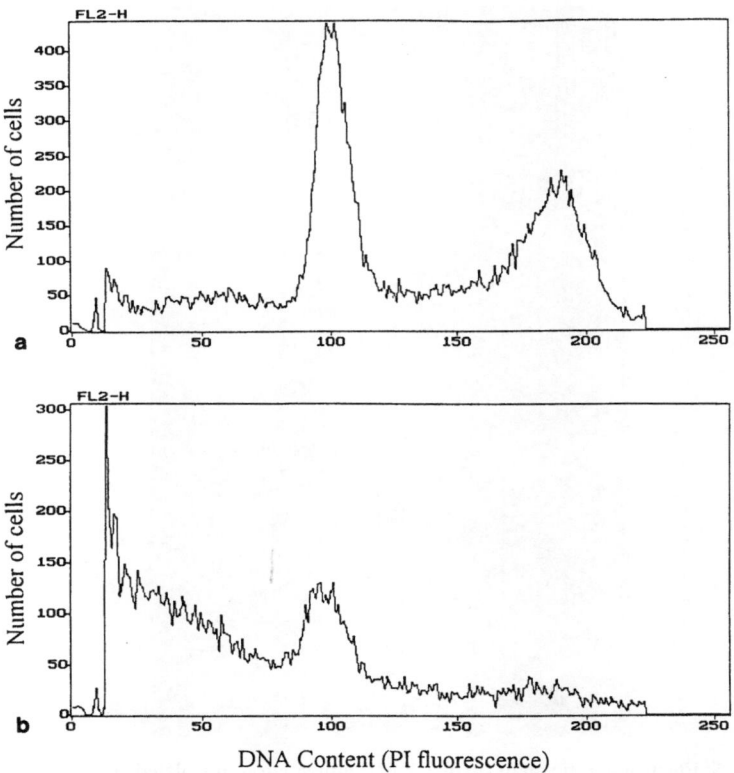

Fig. 4a,b. Spermatogonial stem cells undergo apoptosis in vitro. **a** Flow cytometric analysis of DNA in isolated spermatogonia stained with propidium iodide (*PI*) immediately after differential plating. The peak at fluorescence channel 100 represents normal diploid spermatogonial cells. **b** Spermatogonial stem cells cultured for 24 h in DMEM/F12 alone. An apoptotic peak is apparent in the hypodiploid region at channel 50. There is a concomitant reduction in the number of spermatogonial cells at channel 100

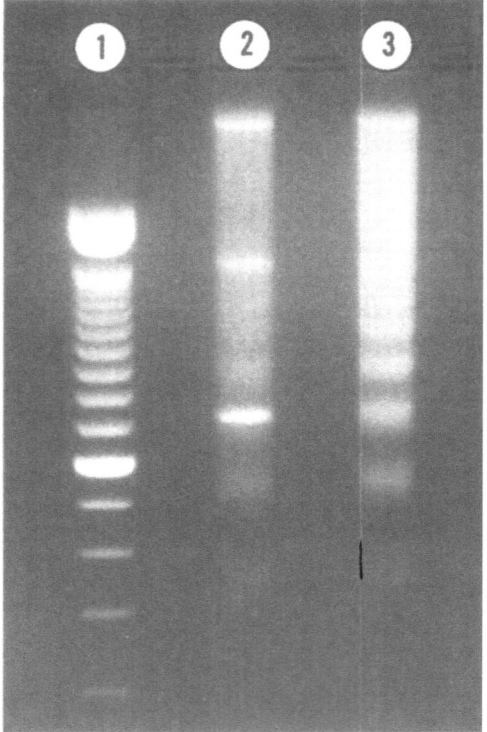

Fig. 5. Electrophoretic analysis of DNA fragmentation in isolated spermatogonia. Low-molecular-weight genomic DNA was isolated from spermatogonial
cells (5×10^6 cells) and subjected to electrophoresis on a 1.8% agarose gel.
Lane 1, 100-bp DNA marker; *lane 2*, DNA from spermatogonia immediately
after differential plating; *lane 3*, DNA from spermatogonia after differential
plating and culture for 24 h in Dulbecco's modified Eagle's and Ham F12
(DMEM/F12) medium alone. DNA laddering is apparent under both conditions, but the extent of internucleosomal DNA degradation is more pronounced
in the spermatogonia cultured for 24 h

to electrophoresis on a 1.8% agarose gel. A DNA ladder was observed
under both conditions, with the DNA degradation being more pronounced in the cells cultured for 24 h in DMEM/F12 than in the cells
obtained immediately after differential plating (Fig. 5).

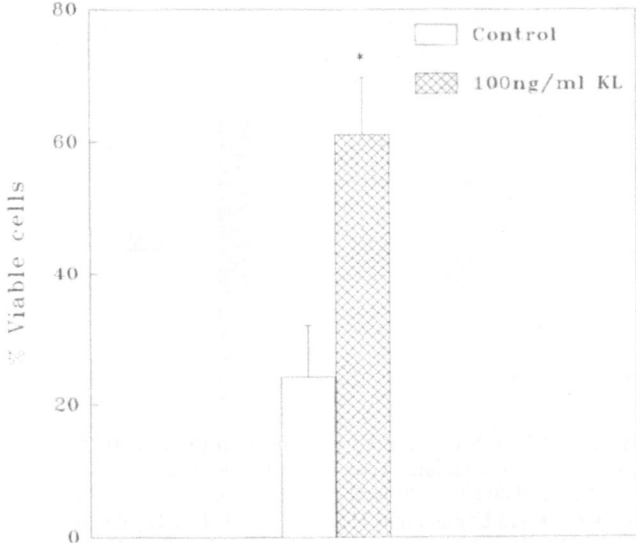

Fig. 6. Effect of the soluble form of the rat kit ligand (*KL*) on the viability of type A spermatogonia in culture. Isolated type A spermatogonial cells were seeded at a density of 10^5 cells/well in 96-well plates, and cultured for 24 h at 34°C in Dulbecco's modified Eagle's and Ham F12 (DMEM/F12) medium in the absence or presence of kit ligand (100 ng/ml). The percent viability of spermatogonial cells cultured in the presence of KL was significantly higher (*$p<0.05$) than in cells cultured in DMEM/F12 alone

8.3.4 Soluble Form of KL Enhances the Survival of Type A Spermatogonial Stem Cells in Culture

The spermatogonial stem cells were cultured in DMEM/F12 medium containing rat KL at a concentration of 100 ng/ml (Fig. 6). In controls, where spermatogonia were cultured in DMEM/F12 alone, viability decreased to almost 25% by 24 h. In contrast, 60%–70% of cells were viable in cells cultured in DMEM/F12 containing KL for 24 h ($p<0.05$).

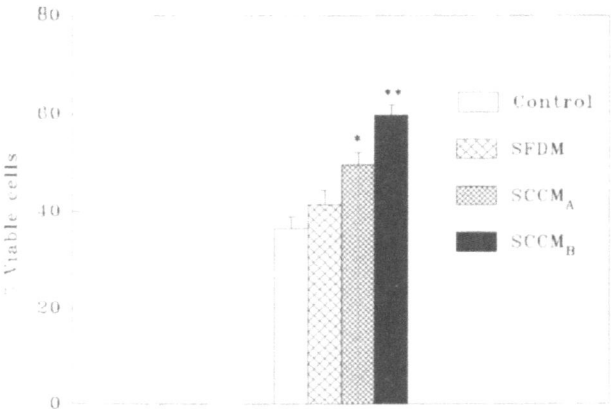

Fig. 7. Effect of Sertoli cell conditioned medium (*SCCM*) on the viability of type A spermatogonia. Isolated type A spermatogonial cells were seeded at a density of 10^5 cells/well in 96-well plates, and cultured for 24 h at 34°C in Dulbecco's modified Eagle's and Ham F12 (DMEM/F12) medium containing 10 µl of SCCM (10 µg total protein) obtained from Sertoli cells cultured in DMEM/F12 alone ($SCCM_A$) or in serum-free defined medium (*SFDM*) ($SCCM_B$). The same volume (10 µl) of concentrated/dialyzed SFDM collected from cell-free dishes was added as a control to distinguish between the effect of the Sertoli cell-secreted factors and the components of SFDM. The percent viability of spermatogonia was significantly higher in cells cultured in the presence of $SCCM_A$ (*$p<0.05$) or $SCCM_B$ (**$p<0.01$) than in cells cultured in DMEM/F12 alone

8.3.5 Effects of Sertoli Cell-Conditioned Media on the Viability of Spermatogonia in Culture

Figure 7 depicts the effects of $SCCM_A$ (derived from Sertoli cells cultured in DMEM/F12 alone), $SCCM_B$ (derived from Sertoli cells cultured in DMEM/F12 supplemented with hormones and growth factors, SFDM), and SFDM alone on the viability of spermatogonia in culture after a 24-h incubation. The percentage of viable spermatogonia was significantly higher in cells cultured in medium containing $SCCM_A$ ($p<0.05$) and $SCCM_B$ ($p<0.01$) (Fig. 7).

To rule out the possibility that hormones and growth factors added to DMEM/F12 for culturing Sertoli cells (in $SCCM_B$) might enhance the

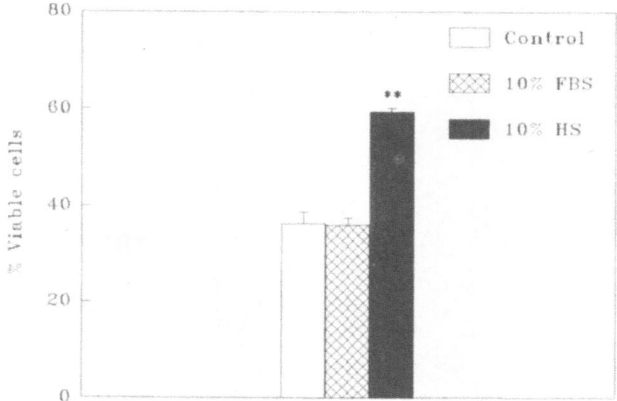

Fig. 8. Effect of fetal bovine serum (*FBS*) and horse serum (*HS*) on the viability of isolated type A spermatogonia. Isolated type A spermatogonial cells were seeded at a density of 10^5 cells/well in 96-well plates, and cultured at 34°C for 24 h in Dulbecco's modified Eagle's and Ham F12 (DMEM/F12) medium containing 10% FBS or 10% HS. Notice that FBS was unable to maintain the viability of spermatogonial cells. In contrast, a significantly higher percentage of viable spermatogonial cells is apparent in the cells cultured in the presence of HS (**$p<0.01$)

viability of spermatogonia rather than Sertoli cell factors, spermatogonia were cultured in DMEM/F12 supplemented with 10 µl of dialyzed/concentrated SFDM. SFDM had no significant effect on the viability of the spermatogonial stem cells cultured for 24 h (Fig. 7).

8.3.6 Effect of FBS and HS on the Viability of Spermatogonial Stem Cells

The culture of the spermatogonia in 10% FBS for 24 h had no significant effect on cell viability compared with the cells cultured in DMEM/F12 alone; less than 40% of spermatogonia remained viable under these conditions. In contrast, 60% of spermatogonia cultured in the presence of 10% HS were viable at the end of 24 h ($p<0.01$) (Fig. 8). In a time-course study using DMEM/F12 medium supplemented with

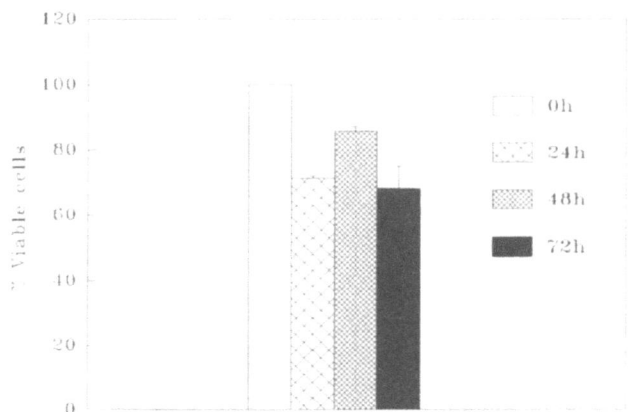

Fig. 9. Time-course study on the viability of spermatogonial cells cultured in Dulbecco's modified Eagle's and Ham F12 (DMEM/F12) medium containing 10% horse serum (HS). Isolated type A spermatogonial cells were seeded at a density of 10^5 cells/well in 96-well plates and cultured at 34°C for 24, 48, and 72 h in DMEM/F12 containing 10% HS. Seventy to eighty percent of spermatogonial cells were viable when cultured for up to 72 h

10% horse serum, 70%–80% of spermatogonia survived after culture for up to 72 h (Fig. 9).

8.3.7 HS and SCCM Maintain the Viability of Isolated Spermatogonial Stem Cells in Culture

Figure 10 depicts the viability of spermatogonial stem cells in culture in the presence of HS and SCCM. Both SCCM$_A$ (derived from Sertoli cells cultured in DMEM/F12 alone, 10 μg total protein) and SCCM$_B$ (obtained from Sertoli cells cultured in SFDM, 10 μg total protein) in combination with HS (10%) were able to maintain the viability of 80%–90% of spermatogonia when cultured for up to 24 h ($p<0.01$ compared with DMEM/F12 alone) (Fig. 10).

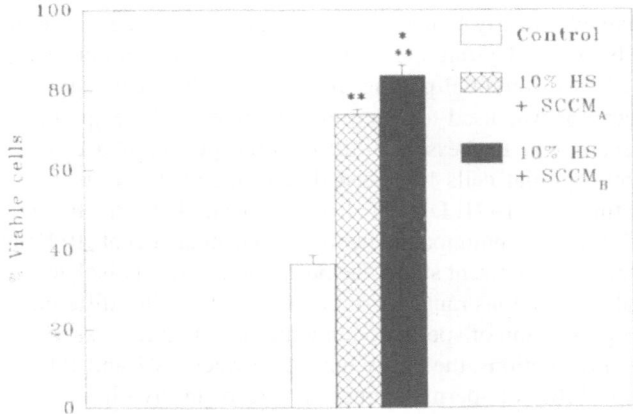

Fig. 10. Effect of horse serum (*HS*) and Sertoli cell-conditioned medium (*SCCM*) on the survival of spermatogonial stem cells in culture. Isolated type A spermatogonial cells were seeded at a density of 10^5 cells/well in 96-well plates, and cultured for 24 h at 34°C in Dulbecco's modified Eagle's and Ham F12 (DMEM/F12) medium in the presence or absence of SCCM$_A$ and SCCM$_B$. The increase in the percent viability of spermatogonia, which is apparent in the cells cultured in the presence of HS (see Fig. 8), is potentiated by addition of SCCM to the culture medium (**p<0.01)

8.4 Discussion

The regulation of the spermatogonial stem cell population in the testis remains one of the last frontiers in male reproductive biology to be addressed. In vitro culture of spermatogonia for long periods of time could prove highly useful for establishing the role of growth and differentiating factors in spermatogonial renewal and differentiation. In addition, this in vitro system may have many potential applications in gene therapy and treatment of infertility which will involve the expansion of the spermatogonial stem cells in culture (Dym 1994). Although velocity sedimentation methods have been used successfully for the separation of mouse spermatogonial cells (Lam et al. 1970; Meistrich 1972; Romrell et al. 1976; Bellvé et al. 1977), purification from other contaminating testicular cells, and culture in vitro has not been possible. By modifying our previously published procedure (Bellvé et al. 1977),

we obtained a nearly homogeneous population of type A spermatogonial cells from 9-day-old rats (Dym et al. 1995). Further purification was
achieved by differential plating. Immunocytochemical staining for the
c-kit receptor was used to determine the purity of the spermatogonial
cell preparations. Expression of the *c-kit* receptor in mouse and rat type
A spermatogonial cells has been demonstrated by Northern analysis
(Sorrentino et al. 1991; Dym et al. 1995), in situ hybridization (Manova
et al. 1990), and immunocytochemistry (Yoshinaga et al. 1991; Dym et
al. 1995). In our present study, the purity of the freshly isolated spermatogonial preparations ranged from 80% to 85%. After differential plating, the population of spermatogonia that we obtained was >95% pure.
In some preparations, the purity ranged between 98% and 100%.

The viability of spermatogonia in vitro or in vivo has always been
assessed based on their ability to differentiate into an advanced stage in
the process of spermatogenesis, i.e., spermatocytes and spermatids (Abe
1987). Since one of the aims of the present study was to maintain
spermatogonia in an undifferentiated state in an artificial culture medium for longer periods of time, a colorimetric assay for the detection of
viable cells was used. The MTT colorimetric assay has previously been
used for the quantitative determination of cellular proliferation in response to growth factors and cytokines (Mosmann 1983; Vistica et al.
1991; Mosman and Fong 1989; Ohno and Abe 1995) and to assess the
viability of Sertoli cells (Dirami et al. 1995). Using the MTT assay, it
was observed that the viability of spermatogonia cultured in plain
DMEM/F12 medium decreased by more than 50% within 24 h, and that
by 96 h, less than 20% of the cells were viable. The nature of cell death
observed in spermatogonial stem cells when cultured in DMEM/F12
alone was investigated by two classical approaches. In the first approach, spermatogonial cells stained with a fluorochrome, propidium
iodide, were analyzed by flow cytometry. Based on the fact that degraded DNA diffuses out of the cells after fixation and permeabilization,
resulting in a decrease in propidium iodide-bound DNA (Telford et al.
1992), apoptotic spermatogonial cells appeared as a broad peak to the
left of the normal diploid peak. In the second approach, internucleosomal DNA degradation was detected by agarose gel electrophoresis in
spermatogonial cells cultured for 24 h. Multiple fragments of the low-
molecular-weight DNA (<15 kb), characteristic of an apoptotic form of
cell death (Compton 1992), were observed. The internucleosomal DNA

degradation observed in the spermatogonial cells obtained just immediately after differential plating for 4 h in DMEM/F12 containing 5% FBS is not surprising, because spermatogonia do undergo spontaneous degeneration in vivo during normal spermatogenesis (Huckins 1978; Allan et al. 1992).

Attempts have been made by many investigators to promote spermatogonial cell survival in vitro by coculture with Sertoli cells (Tres and Kierszenbaum 1983; Tres et al. 1986; Hadley et al. 1985) in medium containing serum or several growth factors. The spermatogonia are present in the basal compartment of the seminiferous tubule and have extensive contacts with Sertoli cells (Dym and Fawcett 1970; Russell 1995). However, desmosome-gap junctions are rare between Sertoli and spermatogonial cells (Russell 1980), suggesting that direct cell–cell contact may not be involved in spermatogonial proliferation and differentiation. Instead, Sertoli cell secretory products including growth factors may regulate spermatogonial proliferation and differentiation (Skinner 1993; Rossi et al. 1993). In our study, a higher percentage of spermatogonia were viable when maintained in culture in the presence of Sertoli cell-conditioned medium. The enhanced viability of cells seen with conditioned medium, and the ineffectiveness of SFDM to maintain viability suggests that some Sertoli cell-secreted factors can maintain the viability of spermatogonia under these culture conditions.

Since several groups have demonstrated the importance of KL for the survival of primordial germ cells, mast cells, and intestinal stem cells (Pesce et al. 1993; Yee et al. 1994; Leigh et al. 1995), we analyzed the effect of this growth factor on spermatogonia. Type A spermatogonia from both mouse (Manova et al. 1990; Yoshinaga et al. 1991; Sorrentino et al. 1991) and rat (Dym et al. 1995) express the c-kit receptor. The ligand for the c-kit receptor is the KL (steel factor, stem cell factor, mast cell growth factor), which is present only in Sertoli cells in the testis and has been cloned and characterized (Williams et al. 1990; Huang et al. 1990). KL exists in two forms, membrane bound and soluble. While the membrane-bound form acts as a survival factor for primordial germ cells in culture (Dolci et al. 1991), the soluble form enhances their proliferation slightly. Since cultured mouse Sertoli cells secrete the soluble form of KL and promote DNA synthesis in type A spermatogonia (Rossi et al. 1991), and the expression of the membrane-bound form of KL appears to change into the soluble form during the postnatal development of testis (Rossi et al. 1993), it was presumed that the soluble form of KL would support the survival of spermatogonia. In agreement with this hypothesis, the soluble form of rat KL was able to prevent the death of rat spermatogonia to a significant extent.

Serum from animals and humans has been successfully used to cultivate somatic cells. The spermatogonia reside in the basal compartment of the blood–testis barrier (Dym and Fawcett 1970) and thus are exposed directly to circulating substances. The Steinbergers (Steinberger and Steinberger 1966) used modified Eagle's medium (MEM) supplemented with 10% calf serum to culture testicular cell suspensions and found that spermatogonia and spermatocytes survived for 3–4 weeks at 31°C. Based on this study, we used DMEM/F12 supplemented with serum from bovine fetus and horse. While FBS was ineffective in maintaining the viability of spermatogonia, HS was able to maintain the viability of 60%–70% of the cells when cultured for up to 72 h. Addition of SCCM enhanced the effect of HS on the survival of spermatogonial stem cells in culture. In agreement with this finding, addition of autologous serum has been shown to increase expansion of hematopoietic progenitor cells (McNiece and Briddell 1995). Currently, we are investigating whether spermatogonia maintained under the conditions described above are proliferating and/or differentiating into advanced stages in the process of spermatogenesis.

In summary, the present study has demonstrated that rat type A spermatogonial cells could be purified to homogeneity and maintained under viable conditions for up to 72 h in medium containingHS. SCCM potentiated the effect of HS on spermatogonial cell survival. Using this model system, it is now possible to study the effect of individual growth factors and hormones on spermatogonial proliferation and differentiation and establish the conditions for the maintenance of spermatogonia for long periods of time in an undifferentiated state for transplantation purposes.

8.5 Summary

Type A spermatogonial cells isolated from 9-day-old rats were purified to near homogeneity by sedimentation velocity at unit gravity followed by differential plating in a 1:1 mixture of DMEM/F12 containing 5% FBS for 4 h. Following this procedure, spermatogonial cells were cultured either in DMEM/F12 alone for various lengths of time, or in DMEM/F12 supplemented with FSH, testosterone, retinoic acid, human transferrin, insulin, and epidermal growth factor (EGF), SFDM, or in DMEM/F12 supplemented with SCCM, or in DMEM/F12 plus KL. In other experiments, the spermatogonial cells were cultured in DMEM/F12 in the presence or absence of 10% FBS for 24 h or 10% HS for up to 72 h. The viability of the spermatogonia was determined using an MTT colorimetric assay. The spermatogonial cells cultured in DMEM/F12 alone exhibited a time-dependent decrease in cell viability with less than 20% of the cells being viable by 96 h. Analysis of low-molecular-weight DNA extracted from the spermatogonial cells cultured in DMEM/F12 alone for 24 h revealed internucleosomal DNA breakdown, characteristic of apoptosis. Flow cytometric analysis also revealed an apoptotic hypodiploid peak. DMEM/F12 supplemented with the soluble form of KL was able to maintain the viability of 60%–70% of spermatogonial cells cultured for 24 h. Likewise, when the cells were cultured in DMEM/F12 containing SCCM, 50%–60% of the spermatogonial cells were viable. While culturing of spermatogonia in 10% FBS in DMEM/F12 did not improve the cell viability compared with the cells cultured in plain DMEM/F12, 10% HS in DMEM/F12 maintained 60%–70% of spermatogonia in a viable condition after culture for up to 72 h. A combination of 10% HS and SCCM further improved the percent viability of spermatogonia to 80%–90%. The results of the present study show that isolated type A spermatogonia maintained in plain DMEM/F12 undergo an apoptotic form of cell death in vitro, and the apoptosis of spermatogonia can be significantly prevented by supplementing the medium with KL, SCCM, or HS. These results provide the first system for the culture of isolated mammalian type A spermatogonia.

Acknowledgments. The work was supported by NIH grant PO1-24633 to M. Dym

References

Abe SI (1987) Differentiation of spermatogenic cells from vertebrates in vitro. Int Rev Cytol 109:159–209

Aizawa S, Nishimune Y (1979) In-vitro differentiation of type A spermatogonia in mouse cryporchid testis. J Reprod Fertil 56:99–104

Allan DJ, Harmon BV, Roberts SA (1992) Spermatogonial apoptosis has three morphologically recognizable phases and shows no circadian rhythm during normal spermatogenesis in the rat. Cell Prolif 25:241–250

Bellvé AR, Cavicchia JC, Millette CF, O'Brien DA, Bhatnagar YM, Dym M (1977) Spermatogenic cells of the prepuberal mouse: isolation and morphological characterization. J Cell Biol 74:68–85

Boitani C, Politi MG, Menna T (1993) Spermatogonial cell proliferation in organ culture of immature rat testis. Biol Reprod 48:761–767

Bradford MM (1976) A rapid and sensitive method for the quantitation of microgram quantities of protein utilizing the principle of protein-dye binding. Anal Biochem 72:248–254

Clermont Y (1966) Renewal of spermatogonia in man. Am J Anat 118:509–524

Clermont Y (1969) Two classes of spermatogonial stem cells in the monkey (Cercopithecus aethiops). Am J Anat 126:57–72

Compton MM (1992) A biochemical hallmark of apoptosis: internucleosomal degradation of the genome. Cancer Metastasis Rev 11:105–119

Curtis D (1981) In-vitro differentiation of diakinesis figures in human testis. Hum Genet 59:406–411

Dirami G, Ravindranath N, Kleinman HK, Dym M (1995) Evidence that basement membrane prevents apoptosis of Sertoli cells in vitro in the absence of known regulators of Sertoli cell function. Endocrinology 136:4439–4447

Dolci S, Williams DE, Ernst MK, Resnick JL, Brannan CI, Lock LF, Lyman SD, Boswell HS, Donovan PJ (1991) Requirement for mast cell growth factor for primordial germ cell survival in culture. Nature 352:809–811

Dym M (1983) The male reproductive system. In: Weiss L (ed) Histology: cell and tissue biology. Elsevier Biomedical, New York, pp 1000–1053

Dym M (1994) Spermatogonial stem cells of the testis. Proc Natl Acad Sci USA 91:11287–11289

Dym M, Clermont Y (1970) Role of spermatogonia in the repair of the seminiferous epithelium following X-irradiation of the rat testis. Am J Anat 128:265–282

Dym M, Fawcett DW (1970) The blood-testis barrier in the rat and the physiological compartmentation of the seminiferous epithelium. Biol Reprod 3:308–326

Dym M, Jia MC, Dirami G, Price JM, Rabin SJ, Mocchetti I, Ravindranath N (1995) Expression of c-kit receptor and its phosphorylation in immature rat type A spermatogonia. Biol Reprod 52:8–19

Ghatnekar R, Lima-De-Faria A, Rubin S, Menander K (1974) Development of human male meiosis in vitro. Hereditas 78:265–272

Hadley MA, Byers SW, Suarez-Quian CA, Kleinman HK, Dym M (1985) Extracellular matrix regulates Sertoli cell differentiation, testicular cord formation, and germ cell development in vitro. J Cell Biol 101:1511–1522

Huang E, Nocka K, Beier DR, Chu T-Y, Buck J, Lahm H-W, Wellner D, Leder P, Besmer P (1990) The hematopoietic growth factor KL is encoded by the Sl locus and is the ligand of the c-kit receptor, the gene product of the W locus. Cell 63:225–233

Huckins C (1971) The spermatogonial stem cell population in adult rats. 1. Their morphology, proliferation and maturation. Anat Rec 169:533–558

Huckins C (1978) The morphology and kinetics of spermatogonial degeneration in normal adult rats: an analysis using a simplified classification of the germinal epithelium. Anat Rec 190:905–926

Lam D, Furrer R, Bruce WR (1970) The separation, physical characterization, and differentiation kinetics of spermatogonial cells of the mouse. Proc Natl Acad Sci USA 65:192–199

Leigh BR, Khan W, Hancock SL, Knox SJ (1995) Stem cell factor enhances the survival of murine intestinal stem cells after photon irradiation. Radiat Res 142:12–15

Manova K, Nocka K, Besmer P, Bachvarova RF (1990) Gonadal expression of c-kit encoded at the W locus of the mouse. Development 110:1057–1069

Martinovitch PN (1937) Development in-vitro of mamalian gonad. Nature 139:413–415

Martinovitch PN (1939) Development in-vitro of mamalian gonad. Arch Exp Zellforsch 22:74–76

McNiece IK, Briddell RA (1995) Stem cell factor. J Leukoc Biol 57:14–22

Meistrich ML (1972) Separation of mouse spermatogenic cells by velocity sedimentation. J Cell Physiol 80:299–312

Mosman TR, Fong TAT (1989) Specific assays for cytokine production by T cells. J Immunol Methods 116:151–158

Mosmann T (1983) Rapid colorimetric assay for cellular growth and survival. J Immunol Methods 65:55–63

Oakberg EF (1971) Spermatogonial stem-cell renewal in the mouse. Am J Anat 169:515–532

Ohno M, Abe T (1995) Rapid colonmetric assay for the quantification of leukemia inhibility factor (LIF) and interleukin-6 (IL-6). J Immunol Methods 145:199–203

Parvinen M, Wright WW, Phillips DM, Mather JP, Musto NA, Bardin CW (1983) Spermatogenesis in vitro: completion of meiosis and early spermiogenesis. Endocrinology 112:1150–1152

Pesce M, Farrace MG, Piacentini M, Dolci S, De Felici M (1993) Stem cell factor and leukemia inhibitory factor promote primordial germ cell survival by suppressing programmed cell death. Development 118:1089–1094

Raj HGM, Dym M (1976) The effects of selective withdrawal of FSH or LH on spermatogenesis in the immature rat. Biol Reprod 14:489–494

Romrell LJ, Bellve AR, Fawcett DW (1976) Separation of mouse spermatogenic cells by sedimentation velocity. A morphological characterization. Dev Biol 49:119–131

Rossi P, Albanesi C, Grimaldi P, Geremia R (1991) Expression of the mRNA for the ligand of c-kit in mouse Sertoli cells. Biochem Biophys Res Commun 176:910–914

Rossi P, Dolci S, Albanesi C, Grimaldi P, Ricca R, Geremia R (1993) Follicle-stimulating hormone induction of steel factor (SLF) mRNA in mouse Sertoli cells and stimulation of DNA synthesis in spermatogonia by soluble SLF. Dev Biol 155:68–74

Russell LD (1980) Sertoli-germ cell interrelations: a review. Gamete Res 3:179–302

Russell LD (1995) Morphological and functional evidence for Sertoli-germ cell relationships. In: Russell LD, Griswold MD (eds) The Sertoli cell. Cache River Press, Clearwater, pp 365–390

Russell LD, Clermont Y (1977) Degeneration of germ cells in normal, hypophysectomized, and hormone treated hypophysectomized rats. Anat Rec 187:347–366

Skinner MK (1993) Secretion of growth factors and other regulator factors. In: Russel LD, Griswold MD (eds) The Sertoli cells. Cache River Press, Clearwater, pp 237–248

Sorrentino V, Giorgi M, Geremia R, Besmer P, Rossi P (1991) Expression of the c-kit proto-oncogene in the murine male germ cells. Oncogene 6:149–151

Steinberger A, Steinberger E (1966) In-vitro culture of rat testicular cells. Exp Cell Res 44:443–452

Steinberger A, Steinberger E, Perloff WH (1964) Mammalian testes in organ culture. Exp Cell Res 36:19–27

Telford WG, King LE, Franker PJ (1992) Comparative evaluation of several DNA binding dyes in the detection of apoptosis-associated chromatin degradation by flow cytometry. Cytometry 13:137–143

Tres LL, Kierszenbaum AL (1983) Viability of rat spermatogenic cells is facilitated by their coculture with Sertoli cells in serum-free hormone supplemented medium. Proc Natl Acad Sci USA 80:3377–3381

Tres LL, Smith EP, VanWyk JJ, Kierszenbaum AL (1986) Immunoreactive sites and accumulation of somatomedin-C in rat Sertoli-spermatogenic cell co-cultures. Exp Cell Res 162:33–50

Vistica DT, Skehan P, Scudiero D, Monks A, Pittman A, Boyd MR (1991) Tetrazolium-based assays for cellular viability: a critical examination of selected parameters affecting formazan production. Cancer Res 51:2515–2520

Williams DE, Eisenman J, Baird A, Rauch C, VanNess K, March CJ, Park LS, Martin U, Mochizuki DY, Boswell HS, Burgess GS, Cosman D, Lyman SD (1990) Identification of a ligand for the c-kit proto-oncogene. Cell 63:167–174

Yee NS, Paek I, Besmer P (1994) Role of kit-ligand in proliferation and suppression of apoptosis in mast cells: basis for radiosurvivability of white spotting and steel mutant mice. J Exp Med 179:1777–1787

Yoshinaga K, Nishikawa S, Ogawa M, Hayashi S, Kunisada T, Fujimoto T (1991) Role of c-kit in mouse spermatogenesis: identification of spermatogonia as a specific site of c-kit expression and function. Development 113:689–699

9 Androgen Receptor in Transcriptional Regulation

P.J. Kallio, T. Ikonen, A. Moilanen, H. Poukka, P. Reinikainen,
J.J. Palvimo, and O.A. Jänne

9.1   Introduction 167
9.2   Genetics of the Androgen Receptor 168
9.3   Hormone Response Elements 171
9.4   Complex Response Elements 172
9.5   Factors Modulating DNA Binding of the Receptor 172
9.6   Interaction of the Receptor with Chromatin 173
9.7   Transcriptional Regulation by the Androgen Receptor 174
9.8   Transcriptional Repression and Cross-Modulation 175
9.9   Role of Phosphorylation in Androgen Receptor Function 178
9.10   Future Directions 179
References 180

9.1 Introduction

Male sex steroids (androgens) sculpture a male body in a number of ways, such as development of male sex organs; growth of facial, body, and pubic hair; enlargement of vocal cords (deepening of the voice); loss of hair at temples; production of sperm; development of muscle strength; growth of prostate, and development of masculine behavior. Each of these events is regulated by tissue-specific mechanisms through the androgen receptor that activates and/or represses gene networks to elicit its distinct physiological actions. The principal events leading to hyperplastic and/or hypertrophic responses to androgens are, however, believed to be similar, if not identical, in reproductive and nonreproductive tissues (Berger and Watson 1989). Recent studies in a number of laboratories have delineated the ways by which androgen receptor interacts with specific DNA elements – located within and/or around responsive genes – to increase the rate of gene transcription. Much less information is available, however, about mechanisms by which androgens bring about gene repression. In order to elicit defined biological (androgenic) responses, the receptor protein ought to communicate not only with DNA motifs, but also with other transcription factors or coactivators. Finally, practically nothing is known about the role of androgen receptor protein in the stabilization of specific mRNA species.

9.2 Genetics of the Androgen Receptor

The human androgen receptor gene comprises eight exons and encompasses ~80 kb of DNA located at a very conserved region on Xq11-12. Two mRNA species (11 and 7.5 kb in size) are transcribed from this gene through utilization of alternative polyadenylation signals at the 3'-untranslated region, with the longer mRNA species being by far more abundant in most tissues (see Jänne and Shan 1991). The expression of androgen receptor gene and accumulation of the receptor protein are regulated at multiple levels by transcriptional, posttranscriptional, and posttranslational mechanisms, and they can be modulated by homologous and heterologous steroids (ligands) in a tissue-specific fashion (Wolf et al. 1993). Accumulation of androgen receptor mRNA is downregulated by male sex steroids in several but not all tissues (see Jänne and Shan 1991; Wolf et al. 1993; Quigley et al. 1995). The downregulation has been shown to take place, at least in part, at the level of receptor gene transcription. The receptor protein itself appears to be stabilized by the presence of the cognate ligand (Kemppainen et al. 1992) and its concentration is, therefore, not always regulated in a fashion identical with that of the cognate mRNA (see Jänne and Shan 1991). Stabilization of the receptor by androgens is steroid specific, in that 5α-dihydrotestosterone is some fivefold more potent in this respect than testosterone, which is one of the reasons for the greater biological potency of the former steroid (Zhou et al. 1995).

Androgen receptor protein is polymorphic due to the homopolymeric glutamine repeat (CAG repeat) in its amino-terminal region. The consequences of this polymorphism on receptor size are poorly understood; however, the genetic lesion behind Kennedy's disease (an adult-onset, slowly progressing motoneuron disease) was linked to this region. In this syndrome, there is an absolute correlation between the increased size of the CAG repeat and the severity of the disease (LaSpada et al. 1992; summarized by Quigley et al. 1995). Affected males also develop gynecomastia and may have reduced fertility, suggesting that expansion of the CAG repeat generates a more general defect in receptor function. The transcriptional activation capacity of the androgen receptor may be somewhat reduced with a progressive expansion of the repeat (Mhatre et al. 1993), even though doubling of the CAG repeat length did not influence the transcriptional repression elicited by the androgen receptor on some promoters (Kallio et al. 1995). A transgenic mouse model with an expanded CAG repeat did not present a clear phenotype, possibly due to a lack of physiological expression pattern (Bingham et al. 1995). Unlike in man, the repeat length showed no meiotic instability in mice, demonstrating the importance of the genetic environment. An additional androgen receptor isoform (87 kDa), devoid of the first ~150 residues at the amino terminus, has been identified is some tissues, but whether this form (the so-called A-form) is present in some cells simultaneously with the wild-type receptor protein is currently unknown. The formation of the A form appears to originate from translation initiation at a downstream methionine codon (Wilson and McPhaul 1994). The physiological functions of the A form itself and/or through interaction with the 110-kDa receptor protein remain to be clarified.

Valuable information concerning the biology of the androgen receptor has been obtained from naturally occurring gene "knockout" models seen in human disorders (summarized by Quigley et al. 1995). Over 200 mutations in the androgen receptor gene have been described to date, thus making the receptor protein the most often mutated transcription factor known thus far. The majority of mutations described in the literature have been single amino acid substitutions affecting hormone binding. The mutations are scattered throughout the ligand-binding domain, with some preferential clustering to exons 5 and 7. These may represent up to two thirds of coding-region mutations of the androgen receptor gene (Quigley et al. 1995). The mutations may change hormone binding of the receptor in at least three different ways: abolish steroid binding completely, modify ligand specificity, or decrease affinity of steroid binding.

Only very few mutations have been identified in the amino-terminal half of the receptor (Quigley et al. 1995). This could be due to less stringent conformational requirements for the proper function of this region, in that single amino acid substitutions may not be sufficient to interfere with the structure needed for protein–protein interaction through the amino-terminal half. An alternative explanation is that the patient populations studied thus far have been selected towards more severe phenotypes. The possibility that the "natural" polymorphism in the amino terminus of the androgen receptor would explain differences among various ethnic populations in their secondary sex characteristics, such as the amount and distribution of body hair, should not be ruled out. No strict genotype–phenotype rules can be established for patients with androgen insensitivity syndrome; rather, the genetic (and biochemical) environment will eventually determine the phenotype of affected individuals (Quigley et al. 1995). There are also several patients with the clinical presentation of typical androgen insensitivity, but in whom no mutations of the androgen receptor gene have been demonstrated, suggesting the presence of postreceptor defects that may involve androgen receptor-specific coactivators or corepressors.

In addition to various forms of androgen insensitivity and Kennedy's syndrome, at least two other human diseases involve the androgen receptor, namely, male breast cancer and prostate cancer. Two recent reports have described androgen receptor gene mutations in male breast cancer (Wooster at al. 1992; Lobaccaro et al. 1993). The mutations were located in the second zinc finger, changing arginine 607 and arginine 608 codons to glutamine and lysine, respectively, and resulting in loss of some yet unknown protective actions of androgens in breast cells. Alternatively, the mutant receptors might stimulate, due to their altered DNA-binding characteristics, genes or gene networks that are normally estrogen responsive (Wooster at al. 1992; Lobaccaro et al. 1993).

The progression of prostate cancer is a multistep process, involving a variety of genetic alterations of oncogenes, tumor suppressor genes and the androgen receptor gene in the cellular environment. The first reports on mutated androgen receptors – at the level of DNA sequence – in primary prostate tumors appeared some 3 years ago (see Klocker et al.

1994) and subsequent work has revealed that the incidence of receptor mutations is much higher in metastatic than in primary lesions (Taplin et al. 1995). In addition, recent data suggest that amplification of the androgen receptor gene plays a role in the progression of some recurrent, hormone-refractory tumors (Visakorpi et al. 1995). Collectively, these results imply that androgen receptor function is mandatory for the development, maintenance, and progression of prostate cancer. This issue continues to be an important topic of future studies.

9.3 Hormone Response Elements

DNA sequences responsible for regulation by steroid hormones have been found in the regulatory regions of numerous genes using both gene transfer and in vitro DNA-binding studies. These hormone response elements (HREs) have generally two 6-bp, nearly palindromic sequences separated by a variable number of intervening "spacing" nucleotides. The HREs are classified into subclasses depending on (a) the sequence, (b) the spacing in between, and (c) the orientation of the half-sites. No strict rules have emerged that could specify the androgen receptor's interaction with DNA; rather, with rare exceptions, androgen-responsive elements (AREs) fall in the category of motifs recognized by all members of the glucocorticoid receptor subfamily. For example, a search for the consensus ARE from a pool of random oligonucleotides yielded a sequence that is similar to that of a glucocorticoid response element (GRE) (Roche et al. 1992). Moreover, the purines in AREs that make contacts with the receptor protein are similar, if not identical, to those in glucocorticoid receptor–GRE complexes (Kallio et al. 1994). In many genes, several motifs together often form a cluster known as a hormone response unit. These are highly active units that may represent a combination of several imperfect elements which themselves are only weakly active, suggesting cooperativity among the different AREs (Kasper et al. 1994).

9.4 Complex Response Elements

Complex response elements with selectivity towards androgen regulation have been described, including those in the genes encoding rat
probasin and 20-kDa proteins as well as mouse sex-limited protein.
Maximal induction of the rat probasin gene requires the presence of two
androgen receptor-binding sites (Rennie et al. 1993) which behave in a
cooperative manner to yield preferentially androgen-specific expression
in transfected cells (Kasper et al. 1994; Rennie et al. 1993). In transgenic
mice, the expression of a reporter gene driven by ~450 nucleotides of
the probasin promoter was strictly prostate specific and only regulated
by androgens (Greenberg et al. 1994).

The specificity of sex-limited protein gene regulation requires, in
addition to a consensus GRE/ARE, other auxiliary motifs present in the
flanking 120 nucleotides of the promoter, implying that androgen-specific *trans*-activation is derived from the interactions governed by the
whole context of the androgen receptor-binding site (Adler et al. 1992).
Similar results were reported for the androgen-regulated gene encoding
the 20-kDa secretory protein in rat ventral prostate. Androgen receptor-
specific elements were located in intron 1 of the gene; however, other
elements besides GRE/AREs were required for specific regulation. In
addition, androgen specificity was dependent on the cell line used (Ho
et al. 1993).

9.5 Factors Modulating DNA Binding of the Receptor

DNA binding of steroid receptors is enhanced by nuclear proteins,
whose cell-specific expression may provide some selectivity for steroid
hormone action. For example, the DNA-bending protein HMG-1 enhances dramatically progesterone receptor–DNA interactions, possibly
by inducing a structural change in the target DNA that favors binding of
progesterone receptor (Onate et al. 1994). This stimulatory effect is
selective, as a number of nonspecific proteins failed to enhance progesterone receptor–DNA interaction. Insulin-degrading enzyme (IDE), a
metalloendoproteinase involved in insulin degradation, facilitates DNA
binding of truncated androgen and glucocorticoid receptor proteins
through formation of heteromeric complexes (Kupfer et al. 1994). It is

of note, however, that enhancement of androgen receptor–ARE interaction was observed in this study only with truncated receptor forms and not with the wild-type protein. In view of this, the biological relevance of androgen receptor–IDE interaction requires further clarification.

Calreticulin and a 60-kDa related protein with amino-terminal sequence homology with calreticulin were shown to inhibit not only DNA binding of androgen receptor, but also androgen-induced gene expression (Dedhar et al. 1994). Similar inhibition was observed with some other nuclear receptors such as the glucocorticoid receptor. Calreticulin elicited its effect through interaction with the conserved Lys-X-Gly-Phe-Phe-Lys-Arg sequence present in the DNA-binding domain of all steroid receptors. However, in view the role of calreticulin in storage of Ca^{2+} in the lumen of endoplasmic reticulum and its interaction with the cytoplasmic domains of all integrin α-subunits, the significance of these findings with nuclear receptors remains to be established.

9.6 Interaction of the Receptor with Chromatin

The access of the transcription apparatus to DNA is modulated by chromatin structure; for example, the affinity of glucocorticoid receptor for its target sequence is affected by the position of the GRE on nucleosomes (Li and Wrange 1993). The highly reproducible nucleoprotein organization associated with stably transfected MMTV-LTR in rodent cells is a useful model for steroid-responsive promoters. Binding of the glucocorticoid receptor to its *cis* element on nucleosomal MMTV remodels chromatin structure, allowing additional transcription factors such as NF-1 to be recruited (Archer et al. 1992). Whereas stimulation by glucocorticoids leads to a rapid increase in transcription initiation, the liganded progesterone receptor fails to induce a comparable effect on stable MMTV chromatin templates (Archer et al. 1994). Thus, chromatin structure provides some selectivity among various steroid receptors present in the same cell. When the MMTV promoter is stably introduced to human T47D cells with a high level of progesterone receptor expression, the organization of chromatin is constitutively in a more open configuration than in rodent cells and displays steroid-independent loading of transcription factors (Mymryk et al. 1995). This implies that the assembly of chromatin on a given promoter is indeed influenced by the cell type and its transcription factor complement. In concert with this notion, a group of proteins – SWI1, SWI2/SNF2, and SWI3 – initially identified as chromatin components in yeast were shown to be essential coactivators of nuclear receptor-induced transcription (Yoshinaga et al. 1992). Future studies on androgen receptor-regulated genes in their native environment with chromatin will help us understand how only a selected population of potentially hormone-responsive genes is activated in target cells in a hormone-specific manner.

9.7 Transcriptional Regulation by the Androgen Receptor

Transcription initiation by RNA polymerase II (RNA pol II) involves a hierarchy of interactions. Factors bound to upstream elements interact with basal factors, which, in turn, make direct contacts with RNA pol II. The transcription factor IID (TFIID) complex has been recently implicated as a central player in the communication between transcriptional activators and the enzyme, and its function also requires the presence of different coactivators (TAFs). Several mechanisms have been suggested for the action of sequence-specific transcriptional factors, most of them supporting the hypothesis of an increased basal factor recruitment to the preinitiation complex (see Roeder 1991; Tijan and Maniatis 1994). Additionally, activators can also act at subsequent steps in the transcription process, such as by enhancing the rate of initiation or elongation by RNA pol II.

The defined regions of androgen receptor responsible for transcriptional activation are not known, and it is likely that the regions differ among various promoters. The regulatory domains identified so far in nuclear receptors do not conform with recognizable activation sequences in other transcription factors. In several steroid receptors, including the androgen receptor, the principal activation function (AF-1) has been localized to amino-terminal domain in the region encompassing amino acid residues 150–300 (Palvimo et al. 1993). A second activation domain (AF-2) has been mapped to the ligand-binding region of many receptors, and a similar function may also exists in the comparable region of the androgen receptor (Kallio et al. 1995). AF-1 and AF-2 activities vary, depending upon the promoter and the cell type, and these two regions may also act synergistically to yield maximal transcriptional response.

Almost nothing is known about interactions between androgen receptor and the basal transcription apparatus. Many other nuclear receptors have been shown to interact with the general transcription factor IIB (TFIIB) (Ing et al. 1992; MacDonald et al. 1995). One TFIID subunit is also a target for steroid receptors, as $TAF_{II}30$ has been shown to interact with the AF-2 region of estrogen receptor (Jacq et al. 1994). Regulatory interactions with other, less well characterized proteins have also been described. A 160-kDa protein (termed ERAP160) with estrogen-dependent binding to the estrogen receptor has been characterized (Cavaillés et al. 1994). Interacting partners have also been delineated by using the yeast two-hybrid system for the thyroid hormone receptor-$\beta 1$ and the retinoid receptor RXR (Lee et al. 1995a, b). One of these proteins shares a striking sequence homology with the yeast transcriptional mediator Sug1, and its overexpression specifically inhibited *trans*-activation by both the thyroid receptor and the retinoid receptor RXR (Lee et al. 1995b).

9.8 Transcriptional Repression and Cross-Modulation

Mechanisms for transcriptional repression by steroids are poorly understood. In some instances, the presence of so-called negative hormone response elements has been suggested, but whether they are negative elements per se or simply overlap with DNA elements for other (positively acting?) factors remains to be elucidated. Alternatively, repression would emerge when a sequence-specific activator is prevented from making contacts with transcriptional apparatus due to competitive protein–protein interactions. One class of genes that are repressed by steroid hormones are those under the positive control by members of the activating protein-1 (AP-1) family (see Pfahl 1993). For example, the glucocorticoid receptor and AP-1 family members mutually influence the activities of each other both in vivo and in vitro. The modulation appears to involve direct interaction between the glucocorticoid receptor and AP-1 subunits. The basic zipper region of c-Jun and c-Fos proteins is at least a part of the target for glucocorticoid-mediated transcriptional interference. Depending on the receptor, cell line, and promoter type,

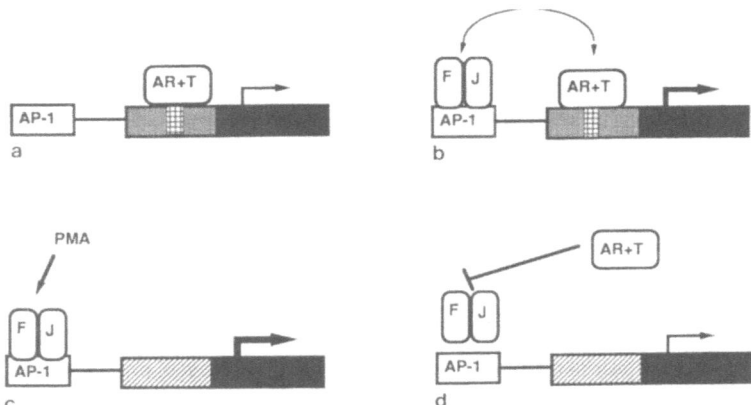

Fig. 1a–d. Schematic representation of the effects of stimulated activating pro-
tein-1 (*AP-1*) activity on the function of androgen receptor. **a** In the presence
of testosterone, androgen receptor binds to androgen response elements
(AREs) on the promoter and stimulates transcription. **b** In the presence of
both ARE and an AP-1 element in the promoter, the androgen receptor (*AR*)
and activated AP-1 components will *trans*-activate in a synergistic fashion.
c,d *Trans*-repression by the receptor in the absence of ARE. Repression does
not require DNA binding of the androgen receptor; rather, the receptor inhibits
trans-activation by interfering with factors governing the basal (and stimulated) expression of the gene, as shown for AP-1 components here. The effect
of promoter context and/or the presence or absence of additional transcription
factors may also have to be considered. *F*, c-Fos; *J*, c-Jun; *PMA*, phorbol ester;
T, testosterone

both positive and negative regulatory interactions between c-Fos/c-Jun
and nuclear hormone receptors have been described (Shemshedini et al.
1991). In addition, specific ligands that can dissociate their *trans*-acti-
vating and *trans*-repressing capabilities have already been designed for
some nuclear receptors (Chen et al. 1995).

Our experiments have shown that androgen receptor is capable of
suppressing a p75 promoter-driven reporter gene expression in a ligand-
dependent manner (Kallio et al. 1995). However, no requisite DNA
motifs were identified in the p75 promoter, suggesting that the negative
regulation could occur via mechanisms not involving direct interaction
between androgen receptor and DNA. When deletion constructs of the
p75 promoter were analyzed in detail, it was realized that transcriptional

repression by the receptor was mediated through an AP-1 element located in the backbone of the reporter plasmid. Expression of p75 promoter-driven CAT constructs (containing the vector AP-1 element) was enhanced by AP-1 activity, and androgen receptor was able to blunt the stimulatory effect in the presence of androgen (Fig. 1). Extensively purified receptor protein was capable of inhibiting DNA binding of c-Jun under cell-free conditions (Kallio et al. 1995). Other studies have previously shown that transcriptional stimulation by c-Fos and c-Jun of a reporter gene driven by five copies of the AP-1 element was severely inhibited by androgen receptor (Shemshedini et al. 1991). A functional AP-1 site in the pUC-based plasmids is also able to mediate transcriptional repression of several reporter constructs by the thyroid receptor (Kushner et al. 1994).

In contrast to the situation with the p75 promoter, other promoters with recognition sites for both androgen receptor and AP-1 proteins behaved in such a way that AP-1 elicited synergistic effects with the receptor in transcriptional activation (Fig. 1). This result and the observation that c-Jun, even at relatively high concentrations, did not inhibit androgen receptor–ARE interaction under cell-free conditions indicate together that, unlike in the case with glucocorticoid receptor, androgen receptor/AP-1 repression is not mutual. In agreement with this notion, stimulation of androgen receptor-mediated *trans*-activation by c-Jun has been previously described (Shemshedini et al. 1991). The effects of c-Jun and c-Fos coexpression were cell and promoter specific, implying that *trans* factors and *cis* elements can inhibit or amplify the response to steroids, thereby providing additional selectivity to transcriptional fine-tuning.

Besides the cross-modulation by AP-1, other regulatory pathways affected by nuclear receptors have been described. *Trans*-activation by nuclear factor-κB (NF-κB), an important regulator of a number of cytokine genes, is antagonized by the activated glucocorticoid receptor (Ray and Prefontaine 1994; Scheinman et al. 1995b). Conversely, stimulation of glucocorticoid responsive genes is inhibited by overexpression of NF-κB. The mutual inhibition is likely to involve a direct interaction between glucocorticoid receptor and the p65 subunit of NF-κB. An additional feature of this interplay is the ability of glucocorticoids to induce transcription of the IκBα gene, which results in an increased rate of synthesis of IκBα protein, an inhibitor of NF-κB function (Scheinman et al. 1995a; Auphan et al. 1995). Whether similar phenomena also hold true for the androgen receptor remains to be established. Other *trans* factors whose function may be influenced by steroid receptors include the cAMP-response element-binding protein CREB, the octamer transcription factor-1 and the Spi.1/PU.1 oncoprotein.

9.9 Role of Phosphorylation in Androgen Receptor Function

The effect of modulators of protein phosphorylation on transcriptional activity of androgen receptor has been studied in our laboratory under transient expression conditions (Ikonen et al. 1994). Activators of protein kinase A (8-Br-cAMP) and protein kinase C (phorbol 12-myristate 13-acetate), or an inhibitor of protein phosphatase 1 and 2A (okadaic acid) influenced minimally pMMTV-driven reporter gene activity in CV-1 or HeLa cells cotransfected with an androgen receptor expression plasmid in the absence of androgen. In this respect, the androgen receptor behaved differently from some other nuclear receptors (Power et al. 1991; Aronica and Katzenellenbogen 1993). In the presence of androgen, however, all compounds enhanced receptor-mediated *trans*-activation by two- to fourfold. Intact DNA- and ligand-binding domains – but not the N-terminal amino acid residues 40–147 – of the androgen receptor were mandatory for the synergism between protein kinase A activators and androgen. Alterations in cellular phosphorylation status did not bring about quantitative or qualitative changes in DNA- and steroid-binding characteristics of the androgen receptor. The results from these and other studies (Reinikainen et al., unpublished data) imply that the synergistic stimulation of androgen receptor-dependent *trans*-activation by androgen and protein kinase activators seems to result from altered interaction of the ligand-activated receptor with other proteins in the transcription machinery. The nature of these proteins is, however, currently unknown.

9.10 Future Directions

The principal regulatory actions elicited by androgens occur at the level of transcription initiation; however, posttranscriptional regulation has also been described. Very little is known about the targets and mechanisms employed by androgens at this latter level, and future studies will be directed to these aspects. At least the following issues should be addressed. Can androgens modulate mRNA stability or translatability? Alternatively, are novel and less well characterized regulatory events involved, such as influence of androgen receptor on RNA pol II elongation rate and on mRNA editing?

The function of androgen receptor protein itself will undoubtedly be a target of exciting work in years to come. For example, what other signaling pathways and ligands can modulate androgen receptor activity and can these be employed to treat disorders of androgen resistance? Could cell-to-cell communication or the tissue-specific contacts with the nuclear matrix affect androgen receptor-mediated transcriptional regulation? Is heterodimerization with other steroid receptors one way to modulate androgen receptor function, similar to the case between mineralocorticoid and glucocorticoid receptors (Trapp et al. 1994)? Does androgen receptor have nongenomic actions in a fashion similar to that of the estrogen receptor (Aronica et al. 1994)? Finally, one major issue that is just beginning to emerge is the characterization of specific TAFs (or inhibitory cofactors) that may interact with various regions of the androgen receptor.

Acknowledgments. The studies performed in the authors' laboratory have been supported by grants from the Medical Research Council (Academy of Finland), the Finnish Cancer Research Foundation, the Sigrid Jusélius Foundation, and the University of Helsinki.

References

Adler AJ, Danielsen M, Robins DM (1992) Androgen-specific gene activation via a consensus glucocorticoid response element is determined by interaction with nonreceptor factors. Proc Natl Acad Sci USA 89:11660–11663

Archer TK, Lefebvre P, Wolford RG, Hager GL (1992) Transcription factor loading on the MMTV promoter: a bimodal mechanism for promoter activation. Science 255:1573–1576

Archer TK, Lee H-L, Cordingley MG, Mymryk JS, Fragoso G, Berard DS, Hager GL (1994) Differential steroid hormone induction of transcription from the mouse mammary tumor virus promoter. Mol Endocrinol 8:568–576

Aronica SM, Katzenellenbogen BS (1993) Stimulation of estrogen receptor-mediated transcription and alteration in the phosphorylation state of the rat uterine estrogen receptor by estrogen, cyclic adenosine monophosphate, and insulin-like growth factor-1. Mol Endocrinol 7: 743–752

Aronica SM, Kraus WL, Katzenellenbogen BS (1994) Estrogen action via the cAMP signalling pathway: stimulation of adenylate cyclase and cAMP-regulated gene transcription. Proc Natl Acad Sci USA 91:8517–8521

Auphan N, DiDonato JA, Rosette C, Helmberg A, Karin M (1995) Immuno-suppression by glucocorticoids: inhibition of NFκB activity through induction of IκB synthesis. Science 270:286–290

Berger FG, Watson G (1989) Androgen-regulated gene expression. Annu Rev Physiol 51:51–65

Bingham PM, Scott MO, Wang S, McPhaul MJ, Wilson EM, Garbern JY, Merry DE, Fischbeck KH (1995) Stability of an expanded trinucleotide repeat in the androgen receptor gene in transgenic mice. Nature Genet 9:191–196

Cavaillés V, Dauvois S, Danielian PS, Parker MG (1994) Interaction of proteins with transcriptionally active estrogen receptors. Proc Natl Acad Sci USA 91:10009–10013

Chen J-Y, Penco S, Ostrowski J, Balaguer P, Pons M, Starrett JE, Reczek P, Chambon P, Gronemeyer H (1995) RAR-specific agonist/antagonists which dissociate transactivation and AP1 transrepression inhibit anchorage-independent cell proliferation. EMBO J 14:1187–1197

Dedhar S, Rennie PS, Shago M, Hagestejn C-YL, Yang H, Filmus J, Hawlwy RG, Bruchovsky N, Cheng H, Matusik RJ, Giguére V (1994) Inhibition of nuclear hormone receptor activity by calreticulin. Nature 367:480–483

Greenberg NM, DeMayo FJ, Sheppard PC, Barrios R, Lebovitz R, Finegold M, Angelopolou R, Dodd JG, Duckworth ML, Rosen JM, Matusik RJ (1994) The rat probasin gene promoter directs hormonally and developmentally regulated expression of a heterologous gene specifically to the prostate in transgenic mice. Mol Endocrinol 8:230–239

Ho K-C, Marschke KB, Tan J, Power SGA, Wilson EM, French FS (1993) A complex response element in the intron 1 of the androgen-regulated 20-kDa protein gene displays cell type-dependent androgen receptor specificity. J Biol Chem 268:27226–27235

Ikonen T, Palvimo JJ, Kallio PJ, Reinikainen P, Jänne OA (1994) Stimulation of androgen-regulated transactivation by modulators of protein phosphorylation. Endocrinology 135:1359–1366

Ing NH, Beekman JM, Tsai SY, Tsai M-J, O'Malley BW (1992) Members of the steroid hormone receptor superfamily interact with TFIIB (S300-II). J Biol Chem 267:17617–17623

Jacq X, Brou C, Lutz Y, Davidson I, Chambon P, Tora L (1994) Human TAF$_{II}$30 is present in a distinct TFIID complex and is required for transcriptional activation by the estrogen receptor. Cell 79:107–117

Jänne OA, Shan L-X (1991) Structure and function of the androgen receptor. Ann N Y Acad Sci 626:81–91

Kallio PJ, Palvimo JJ, Mehto M, Jänne OA (1994) Analysis of androgen receptor-DNA interactions with receptor proteins produced in insect cells. J Biol Chem 269:11514–11522

Kallio PJ, Poukka H, Moilanen A, Jänne OA, Palvimo JJ (1995) Androgen receptor-mediated transcriptional regulation in the absence of direct interaction with a specific DNA element. Mol Endocrinol 9:1017–1028

Kasper S, Rennie PS, Bruchovsky N, Sheppard PC, Cheng H, Lin L, Shiu RPC, Snoek R, Matusik RJ (1994) Cooperative binding of androgen receptors to two DNA sequences is required for androgen induction of the probasin gene. J Biol Chem 269:31763–31769

Kemppainen JA, Lane MV, Sar M, Wilson EM (1992) Androgen receptor phosphorylation, turnover, nuclear transport, and transcriptional activation. Specificity for steroids and antihormones. J Biol Chem 267:968–974

Klocker H, Culig Z, Hobisch A, Cato ACB, Bartsch G (1994) Androgen receptor alterations in prostatic carcinoma. Prostate 35:266–273

Kupfer SR, Wilson EM, French FS (1994) Androgen and glucocorticoid receptors interact with insulin degrading enzyme. J Biol Chem 269:20622–20628

Kushner PJ, Baxter JD, Duncan KG, Lopez GN, Schaufele F, Uht RM, Webb P, West BL (1994) Eukaryotic regulatory elements lurking in plasmid DNA: the activator protein-1 site in pUC. Mol Endocrinol 8:405–407

LaSpada AR, Roiling DB, Harding AE, Warner CL, Spiegel R, Hausmanowa-Petrusewicz I, Yee W-C, Fischbeck KH (1992) Meiotic stability and genotype-phenotype correlation of the trinucleotide repeat in X-linked spinal and bulbar muscular atrophy. Nature Genet 2:301–304

Lee JW, Chois HS, Gyuris J, Brent R, Moore DD (1995a) Two classes of proteins dependent on either the presence or absence of thyroid hormone for interaction with the thyroid hormone receptor. Mol Endocrinol 9:243–254

Lee JW, Ryan F, Swaffield JC, Johnston SA, Moore DD (1995b) Interaction of thyroid hormone receptor with a conserved transcriptional mediator. Nature 374:91–94

Li Q, Wrange Ö (1993) Translational positioning of a nucleosomal glucocorticoid response element modulates glucocorticoid receptor affinity. Genes Dev 7:2471–2482

Lobaccaro J-M, Lumbroso S, Balon C, Galtier-Dereure F, Bringer J, Lesimple T, Namer M, Cutuli BF, Pujol H, Sultan C (1993) Androgen receptor gene mutation in male breast cancer. Hum Mol Genet 2:1799–1802

MacDonald PN, Sherman DR, Dowd DR, Jefcoat SC, Delisle RK (1995) The vitamin D receptor interacts with general transcription factor IIB. J Biol Chem 270:4748–4752

Mhatre AN, Trifiro MA, Kaufman M, Kazemi-Esfarjani P, Figlewicz D, Rouleau G, Pinsky L (1993) Reduced transcriptional regulatory competence of the androgen receptor in X-linked spinal and bulbar muscular atrophy. Nature Genet 5:184–188

Mymryk JS, Berard D, Hager GL, Archer TK (1995) Mouse mammary tumor virus chromatin in human breast cancer cells is constitutively hypersensitive and exhibits steroid hormone-independent loading of transcription factors in vivo. Mol Cell Biol 15:26–34

Onate SA, Prendergast P, Wagner JP, Nissen M, Reeves R, Pettijohn DE, Edwards DP (1994) The DNA-bending protein HMG-1 enhances progesterone receptor binding to its target DNA sequences. Mol Cell Biol 14:3376–3391

Palvimo JJ, Kallio PJ, Ikonen T, Mehto M, Jänne OA (1993) Dominant negative regulation of trans-activation by the rat androgen receptor: roles of the N-terminal domain and heterodimer formation. Mol Endocrinol 7:1399–1407

Pfahl M (1993) Nuclear receptor/AP-1 interaction. Endocr Rev 14:651–658

Power RF, Mani SK, Codina J, Conneely OM, O'Malley BW (1991) Dopaminergic and ligand-independent activation of steroid hormone receptors. Science 254:1636–1639

Quigley CA, De Bellis A, Marschke KB, El-Awady MK, Wilson EM, French FS (1995) Androgen receptor defects: historical, clinical, and molecular perspectives. Endocr Rev 16:271–321

Ray A, Prefontaine KE (1994) Physical association and functional antagonism between the p65 subunit of transcription factor NF-κB and the glucocorticoid receptor. Proc Natl Acad Sci USA 91:752–756

Rennie PS, Bruchovsky N, Leco KJ, Sheppard PC, McQueen SA, Cheng H, Snoek R, Hamel A, Bock ME, MacDonald BS, Nickel BE, Chang C, Liao S, Cattini PA, Matusik RJ (1993) Characterization of two cis-acting DNA elements involved in the androgen regulation of the probasin gene. Mol Endocrinol 7:23–36

Roche PJ, Hoare SA, Parker MG (1992) A consensus DNA-binding site for the androgen receptor. Mol Endocrinol 6:2229–2235

Roeder RG (1991) The complexities of eukaryotic transcription initiation: regulation of preinitiation complex assembly. Trends Biochem Sci 16:402–407

Scheinman RI, Cogswell PC, Lofquist AK, Baldwin AS Jr (1995a) Role of transcriptional activation of IκBα in mediation of immunosuppression by glucocorticoids. Science 270:283–286

Scheinman RI, Gualberto A, Jewell CM, Cidlowski JA, Baldwin AS Jr (1995b) Characterization of mechanisms involved in transrepression of NF-κB by activated glucocorticoid receptors. Mol Cell Biol 15:943–953

Shemshedini L, Knauthe R, Sassone-Corsi P, Pornon A, Gronemeyer H (1991) Cell-specific inhibitory and stimulatory effects of Fos and Jun on transcription activation by nuclear receptors. EMBO J 10:3839–3849

Taplin M-E, Burley GJ, Shuster TD, Frantz ME, Spooner AE, Ogata GK, Keer HN, Balk SP (1995) Mutation of the androgen-receptor gene in metastatic androgen-independent prostate cancer. N Engl J Med 322:1393–1398

Tjian R, Maniatis T (1994) Transcriptional activation: a complex puzzle with few easy pieces. Cell 77:5–8

Trapp T, Rupprecht R, Castrén M, Reul JMHM, Holsboer F (1994) Heterodimerization between mineralocorticoid and glucocorticoid receptor: a new principle of glucocorticoid action in the CNS. Neuron 13:1–20

Visakorpi T, Hyytinen E, Koivisto P, Tanner M, Keinänen R, Palmberg C, Palotie A, Tammela T, Isola J, Kallioniemi O-P (1995) In vivo amplification of the androgen receptor gene and progression of human prostate cancer. Nature Genet 9:401–406

Wilson CM, McPhaul MJ (1994) A and B forms of the androgen receptor are present in human genital skin fibroblasts. Proc Natl Acad Sci USA 91:1234–1238

Wolf DA, Herzinger T, Hermeking H, Blaschke D, Hörz W (1993) Transcriptional and posttranscriptional regulation of human androgen receptor expression by androgen. Mol Endocrinol 7:924–936

Wooster R, Mangion J, Eeles R, Smith S, Dowsett M, Averill D, Barret-Lee P, Easton DF, Ponder BAJ, Stratton MR (1992) A germline mutation in the androgen receptor gene in two brothers with breast cancer and Reifenstein syndrome. Nature Genet 2:132–134

Yoshinaga SK, Peterson CL, Herskowitz I, Yamamoto KR (1992) Roles of SWI1, SWI2, and SWI3 proteins for transcriptional enhancement by steroid receptors. Science 258:1598–1604

Zhou Z-X, Lane MV, Kemppainen JA, French FS, Wilson EM (1995) Specificity of ligand-dependent androgen receptor stabilization: receptor domain interactions influence ligand dissociation and receptor stability. Mol Endocrinol 9:208–218

10 The 3β-Hydroxysteroid Dehydrogenase/Isomerase Gene Family: Lessons from Type II 3β-HSD Congenital Deficiency

F. Labrie, J. Simard, V. Luu-The, A. Bélanger, G. Pelletier,
Y.Morel, F. Mebarki, R. Sanchez, F. Durocher, C. Turgeon,
Y. Labrie, E. Rheaume, C. Labrie, and Y. Lachance

10.1   Introduction 186
10.2   3β-HSDs and Intracrine Androgen Formation 188
10.3   Structure and Expression of Human Types I
        and II 3β-HSD Isoenzymes 189
10.4   Human Types I and II Genes and Pseudogenes 193
10.5   Structure and Expression of Members
        of the Rodent 3β-HSD Gene Family 194
10.6   Role of 3-Ketosteroid Reductase Activity of Rat Type III
        and Mouse Types IV and V 3β-HSDs in the Control
        of DHT Bioavailability 195
10.7   Role of 17β-HSD Activity of Rat Types I and IV 3β-HSDs
        in the Control of DHT Bioavailability 197
10.8   Localization, Ontogeny, and Regulation of 3β-HSD Expression
        in the Testis 197
10.9   Localization, Ontogeny, and Regulation of 3β-HSD Expression
        in the Adrenal 199
10.10   Molecular Genetics of Human 3β-HSD Deficiency 200
10.10.1 Molecular Basis of the Salt-Losing Form
        of Classical 3β-HSD Deficiency 202
10.10.2 Molecular Basis of the Nonsalt-Losing Form
        of Classical 3β-HSD Deficiency 206
References 208

10.1 Introduction

The membrane-bound nicotinamide adenine dinucleotide (NAD^+)-dependent 3β-hydroxysteroid dehydrogenase /Δ5-Δ4-isomerase (3β-HSD), located in the endoplasmic reticulum and in mitochondrial membrane (Chapman et al. 1992; Cherradi et al. 1993, 1994; Luu-The et al. 1989, 1990; Sauer et al. 1994; Simard et al. 1991a; Thomas et al. 1989), catalyzes the conversion of Δ5–3β-hydroxysteroids into the corresponding Δ4–3-ketosteroids (Fig. 1). This activity is essential for the formation of all classes of steroids, namely, progesterone, mineralocorticoids, glucocorticoids, androgens, and estrogens. In addition, the enzymes of the 3β-HSD family also catalyze the formation and/or degradation of the 5α-androstanes and 5α-pregnanes, such as dihydrotestosterone (DHT) and dihydroprogesterone (Fig. 1) (de Launoit et al. 1992a, b; Labrie et al. 1994b; Luu-The et al. 1989; Mason 1993; Rheaume et al. 1991; Sanchez et al. 1994a; Simard et al. 1991a, 1993a, b; Zhao et al. 1991).

In human and rhesus monkey the 3β-HSD activity is not only detectable in the adrenal cortex, gonads, and placenta, but also in several peripheral tissues, including the liver, adipose tissue, skin, endometrium, myometrium, prostate, epididymis, seminal vesicle, intestine, mammary gland, kidney, muscle, lung, heart, pituitary, and brain (Dumont et al. 1992; Dupont et al. 1990a, 1991, 1992; Lachance et al. 1990; Luu-The et al. 1989; Martel et al. 1994; Milewich et al. 1991, 1993; Rheaume et al. 1991; Riley et al. 1992, 1993; Sasano et al. 1990a, b, 1994; Simard et al. 1991b). A widespread tissue distribution of 3β-HSD expression and/or activity has also been observed in other mammalian species, especially in rodents (Abbaszade et al. 1995a; Bain et al. 1991; Dalla Valle et al. 1995; Dupont et al. 1994; Keeney et al. 1993; Simard et al. 1993a; Zhao et al. 1991). Such a distribution of 3β-HSD expression suggests that these enzymes play an important role in the intracrine formation of sex steroids in peripheral target tissues. This role of 3β-HSD isoenzymes is of major importance in humans and some other primates since their adrenal glands secrete large amounts of dehydroepiandrosterone (DHEA) and especially its sulfate (DHEA-S), which are converted into Δ4-androstenedione (Δ4-DIONE), and then into potent androgens and estrogens in peripheral tissues, therefore providing autonomous intracrine control to target tissues which can thus

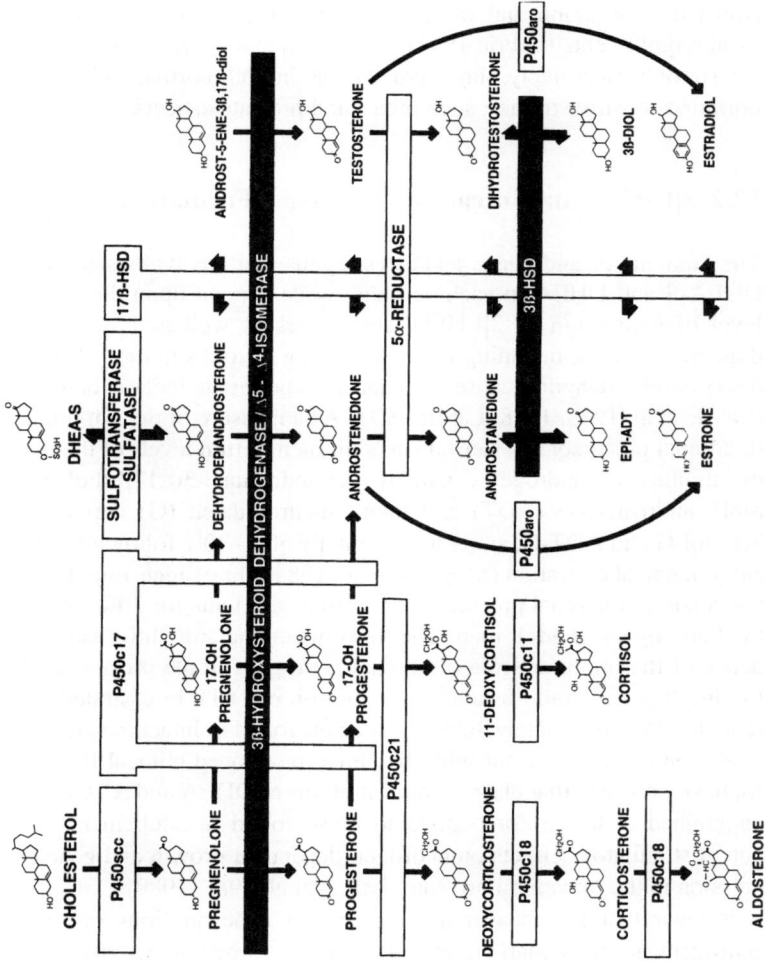

Fig. 1. Schematic representation of the major mammalian steroidogenic pathways. All P450 are cytochrome enzymes. *P450scc*, P450 cholesterol side-chain-cleavage; *3β*-HSD, 3β-hydroxysteroid dehydrogenase/Δ^5-Δ^4 isomerases; *P450c21*, P450 21α-hydroxylase; *P-450c17*, P450 17α-hydroxylase/17–20-lyase ; *P450c11*, P450 11β-hydroxylase; *P450c18*, this enzyme mediates 11β-hydroxylation and the further reactions involved in the biosynthesis of aldos-terone; *17β*-HSD, 17β-hydroxysteroid dehydrogenases; 5α-reductases: *P450Aro*, P450 aromatase; *DHEA-S*, dehydroepiandrosterone-sulfate, *EPI-ADT*, epiandrosterone

adjust the formation and metabolism of active steroids according to local requirements (Labrie 1991). Formation and degradation of active sex steroids most likely play a crucial role in both normal and tumoral hormone-sensitive tissues, such breast and prostate cancers.

10.2 3β-HSDs and Intracrine Androgen Formation

The amounts of androgens and/or estrogens that are synthesized from DHEA-S and DHEA in each cell and tissue depend upon the relative level of expression of 3β-HSD isoenzymes as well as other steroidogenic enzymes, including those catalyzing steroid sulfatase, 17β-hydroxysteroid dehydrogenase, aromatase, and 5α-reductase activities (Labrie et al. 1985, 1988; Labrie 1991) As a measure of the importance of adrenal precursor sex steroids in adult men, serum levels of the main metabolites of androgens, namely 5α-androstane-3α,17β-diol (3α-diol), androsterone (ADT) and their glucuronidated (G) derivatives, 3α-diol-G and ADT-G, are reduced only by 50%–70% following surgical or medical castration (Moghissi et al. 1984), thus suggesting that the conversion of adrenal precursor sex steroids accounts for 30%–50% of total androgens in adult men. The most direct and straightforward evidence of the important role of adrenal androgens in the prostate is the finding that the intraprostatic concentration of DHT in castrated men remains at approximately 40% of the levels found in intact men (Labrie et al. 1985). In agreement with the above-mentioned clinical findings, we have observed that plasma concentrations of DHEA and Δ^4-DIONE, maintained at levels comparable to those found in adult men, exert potent stimulatory effects on androgen-dependent growth and gene expression in the rat ventral prostate (Labrie et al. 1988, 1989).

It is clear that the measurement of serum concentrations of active androgens are poor markers of intracellular androgenic activity which can only be evaluated by the circulating levels of the metabolites of androgens, namely, ADT-G, 3α-diol-G, androstane-3β,17β-diol-G (3β-diol-G), and ADT-sulfate (ADT-S). For example, percutaneous administration of DHEA to men which led to a twofold increase in serum DHEA had no significant effect on the serum levels of testosterone (T), DHT, or estradiol (E_2) while the concentrations of ADT-G, 3α-diol-G, 3β-diol-G, ADT-S, and E_2 sulfate (E_2-S) were increased (Labrie et al., unpublished data). However, these changes in the circulating levels of androgen metabolites reflect the total amount of androgens produced in the whole body and are not particular to any tissue. Specific androgen formation and action must thus be investigated at the level of the cell or tissue and/or a specific cellular function must be measured.

10.3 Structure and Expression of Human Types I and II 3β-HSD Isoenzymes

Despite their essential role in steroidogenesis, the structure of the enzymes of the 3β-HSD gene family has been characterized only recently in human and several other vertebrate species (Fig. 2; Table 1).The type I 3β-HSD cDNA was isolated and characterized in our laboratory following purification of 3β-HSD from human placenta (Luu-The et al. 1988, 1989, 1990; Fig. 2). This sequence was later confirmed by others (Lorence et al. 1990b; Nickson et al. 1991). The second 3β-HSD type, chronologically designated as type II, was isolated from a human adrenal cDNA library (Rheaume et al. 1991). The type I 3β-HSD gene encodes a protein of 372 amino acids and is predominantly expressed in the placenta and peripheral tissues, such as the skin and mammary gland, while the type II gene, which encodes a protein of 371 amino acids sharing 93.5% identity with the type I, is almost exclusively expressed in the adrenals and gonads (Rheaume et al. 1991; Simard et al. 1995).

Transient expression of human type I and II (Lachance et al. 1990; Lorence et al. 1990b; Rheaume et al. 1991) isoenzymes provided the first direct evidence that the 3β-HSD and Δ^5-Δ^4 isomerase activities reside within a single protein. However, data obtained from affinity alkylation (Thomas et al. 1990) and inhibition experiments (Luu-The et al. 1990) that suggested separate 3β-HSD and isomerase sites are also consistent with a bifunctional catalytic site adopting a different conformation for each activity as suggested by affinity labeling (Thomas et al. 1992). The type I displays an ~ tenfold higher substrate affinity than the type II, whereas the V_{max} of both types are comparable (Rheaume et al. 1991). The higher affinity of type I 3β-HSD could facilitate steroid formation from relatively low concentrations of substrates usually present in peripheral tissues.

```
                      10         20         30         40         50         60
HUMAN I       TGWSCLVTGA GGFLGQRIIR LLVKEKELKE IRVLDKAFGP ELREEFSKLQ NKTKLTVLEG
HUMAN II      .......... ...L.....V ...E...... ...A.....R. .......... .R........
MACAQUE       .......... ......V... ...E...... .........R. .......... ..........
BOVINE        .......... ........C ...E..D.Q. ......V.R. .V........ S.I...L...
MOUSE I       A........G .........K M..Q....Q. V.A...V.R. .TK....... T..V....
MOUSE II      A......... ...V.....K M..Q....Q. V.A...V.R. .TK....FNLE TSI.V....
MOUSE III     P......... .........Q ..Q.ED.E. ......V.R. .T.K.FNLE TSI.V....
MOUSE IV      P......... ........V. M..Q.E..Q ..A.FRT..R KQE..L... T...V...K.
MOUSE V       P......... ........V. M..Q.E..Q ..A.FRT..R KHE...L... T.A.VR..K.
RAT I         P......... ...V..... M..Q....Q. V.A...V.R. .TK....... T.A.V.M...
RAT II        P......... ...V..... M..Q....Q. V.A...V.R. .TK....... T.A.V.M...
RAT III       P......... ....VQ M..Q....Q. V...YRT.S. KHK..L... T.A.V...R.
RAT IV        P......... ....VQ ..Q.D... V...V.R. .T....FN.G TSI.V....
RAINBOW TROUT SLQ.DV.V.. C.....E.LV. ..LE.DK.T. ..M..INVR. Q.IQCLEEIR GD.LVS.F..

                      70         80         90        100        110        120
HUMAN I       DILDEPFLKR ACQDVSVIIH TACIIDVFGV THRESIMNVN VKGTQLLLEA CVQASVPVFI
HUMAN II      .......... .......V.. .......... .......... .......... ..........
MACAQUE       .......... .......V.. .......... .......... .......... ..........
BOVINE        ....QC..G ...GT..V.. ...SV...RNA VP..T.... .......... ..........
MOUSE I       ....AQC.R. ...GI..V.. ...AV....T. IP.QT.LD.. L....N.... .......A..
MOUSE II      ....TQY.R. ...GI..V.. ...A....T. IP.QT.LD.. L....N.... .I.....A..
MOUSE III     ....TQY.R. ...GI..V.. ...A....T. IP.QT.LD.. L....N.... .I.....A..
MOUSE IV      ....AQC... ...GM.AV.. ...AA...PL.A AS.QT.LD.. L......D. .E.N..T..
MOUSE V       ....AQC... ...GM.AV.. ...AA...PR.A AS.QT.LD.. L......D. .E.....A..
RAT I         ....AQY.R. ...GI..V.. ...AV....SH. LP.QT.LD.. L....NI... .E.....A..
RAT II        ....AQY.R. ...GI..V.. ...SVM.FSR. LP.QT.LD.. L....N.... GIH.....A.
RAT III       ...V.AQ..R. ...GM.... ...AAL.IA.F LP.QT.LD.. .......D. .E.....A..
RAT IV        ....TQC.R. ...GI..V.. ...AL...T. NP.QT.LD.. L....N.... .......A..
RAINBOW TROUT ...S.SEL.R. ..KGA.LVF. ...SL...T.K VLYSELHR.. .........T ...EN.VS..

                     130        140        150        160        170        180
HUMAN I       YTSSIEVAGP NSYKEIIQNG HEEEPLENTW PAPYPHSKKL AEKAVLAANG WNLKNGGTLY
HUMAN II      ...TL..... .......... .......... .T...Y.... .......... .......D..
MACAQUE       ...TL..... ...R....D. R...HH.SA. SS...Y.... .......... .T........
BOVINE        H..T..... ...R....D. R...HH.SA. SS...Y.... .......G... ..A.......
MOUSE I       FC...VD.... ...K.VL... .QNH.S... SD...Y..M ......... SM.......N
MOUSE II      FS...VD.... ......VL... ...CH.S... SD...Y..M ......... SM.......Q
MOUSE III     FS...VD.... ...D.VL... .D.HR.S... SD...Y..M ......... SM.......Q
MOUSE IV      .S...VL.... ......L.A ...HH.S... SN...Y..M ......... SI.......H
MOUSE V       .S...VL.... ......L.A ...HH.S... .N...Y..RM ......T. RL.......H
RAT I         .C.TVD.... ...K.VL... ...HH.S... SDA...Y..RM ......... SI.......H
RAT II        .C.TVD.... ...KT.L.. R...HH.S... SN...Y..M ......... SI.......H
RAT III       .S..TG.... ....T.L.D R...HR.S... SN...Y..M ......... SI......FH
RAT IV        .C.TVD.... ...K.L.. ...HH.S... SN...Y..M ......... SI.......H
RAINBOW TROUT .......... ..ANGDP.I.. D.NT.YTCSL KF..SKT..E ..QVT.Q.Q. EV.Q...R.A

                     190        200        210        220        230        240
HUMAN I       TCALRPMYIY GEGSRFLSAS INEALNNNGI LSSVGKFSTV NPVYVGNVAW AHILALRALQ
HUMAN II      .......T... ...GP..... .......... .......... .......... .........R
MACAQUE       .......... ...GP..... .......... .......... .......... .........R
BOVINE        .......... ...P....Y MHG...... .TNHC...R. .......... .........R
MOUSE I       .......... .R.P.IFNA .IR..K.K.. .CVT....IA ......E.... ..A.G.R
MOUSE II      ......C... .R.PLI.NI .IM..KHK.. .R.F...N.A ......... ..A.G.R
MOUSE III     ......C... .R.Q...NT .IK..K.KF. .RGG.....A ......... ..A.G.R
MOUSE IV      ...LSF.... .ECQVT.TT VKT..K..S. IKKNAT..IA ......A.... ..A.S...
MOUSE V       ...LPF.... .ECQVT.TT VKT..K..S. IKKNAT..IA ......A.... ..A.S...
RAT I         .......... .R.P....VM .LA..K.K.. .NVT.....IA ......... ..A.G.R
RAT II        .......... .RGQ....RI .IM..K.K.V .NVT....I.. ......... ..A.G.R
RAT III       ...LPF.... .E.QII.TM V.R..K.NS. IKRHAT..IA ......A.... ..A.G.R
RAT IV        .......... .R.P....VM .LA..K.K.. .NVT.....IA ......... ..A.G.R
RAINBOW TROUT .......... ...C...LGH MGDGIR.GDM .YRTSREAQ. .......A.L ..LQ.A..R
```

Fig. 2. Legend see p. 191

```
              250        260        270        280        290        300
HUMAN I       DPKKAPSIRG QFYYISDDTP HQSYDNLNYT LSKEFGLRLD SRWSFPLSLM YWIGFLLEIV
HUMAN II      ......V..  .........  .........I  .......... ....L..T.. .........V.
MACAQUE       ......VQ.  .........  .........I  .......C.. ....L..A.. .........V.
BOVINE        ...V.N.Q.  .........  ....D....  ....W.FC.. ..M.L.I..Q ..LA......
MOUSE I       ....ST..Q. .........  ....D....  ....W...PN AS..L..P.L ..LA....T.
MOUSE II      ...S.N.Q.  E........  ...F.DIS.. ....W.FCP. .S..L.VP.L ..LA....T.
MOUSE III     N...S.N.Q. E........  ....D....  ....W.FC.N ...YL.VPIL ..LA....T.
MOUSE IV      ....S...Q. ......T..  ....D.KC.  ....W..... TS..L..P.L ..LA....T.
MOUSE V       ....S...Q. ......N..  ....D....  ....W..C.. .G.RL...L  ..LA....T.
RAT I         ...SQNVQ.  .........  ....D..C.  ....W..... .S..L..P.L ..LA....T.
RAT II        ....SQN.Q. .........  ....D..C.  ....W..... .S..L..P.L ..LA....T.
RAT III       ..E.SQ..Q. .........  ....D....  ....W.FC.. .S..L..P.L ..LA....T.
RAT IV        ....SQNVQ. .........  ....D....  ....W..H.. .S..L..P.L ..LA......
RAINBOW TROUT ..QRRAA.G. N........  PV..SDF.HA VLSPL.FSIQ EKPIL.IPYL .LLC..M.ML

              310        320        330        340        350        360
HUMAN I       SFLLRPIYTY RPPFNRHIVT LSNSVFTFSY KKAQRDLAYK PLYSWEEAKQ KTVEWVGSLV
HUMAN II      ....S...S. Q......T..
MACAQUE       ....S.V.S. Q......T..
BOVINE        ....S...K. N.C....L..            .......G.E ...T...... ..K..I....
MOUSE I       ......V.R. ..L....LI. .....T....  .......G.E ..VN...... ..S..I.TI.
MOUSE II      ....S...R. I......L.. ..G.T.....  .......G.E ..V....... ..S..I.T..
MOUSE III     ....S...R. I......L.. .TA.T.....  .......G.E ..V....... ..S..I.T..
MOUSE IV      ......V.N. ....LLI.   VL........  .......G.E ..V....... ..S..I.T..
MOUSE V       ......V.N. ....T.LLI. VL.....I..  .......G.Q ..V....... ..S..I.T..
RAT I         ......F.N. ......C.L. ...K......  .......G.V ..V....... ..S..I.T..
RAT II        ......F.N. ......C.L. ...K......  .......G.E ..V....... ..S..I.T..
RAT III       ......F.N. ......FM.. IL.....I..  .......G.E ..V....... ..S..I.T..
RAT IV        ..F.H.V.N. ..S....L.. ...K......  .......G.E .......... ..S..I.T..
RAINBOW TROUT QI..C.FKRF T..I..QLL. ML.TP.S... RR....MG.A .R......RK R.MD..A.QL

              370
HUMAN I       DRHKETLKSK TQ
HUMAN II      .......... ..
MACAQUE       .......... ..
BOVINE        KQ......T. 1H
MOUSE I       EQ.R.I.DT. C.
MOUSE II      EQ.R...DT. S.
MOUSE III     EQ.R...DT. S.
MOUSE IV      MQ.R.IGNK. S.
MOUSE V       KQ.R...HK. S.
RAT I         EQ.R...DT. S.
RAT II        EQ.R...DT. S.
RAT III       EQ.R...DT. S.
RAT IV        EQ.R...DT. S.
RAINBOW TROUT PKER.RI.V. --
```

◀ **Fig. 2.** Comparison of the amino acid sequences of human types I and II , macaque ovary, bovine ovary, mouse types I, II, III , IV and V, rat types I, II, III and IV, and rainbow trout ovary members of the 3β-hydroxysteroid dehydrogenase (3β-HSD) enzyme family. Residues common to human type I 3β-HSD are designed by a *dot*. Note that the members of the mammalian 3β-HSD family have been chronologically designated as a function of their elucidation in each species

Little is known about the structure–function relationships of these isoenzymes. The sequence of vertebrate 3β-HSD enzymes revealed that the similarity with members of the short-chain alcohol dehydrogenase superfamily is almost exclusively limited to the NH$_2$-terminal βαβ dinucleotide-binding fold recognized as part of the cofactor binding domain and two characteristic Y-X-X-X-K sequences located from Tyr 155 to Lys 159 and Tyr 270 to Lys 274 (based on human type I 3β-HSD sequence), which is found in the active site of short-chain alcohol dehydrogenases (Gosh et al. 1995; Krosowski 1992; Scrutton et al.

Table 1. Characteristics of members of the vertebrate 3β-HSD gene family

Species	Type	K_m (mM) PREG/DHEA	Cofactor	Major sites of expression	First cloning
Human	I	<1	NAD^+	Placenta, skin and mammary gland	(Luu-The et al. 1989)
	II	1–4	NAD^+	Adrenal and gonads	(Rheaume et al. 1991)
Rat	I	<1	NAD^+	Adrenals and gonads	(Zhao et al. 1991)
	II	>10	NAD^+	Adrenals and gonads	(Zhao et al. 1991)
	III	3-KSR	NADPH	Male liver	(Zhao et al. 1990)
	IV	<1	NAD^+	Placenta and skin	(Simard et al. 1993a)
Mouse	I	<1	NAD^+	Adrenals and gonads	(Bain et al. 1991)
	II	N.D.	N.D.	Kidney and liver	(Bain et al. 1991)
	III	<1	NAD^+	Liver > kidney	(Bain et al. 1991)
	IV	3-KSR	NADPH	Kidney	(Clarke et al. 1993a)
	V	3-KSR	NADPH	Male liver	(Abbaszade et al. 1995a)
	VI	N.D.	NAD^+	Placenta and skin	(Abbaszade et al. 1995b)
Hamster	I	2–5.5	NAD^+	Adrenals and gonads	(Rogerson et al. 1995)
	II	2–9	NAD^+	Kidney and liver	(Rogerson et al. 1995)
	III	3-KSR	NADPH	Male liver	(Rogerson et al. 1995)
Macaque	I	N.D.	N.D.	Adrenals and gonads	(Simard et al. 1991a)
Bovine	I	>10	NAD^+	Adrenals and gonads	(Zhao et al. 1989)
Guinea pig	I	<1	NAD^+	Adrenals and gonads	(Durocher et al. 1994)
Rainbow trout	I	DHEA>PREG	NAD^+	Ovary	(Sakai et al. 1994)

HSD, hydroxysteroid dehydrogenase; N.D., not determined; PREG, pregnenolone; DHEA, dehydroepiandrosterone; NAD^+, nicotinamide adenine dinucleotide; 3-KSR, 3-ketosteroid reductase; NADPH, nicotinamide adenine dinucleotide phosphate, reduced.

1990). Affinity labeling of purified human type I 3β-HSD identified two tryptic peptides, comprising amino acids Asn176 to Arg186 and Gly251 to Lys274 that should contain residues involved in the putative substrate-binding domain (Thomas et al. 1993) (Fig. 2). Thus the exact role of the first YXXXK motif in the 3β-HSD family remains to be confirmed. However, sequence alignment analysis revealed that members of the vertebrate 3β-HSD family share sequence similarity with plant dihydroflavonol reductases, *Escherichia coli* uridine diphosphate (UDP)-galactose-4-epimerase, *Nocardia* cholesterol dehydrogenase, and open reading frames (ORF) present in the fish lymphocystic disease virus and in the vaccinia virus, which have a 3β-HSD activity (Baker and Blasco 1992; Baker et al. 1990; Moore and Smith 1992).

10.4 Human Types I and II Genes and Pseudogenes

The structure of type I (HSD3B1) and type II (HSD3B2) 3β-HSD genes consists of four exons included within a DNA fragment of 7.8 kb (Lachance et al. 1990, 1991, 1992; Lorence et al. 1990a) and were assigned to the chromosome 1p13.1 region at 1–2 cM of the centromeric marker D1Z5 (Bérubé et al. 1989; Morissette et al. 1995; Morrison et al. 1991). Comparison of the nucleotide sequences of the two genes indicates that they share 77.4, 91.8, 94.5, 91.0, 84.0, 80.4, and 74.2% identity in exons I, II, III, and IV as well as in introns I, II, and III, respectively. The 1250-bp long sequence in the 5' flanking region share 81.9% identity. Our data suggest that the HSD3B1 and HSD3B2 genes and the three related pseudogenes (Luu-The et al. 1992) are included within a 0.29-megabase *Sac*II DNA fragment, thus suggesting that the human 3β-HSD gene family exists as a tandem cluster of related genes (Morissette et al. 1995) as observed for the mouse 3β-HSD genes (Bain et al. 1993). The current information concerning the transcriptional control of these genes is almost limited to the demonstration of overlapping *cis*-acting elements located in the first intron of the type I gene involved in its basal transcriptional activity (Guérin et al. 1995).

10.5 Structure and Expression of Members of the Rodent 3β-HSD Gene Family

The structures of four members of the rat 3β-HSD family have been characterized by our group (Simard et al. 1993a; Zhao et al. 1990, 1991) (Fig. 2, Table 1). The rat type I and II 3β-HSD proteins expressed in the adrenals, gonads, kidney, placenta, adipose tissue, and uterus share 93.8% identity. The type III protein shares approximately 80% identity with the type I and II proteins and is a specific 3-ketosteroid-reductase (3-KSR). The type III gene is exclusively expressed in the male liver and its marked sexual dimorphic expression results from a pituitary hormone-induced gene repression in female rat liver (de Launoit et al. 1992b; Zhao et al. 1990). The type IV shares 90.9%, 87.9%, and 78.8% identity with that of type I, II and III proteins, respectively, and is the predominant mRNA species detectable in the placenta and the skin (Simard et al. 1993a). In this regard, it could be suggested that rat type IV and human type I have conserved some *cis*-acting elements in their promoter region involved in a tissue-specific transcriptional control common to skin and placenta. The type IV is also detectable in the ovary and, to a lesser degree, in the adrenal gland (Simard et al. 1993a). The activities of rat types I and IV are similar (Simard et al. 1993a), while the much lower activity of the type II compared to the type I is due to a change of four residues in a putative membrane spanning domain (MSD) between residues 75 and 91, which is predicted in all other mammalian 3β-HSDs, with the exception of bovine 3β-HSD and mouse type V 3-KSR (Simard et al. 1991b).

Six distinct cDNAs encoding members of the 3β-HSD family have been cloned in the mouse (Table 1) (Abbaszade et al. 1995a, b; Bain et al. 1991; Clarke et al. 1993a, b; Keeney et al. 1993). The five published sequences are shown in Fig. 2. Mouse type I is the gene expressed in the adrenal glands and gonads, while the types II and III are expressed in the liver and the kidney, with much higher levels of type III in the liver than in the kidney (Bain et al. 1991), whereas the type IV is expressed in the kidney of both sexes (Clarke et al. 1993a). The newly characterized male liver-specific type V is more related to mouse type IV (93%) and rat type III (84%) than to the other mouse types (I: 74%; II: 72%; III: 72%) (Abbaszade et al. 1995a). Similar to rat type III and mouse type IV, mouse type V functions exclusively as a 3-KSR, using nicotinamide adenine dinucleotide phosphate, reduced (NADPH) as preferred cofactor (Abbaszade et al. 1995a). The type VI is predominantly expressed in the placenta, thus suggesting that this type is the mouse homologue of human type I and rat type IV(Abbaszade et al. 1995b).

10.6 Role of 3-Ketosteroid Reductase Activity of Rat Type III and Mouse Types IV and V 3β-HSDs in the Control of DHT Bioavailability

We have demonstrated that the rat type III protein (Zhao et al. 1990) does not display oxidative activity for the classical substrates, namely pregnenolone (PREG), DHEA, Δ^5-DIOL and 3β-DIOL, but is rather a specific 3-KSR and is responsible for the conversion of 3-keto saturated steroids, such as DHT and 5α-dihydroprogesterone, into inactive steroids using NADPH as preferred cofactor instead of nictonamide adenine dinucleotide, reduced [NAD(H)] (de Launoit et al. 1992b). This liver-specific 3-KSR may thus be considered as an inactivating enzyme.

Examination of the 3β-HSD isoenzymes shows a typical βαβ dinucleotide-binding fold with Asp36 located in the position predicted for the acidic residue that participates in hydrogen bond formation with 2'hydroxyl moiety of all known NAD-dependent dehydrogenases. We recently demonstrated by site-directed mutagenesis that the presence of a Tyr residue at position 36 in this typical βαβ dinucleotide-binding fold of the cofactor binding domain of rat type III instead of Asp is responsible for the difference in cofactor specificity of the rat 3-KSR (type III) protein, but is not sufficient to explain its low activity with Δ^5-3β-hydroxysteroid substrates (Turgeon et al. 1995). The physiological importance of this peculiar member of the rat 3β-HSD family is well supported by the recent finding that mouse types IV and V and hamster type III also possess a specific 3-KSR activity (Table 1) (Abbaszade et al. 1995a; Clarke et al. 1993a; Rogerson et al. 1995). The 3-KSR activity of these three latter enzymes is most likely due to the presence of Phe36 instead of Asp36 as suggested by our data on rat type III.

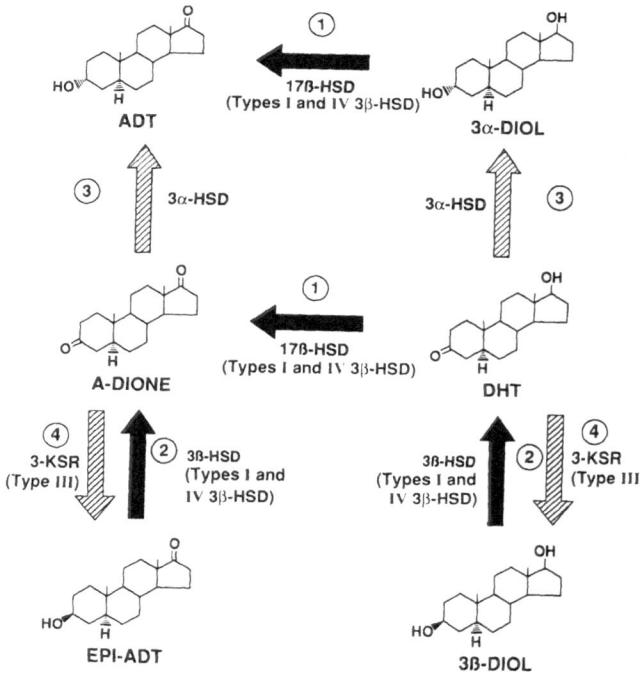

Fig. 3. Enzymatic 17β-hydroxysteroid dehydrogenase (*17*β-HSD) and 3β-HSD activities of rat types I and IV 3β-HSD expressed in intact cells. Reaction *1* corresponds to the androgenic 17β-HSD activity measured in cells expressing the rat types I, IV or guinea pig type I 3β-HSD isoenzymes. Reaction *2* corresponds to the 3β-HSD activity present in cells expressing rat types I, IV or guinea pig type I 3β-HSD enzymes. Reaction *3* corresponds to 3α-HSD activity in some cells. Reaction *4* corresponds to the 3-ketosteroid reductase (*3-KSR*) activity present in liver cells expressing the rat 3-KSR (type III) enzyme. The *black arrows* indicate predominant reactions expected to use primarily NAD, nictonamide adenine dinucleotide (NAD$^+$) as cofactor, while the *hatched arrows* indicate the predominant reactions expected to use primarily nictonamide adenine dinucleotide phosphate, reduced (NADPH) as cofactor. *ADT*, androsterone; *3α-DIOL*, 5α-androstane-3α,17β-diol; *3β-DIOL*, 5α-androstane-3β,17β-diol; *A-DIONE*, 5α-androstane-3,17-dione

10.7 Role of 17β-HSD Activity of Rat Types I and IV 3β-HSDs in the Control of DHT Bioavailability

We first observed that the rat type I 3β-HSD protein has androgenic 17β-HSD activity, having an affinity for DHT, which is similar to the affinity of its 3β-HSD activity for this androgen, but with a velocity much lower than that of 3β-HSD activity when measured in cell homogenates (de Launoit et al. 1992a). However, we have observed that in intact transfected cells, the types I and IV enzymes catalyze almost exclusively the conversion of DHT into androstanedione through its 17β-HSD activity. This intrinsic 17β-HSD activity of rat type I and IV 3β-HSD is specific to 5α-androstane-17β-ol steroids, thus suggesting its key role in controlling the bioavailability of the active androgen DHT.

The predominance of this secondary 17β-HSD activity over the primary 3β-HSD activity in intact cells most likely results from the high bioavailability of NAD^+ in mammalian cells relative to the low levels of the intracellular pool of NADH (Fig. 3). Such secondary activity could be explained by the binding of the steroid in the inverted substrate orientation to the same active site responsible for the primary activity of the enzyme. The physiological relevance of this secondary 17β-HSD activity is also supported by the observation that the rat type IV, the guinea pig (Durocher et al. 1994), and the purified bovine adrenal 3β-HSD enzyme (Cherradi et al. 1994) also possess this 17β-HSD activity (de Launoit et al. 1992a; Sanchez et al. 1994a) (Table 1).

10.8 Localization, Ontogeny, and Regulation of 3β-HSD Expression in the Testis

It is well known that the production of T by the testis and the concentration of plasma T in the fetus start to rise at the end of the second month of gestation and shortly thereafter attain high values that are maintained until late gestation when they decrease (Griffin and Wilson 1988). At the time of birth, plasma T levels are very low and shortly afterwards, they begin to rise and remain elevated for approximately 3 months, falling to low levels by the age 1 year (Frasier et al. 1969; Forest and Cathiard 1975; Winter et al. 1976; Bidlingmainen et al. 1983). The concentration remains low until the onset of puberty, when it again increases to reach adult levels by the age of 17 (Baillie et al. 1965; August et al. 1972).

In order to correlate possible changes in 3β-HSD with the well-known variations in T production during development, we have localized the 3β-HSD by immunocytochemistry during different fetal and postnatal periods of development in the human testis. In the testis of 22-week-old fetuses, immunostaining was observed exclusively in the cytoplasm of interstitial cells, whereas the seminiferous tubular elements remained completely unreactive (Dupont et al. 1991). At 28 weeks of fetal life, strong immunolabeling could be detected in the cytoplasm of interstitial cells. The seminiferous tubules were similar to those of 22-week-old fetuses. Interestingly, the interstitial cells appeared much larger than those observed at 22 weeks of gestation. In fetuses of 31 weeks, immunostaining was also observed in the cytoplasm of interstitial cells. It was of interest to note heterogeneity in labeling, approximately half the interstitial cells being weakly labeled. In 8-month-old infants and during the childhood, no immunostaining for 3β-HSD could be observed in the testis. With puberty, dramatic changes were observed in the testis histology. As observed in sections through a testis of a 15-year-old boy, the seminiferous tubules appeared well developed and the interstitial cells contain immunoreactive material. The same intensity of immunostaining was also observed in adult testes. The present data clearly show that 3β-HSD could be detected in Leydig cells in the fetus and that immunolabeling was absent 8 months and 12 years after birth, to become detectable at the time of puberty. These immunocytochemical results agree well with previous data from Baillie et al. (1965) who used enzyme histochemistry to detect 3β-HSD activity in testes of human fetuses from 8 to 22 weeks of gestation. Our results, which indicate that 3β-HSD is present in fetal testis during the second and third trimester of gestation (22, 28 and 31 weeks), agree well with previous results demonstrating that in human embryo plasma T levels are high during the second and third trimester of gestation and decrease during the last weeks of gestation.

We have thus demonstrated variation in the testicular content of 3β-HSD during pre- and postnatal development in the human. Since the pattern observed in 3β-HSD content is similar to that observed for androgen production, it might be suggested that activation of 3β-HSD by trophic hormones plays an important role in androgen production during fetal life and postnatal development. A similar conclusion was also obtained from studies in the rat (Dupont et al. 1993). In support of this hypothesis, we have demonstrated the marked stimulatory effect of luteinizing hormone/human chorionic gonadotropin (LH/hCG) on 3β-HSD expression in the testis of intact and hypophysectomized rats (Labrie et al. 1994a). Moreover, LH and agents increasing intracellular cAMP levels caused an increase in 3β-HSD expression in immature and adult rat Leydig cells as well as in H450 rat Leydig tumor cells (Keeney and Mason 1992a, b). In mouse Leydig cells, the endogenously produced T appears to negatively regulate cAMP-induced 3β-HSD expression (Payne and Sha 1991). The inhibitory action of androgens on 3β-HSD activity was also observed in cultured testicular cells from hypophysectomized immature rats (de Galarreta et al. 1983). It is also of interest to note that epidermal growth factor specifically stimulates 3β-HSD activity in cultured porcine Leydig cells (Sordoillet et al. 1991). Moreover, insulin and insulin-like growth factor (IGF)-I can partially reverse the inhibitory effect of acidic fibroblast growth factor (FGF; Murono et al. 1993b) and basic FGF (Murono et al. 1993a) on 3β-HSD activity in cultured immature rat Leydig cells, while platelet-derived growth factor (PDGF) exerts an inhibitory effect on this parameter (Murono and Washburn 1990).

10.9 Localization, Ontogeny, and Regulation of 3β-HSD Expression in the Adrenal

The localization and ontogeny of 3β-HSD in the human (Dupont et al. 1990a) and rat adrenal gland were first studied by our MRC group (Dupont et al. 1990a, b). In humans, the 3β-HSD is expressed in the neocortex after 22 to 28 weeks of gestation, while this enzyme is detectable in glomerulosa cells and in some differentiated fasciculata cells in mature fetus (35 weeks). In the 2-month-old infant 3β-HSD is expressed in the zona glomerulosa and zona fasciculata cells, while in a 2-year-old child uniform labeling can be observed throughout the three layers of the adrenal cortex. These data, coupled with those obtained by using other methods (Doody et al. 1990; Mesiano et al. 1993; Voutilainen et al. 1991), clearly indicate that the onset of 3β-HSD expression confers on definitive zone cells the ability to produce aldosterone and on transitional zone cells the ability to synthesize cortisol. In vitro experiments suggest that, in contrast to the other steroidogenic enzymes, the expression of 3β-HSD in human fetal adrenal cells is almost exclusively regulated by adrenocorticotropic hormone (ACTH; Doody et al. 1990; Lebrethon et al. 1994b; Voutilainen et al. 1991). The stimulatory effect of ACTH on 3β-HSD expression was also observed in rat (Trudel et al. 1991) as well as in cultured bovine (Naville et al. 1991b; Rainey et al. 1991) and ovine adrenocortical cells (Naville et al. 1991a).

In the adrenal cortex the relative expression levels of P450scc and especially 3β-HSD and P450c17 play a pivotal role in determining the final zone-specific steroid products secreted by the adrenal cells. For example, in adult human adrenal cells incubated in the presence of ACTH, transforming growth factor (TGF)-β1 increased 3β-HSD mRNA levels, decreased P450c17 mRNA levels, but did not change P450scc expression (Lebrethon et al. 1994b). Moreover, in ovine and bovine adrenocortical cells, although expression of both the 3β-HSD and P450c17 were decreased by TGFβ, this inhibitory effect was much more pronounced on P450c17 (Naville et al. 1991a; Rainey et al. 1991). In human cultured adrenal fasciculata-reticularis cells the stimulatory effects of angiotensin-II (A-II) were additive only on the 3β-HSD expression (Lebrethon et al. 1994a). In contrast, in bovine adrenocortical cells, A-II decreased the ACTH-induced 3β-HSD expression (Rainey et al. 1991). It is now clear that the regulation of 3β-HSD expression plays a key role in adrenal cortex steroidogenesis.

10.10 Molecular Genetics of Human 3β-HSD Deficiency

Congenital adrenal hyperplasia (CAH) is the most frequent cause of ambiguous genitalia and adrenal insufficiency in newborns (New et al. 1989). It comprises a group of syndromes caused by specific enzymatic deficiencies in the adrenal cortex that affect the pathway of cortisol biosynthesis, leading to a compensatory hypersecretion of adrenocorticotropin by the anterior pituitary gland with consequent hyperplasia of the adrenal cortex. In contrast to the two most frequent causes of CAH, 21-hydroxylase and 11β-hydroxylase deficiencies, which are adrenal defects, classic 3β-HSD deficiency impairs steroidogenesis in both the adrenals and the gonads, resulting in the diminished formation of sex steroids in addition to cortisol and aldosterone.

The expected severe inhibition of T biosynthesis by the fetal testis, resulting in a marked decrease in 3β-HSD activity, provides an explanation for the incomplete masculinization of the external genitalia seen in the male patients studied. On the other hand, as frequently seen, complete or partial inhibition of 3β-HSD activity in the adrenals and ovaries was not accompanied by a noticeable alteration of the differentiation of the external genitalia of females patients, as indicated by the absence of ambiguity of external genitalia in the such patients.

Since the first report by Bongiovanni (1962) many patients of both sexes have been described and the heterogeneity of the clinical presentation evidenced. The salt-losing form of classic 3β-HSD deficiency is usually diagnosed during the first few months of life because of insufficient biosynthesis of aldosterone with consequent salt loss (Bongiovanni 1962; Zachmann et al. 1970). In contrast, the nonsalt-losing form of the 3β-HSD deficiency may be diagnosed either at a young age in the presence of indicating factors, such as a family history of death during early infancy (Heinrich et al. 1993), perineal hypospadias in male newborns (Nahoul et al. 1989), or failure to gain weight (Kenny et al. 1971), or the diagnosis may be made at a later age (de Peretti et al. 1980; Pang et al. 1983; Rosenfield et al. 1980). Because sexual differentiation is normal in female newborns affected by nonsalt-losing 3β-HSD deficiency, the proper diagnosis is delayed until adrenarche (Pang et al. 1983) or puberty (Rosenfield et al. 1980; Bongiovanni 1981).

An elevated ratio of Δ^5- to Δ^4-steroids is considered the best biological parameter for the diagnosis of 3β-HSD deficiency (Cara et al. 1985). It is well recognized, however, that levels of 17-OH progesterone and Δ^4-DIONE plasma and other Δ^4 steroids are frequently elevated in 3β-HSD-deficient patients. Such observations suggest functional 3β-HSD that is expressed in peripheral tissues and is responsible for the extraadrenal and extragonadal conversion of 5-ene-hydroxysteroid precursors into the corresponding Δ^4–3-ketosteroids.

We have recently reviewed in greater detail the molecular basis of classical 3β-HSD deficiency (Simard et al. 1995). We will limit our present review to data providing a molecular explanation for the enzymatic heterogeneity ranging from severe salt-losing form to the clinically inapparent salt-wasting form of the disease. The findings providing pertinent information concerning the structure–function relationships of the 3β-HSD enzymes will also be briefly described.

10.10.1 Molecular Basis of the Salt-Losing Form of Classical 3β-HSD Deficiency

The sequences of the type I and/or type II 3β-HSD genes were determined by direct sequencing of polymerase chain reaction (PCR) products to identify the molecular lesions responsible for classic 3β-HSD deficiency. No mutation was detected in the type I gene in five unrelated patients suffering from the salt-losing form of the disease (Table 2) (Rheaume et al. 1992; Sanchez et al. 1994b; Simard et al. 1993b, 1995), as well as in three unrelated patients with the nonsalt-losing form (Table 2) (Mébarki et al. 1995; Rheaume et al. 1994; Simard et al. 1993b). The eight different mutations characterized in the ten patients suffering from the salt-losing form studied by us were all detected in the type II 3β-HSD gene (Fig. 4, Table 2) (Rheaume et al. 1992, 1995;

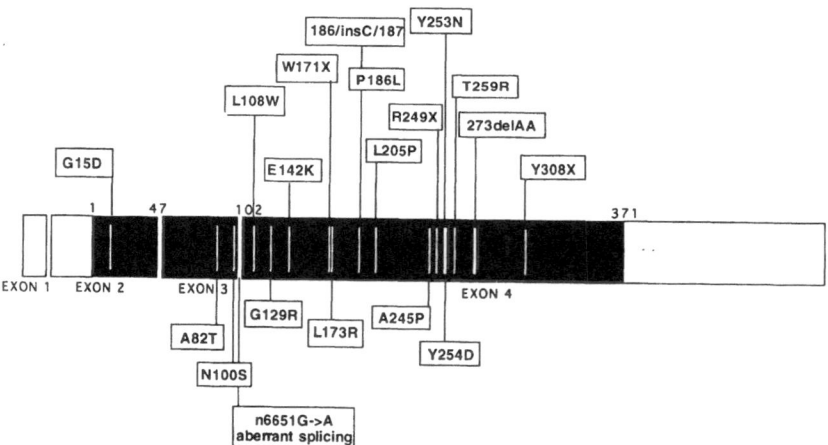

Fig. 4. Schematic representation of the mutations in type II 3β-hydroxysteroid dehydrogenase (3β-HSD) gene found in patients suffering from classic 3β-HSD deficiency. The mutations indicated *above the bar diagram* were found in patients suffering from the salt-losing form of the disease, whereas the mutations illustrated *below the diagram* were detected in nonsalt-losing patients. The coding region is indicated by *black boxes* while the *open boxes* demarcate the 5' and 3' noncoding regions

Table 2. Mutations in the type II 3β-HSD gene in patients with classical 3β-HSD deficiency

Family	Origin	Karyotype	Salt wasting	Mutation(s)	Molecular lesion Type	Mutation report
1	Swiss	46xx	Yes	Trp171Stop	Nonsense	Rheaume et al. 1992
2	Swiss	46xx	Yes	Trp171Stop	Nonsense	Rheaume et al. 1992
3	American	46xy	Yes	Trp171Stop:186/insC/187	Nonsense frameshift	Rheaume et al. 1992
4	American	46xy	Yes	Glu142Lys:Trp171Stop	Missense nonsense	Simard et al. 1993b
5	Dutch	46xy	Yes	186/insC/187:Tyr253Asn	Frameshift missense	Simard et al. 1993b
6	Afghan/Pakistani	46xy	Yes	273ΔAA	Frameshift	Simard et al. 1994
7	Afghan/Pakistani	46xy	Yes	273ΔAA	Frameshift	Simard et al. 1994
8	Afghan/Pakistani	46xy	Yes	273ΔAA	Frameshift	Simard et al. 1994
9	Algerian	46xy	Yes	Gly15Asp	Missense	Rheaume et al. 1995
10	Spanish/Portuguese	46xy	Yes	Leu108Trp:Pro186Leu	Missense missense	Sanchez et al. 1994b
11	Japanese	46xy	Yes	Leu205Pro	Missense	Katsumata et al. 1995
12	Japanese	46xy	Yes	Arg249Stop	Nonsense	Tajima et al. 1995
13	Japanese	46xy	Yes	Arg249Stop	Nonsense	Tajima et al. 1995
14	Japanese	46xy	Yes	Tyr308Stop	Nonsense	Tajima et al. 1995
15	Japanese	46xy	Yes	Thr259Arg	Missense	Tajima et al. 1995
16	Turkish	46xx	Yes	Ala245Pro	Missense	Simard et al. 1993b
17	American	46xx	No	Gly129Arg:6651→A	Missense splicing	Rheaume et al. 1994
18	Algerian	46xy	No	Asn100Ser	Missense	Mébarki et al. 1995
19	American	46xy	No	Tyr254Asp:?	Missense?	Sanchez et al. 1994c
20	Scottish	46xy	No	Leu173Arg	Missense	Russell et al. 1994
21	Scottish	46xy	No	Leu173Arg	Missense	Russell et al. 1994
22	Brazilian	46xy	No	Ala82Thr	Missense	Mendonca et al. 1994
23	Brazilian	46xx	No	Ala82Thr	Missense	Mendonca et al. 1994

3β-HSD, 3β-hydroxysteroid dehydrogenase/Δ^5-Δ^4 isomerase.

Sanchez et al. 1994b; Simard et al. 1993b, 1994). Recently, four additional mutations in this gene were detected in five Japanese families (Table 2) (Katsumata et al. 1995; Tajima et al. 1995). The increased levels of some Δ^4-steroids and their metabolites in patients with classic 3β-HSD deficiency are thus best explained by normal peripheral type I 3β-HSD activity exerting its catalytic activity on the elevated levels of substrates resulting from a deficiency of type II 3β-HSD in the adrenals and gonads.

It is expected that no functional type II 3β-HSD isoenzyme is expressed in the adrenals and gonads of the patients from families 1, 2, 3, 6, 7, 8, 12, 13, and 14 bearing mutations leading to a putative truncated protein (Table 2), which is in agreement with the severity of the disorder in these index cases. Both the mutant E142K and Y253N enzymes exhibited no detectable activity (Simard et al. 1993b). Thus, in the compound heterozygote patients E142K:W171X (family 4) and 186/insc/187:Y253N (family 5), it is also expected that no functional type II 3β-HSD isoenzyme is expressed (Simard et al. 1993b).

In addition to studying the effect of the Gly15 for Asp15 change detected in the homozygous patient of family 9, we evaluated the effect of substituting Gly15 for Ala15 to investigate further the involvement of residue 15 in the βαβ dinucleotide-binding fold (Rheaume et al. 1995). This Gly-X-X-Gly-X-X-Gly fingerprint is similar to the common Gly-X-Gly-X-X-Gly conserved sequence of most NAD(H) binding enzymes (Scrutton et al. 1990). In intact transfected cells, no detectable activity was observed in cells expressing the G15D protein, while a relatively high activity was found with G15A protein. On the other hand, the G15D protein shows an activity similar to that of G15A in homogenates (Table 3). It could be suggested that, in addition to decreasing the apparent affinity for both the substrate and the cofactor, this mutation may alter the proper intracellular localization of this protein or that its association with intact membranes in vivo may exert some strain preventing adoption of its final maximally efficient conformation.

Unexpectedly, we observed the presence of a low but detectable activity for both mutant L108 W and P186L 3β-HSD proteins in intact transfected cells in culture (Table 3) (Sanchez et al. 1994b). The mutant L108 W and P186L proteins possess a marked reduced affinity for the substrate and the cofactor (Table 3). The in vitro overall efficiency, relative to the normal enzyme, was approximated to be ~0.1%–0.3%.

Table 3. Kinetic parameters of native type II 3β-HSD and mutant G15D, G15A, N100S, L108 W, G129R, P186L and A245P proteins

Protein	K_m PREG	Relative V_{max} PREG	Relative V_{max}/K_m	K_m NAD	Relative V_{max} NAD	Relative V_{max}/K_m
Type II 3β-HSD	0.72	100	139	22	100	4.5
G15D	3.2	120	38	113	121	1.1
G15A	3.4	134	39	148	116	0.78
Type II 3β-HSD	1.7	100	59	24	100	4.2
L108W	12.0	16.1	1.3	678	17	0.025
P186L	18.0	20.7	1.2	920	17	0.019
Type II 3β-HSD	3.5	100	29	20	100	5.0
N100S	25	19.3	0.8	650	30	0.05
Type II 3β-HSD	2.6	100	39	–	–	–
A245P	4.6	20.3	4.4	–	–	–
Type II 3β-HSD	1	100	100	–	–	–
G129R	10	0.2	2.0	–	–	–

Relative V_{max} values were calculated assuming that the V_{max} for the human type II enzyme is equal to 100.
3β-HSD, 3β-hydroxysteroid dehydrogenase/Δ^5-Δ^4 isomerase; PREG, pregnenolone; NAD, nictonamide adenine dinucleotide.

The presence of such a low level of activity is thus apparently inadequate to permit the formation of mineralocorticoids in quantities sufficient to avoid severe salt wasting in this patient.

10.10.2 Molecular Basis of the Nonsalt-Losing Form of Classical 3β-HSD Deficiency

The seven different point mutations characterized in the six families studied were all detected in the type II 3β-HSD gene (Fig. 4, Table 2)(Mébarki et al. 1995; Mendonca et al. 1994; Rheaume et al. 1994; Russell et al. 1994; Sanchez et al. 1994c; Simard et al. 1993b). The observation of no detectable 3β-HSD activity in homogenates from transfected cells expressing the mutant A245P enzyme in the absence of glycerol, whereas significant enzymatic activity was measured in intact transfected cells and cell homogenates prepared in the presence of glycerol, a known stabilizing agent, might suggest that this mutation weakens the association with proper intracellular membranes (Simard et al. 1993b). As measured by the V_{max}/K_m ratio, the mutant A245P enzyme had about 11.9% of the activity catalyzed by the native type II 3β-HSD (Table 3). The G129R mutation decreased the activity of the enzyme to about 2.0% of the native type II 3β-HSD, using PREG as substrate (Table 3). It appears likely that this low level of activity is sufficient to prevent salt loss, but it is also possible that part of the enzymatic activity comes from the putative remaining percentage of correctly spliced 6651→A allele in these patients (Rheaume et al. 1994). Thus, the absence of salt wasting in these patients could well be explained by the weak but measurable 3β-HSD activity, which permits formation of mineralocorticoids sufficient to avoid severe salt wasting, in analogy to some nonsalt-losing CAH cases secondary to 21-hydroxylase deficiency (Tusie-Luna et al. 1990).

This hypothesis is also supported by the observation made in the male pseudohermaphrodite in family 18 bearing the homozygous mutation N100S (Mébarki et al. 1995), having a poor male differentiation associated with a lack of salt loss (Table 3). The overall efficiency of N100S protein is closely similar (~0.1%) to that of the L108 W and P186L proteins (Table 3). Our findings suggest that this very weak residual activity of the mutated N100S enzyme is sufficient to prevent salt loss at the price of high renin synthesis, although it was insufficient for normal male sex differentiation in the patient. The functional characterization of these mutant proteins cannot provide an explanation for the heterogeneity responsible for the severe salt-losing form (L108 W:P186L) down to the clinically inapparent form of salt loss (N100S) of 3β-HSD deficiency. Nevertheless, the hormonal profile of the patient with the N100S mutation suggests that salt loss was compensated by a high renin synthesis. The enzymatic properties of the missense 3β-HSD mutants L205P, T259R (Table 2), L173R, and A82T (Table 2) detected by other groups have not yet been reported.

It is of special interest to note that the amino acids Gly15, Ala82, Asn100, Leu108, Gly129, Glu142, Leu173, Tyr253, Tyr254, and Thr259, which are the sites of the missense mutations described above, are conserved in all known members of the vertebrate 3β-HSD isoenzymes family (Fig. 2). However, although amino acid Pro186 is also well conserved in the vertebrate 3β-HSD family, it is not conserved in all members; rat type III and mouse type IV share a Leu at this position (Fig. 2). Moreover, because Leu205 and Ala245 are not always conserved in the 3β-HSD family, it is conceivable that these mutations generating a Pro cause a turn in the polypeptide chain which is responsible for the decreased activity of these mutant enzymes. The characterization of the molecular basis of classic 3β-HSD deficiency thus provides pertinent information on the structure–function relationships of the 3β-HSD family.

The situation in classical or severe 3β-HSD deficiency may be comparable to that in castrated men: in 3β-HSD deficiency, type II 3β-HSD is inactive in the testis, while, in castrated men, testicular activity has been eliminated surgically or medically with a luteinizing hormone releasing hormone (LHRH) superagonist. In both cases, androgen formation is limited to peripheral steroidogenesis from adrenal precursors. It should be mentioned that the 3β-HSD-deficient patients who in the early postnatal period survive the severe deficiency in glucocorticoids and mineralocorticoids have normal adrenarche, hair growth, and secondary sexual characteristics, and in some cases are even fertile (Rheaume et al. 1992). Thus, classical 3β-HSD deficiency represents a good example from nature itself of the major role of adrenal androgen precursors in the formation of androgens by peripheral tissues in man.

References

Abbaszade I, Clarke T, Park C-H, Payne AH (1995a) The mouse 3β-hydroxysteroid dehydrogenase multigene family includes two functionally distinct groups of proteins. Mol Endocrinol 9:1214–1222

Abbaszade L, Arensburg Y, Clarke T, Kasa-Vubu J, Orly J, Payne AH (1995b) Isolation of mouse 3β-HSD isoform that may be critical for maintenance of early pregnancy. Proceedings of the 77th annual meeting of the Endocrinological Society, abstract 619 P3-601

August GP, Grumbach MM, Kaplan SL (1972) Hormonal changes in puberty. III. Correlation of plasma testosterone, LH, FSH, testicular size, and bone age with male pubertal development. J Clin Endocrinol Metab 34:319–326

Baillie AH, Niemi M, Ikanen M (1965) 3β-hydroxysteroid dehydrogenase activity in the human foetal testis. Acta Endocrinol (Copenh) 48:429–438

Bain PA, Yoo M, Clarke T, Hammond SH, Payne AH (1991) Multiple forms of mouse 3β-hydroxysteroid dehydrogenase/Δ5-Δ4 isomerase and differential expression in gonads, adrenal glands, liver, and kidneys of both sexes. Proc Natl Acad Sci USA 88:8870–8874

Bain PA, Meisler MH, Taylor BA, Payne AH (1993) The genes encoding gonadal and nongonadal forms of 3β-hydroxysteroid dehydrogenase/Δ5-Δ4 isomerase are closely linked on mouse chromosome 3. Genomics 16:219–223

Baker ME, Blasco R (1992) Expansion of the mammalian 3β-hydroxysteroid dehydrogenase/plant dihydroflavonol reductase superfamily to include a bacterial cholesterol dehydrogenase, a bacterial UDP-galactose-4-epimerase and open reading frames in vaccinia virus and fish lymphocystis disease virus. FEBS Lett 301:89–93

Baker ME, Luu TY, Simard J, Labrie F (1990) A common ancestor for mammalian 3β-hydroxysteroid dehydrogenase and plant dihydroflavonol reductase (letter). Biochem J 269:558–559

Bérubé D, Luu-The V, Lachance Y, Gagné R, Labrie F (1989) Assignment of the human 3β-hydroxysteroid dehydrogenase gene (HSDB3) to the p13 band of chromosome 1. Cytogenet Cell Genet 52:199–200

Bidlingmaier F, Dorr HG, Eisenmenger W, Kuhnle U, Knorr D (1983) Testosterone and androstenedione concentrations in human testis and epididymis during first two years of life. J Clin Endocrinol Metab 57:311–315

Bongiovanni A (1962) The adrenogenital syndrome with deficiency of 3β-hydroxysteroid dehydrogenase. J Clin Invest 41:2086–2092

Bongiovanni AM (1981) Acquired adrenal hyperplasia: with special reference to 3β-hydroxysteroid dehydrogenase. Fertil Steril 35:599–608

Cara JF, Moshang TJ, Bongiovanni AM, Marx BS (1985) Elevated 17-hydroxyprogesterone and testosterone in a newborn with 3-β-hydroxysteroid dehydrogenase deficiency. N Engl J Med 313:618–621

Chapman JC, Waterhouse TB, Michael SD (1992) Changes in mitochondrial and microsomal 3β-hydroxysteroid dehydrogenase activity in mouse ovary over the course of the estrous cycle. Biol Reprod 47:992–997

Cherradi N, Defaye G, Chambaz EM (1993) Dual subcellular localization of the 3 β-hydroxysteroid dehydrogenase isomerase: characterization of the mitochondrial enzyme in the bovine adrenal cortex. J Steroid Biochem Mol Biol 46:773–779

Cherradi N, Defaye G, Chambaz EM (1994) Characterization of the 3β-hydroxysteroid dehydrogenase activity associated with bovine adrenocortical mitochondria. Endocrinology 134:1358–1364

Clarke TR, Bain PA, Greco TL, Payne AH (1993a) A novel mouse kidney β-hydroxysteroid dehydrogenase complementary DNA encodes a 3-ketosteroid reductase instead of a 3β-hydroxysteroid dehydrogenase/Δ5-Δ4-isomerase. Mol Endocrinol 7:1569–1578

Clarke TR, Bain PA, Sha LL, Payne AH (1993b) Enzyme characteristics of 2 distinct forms of mouse 3-β-hydroxysteroid dehydrogenase/Δ5-Δ4-isomerase complementary deoxyribonucleic acids expressed in COS-1 cells. Endocrinology 132:1971–1976

Dalla Valle L, Couet J, Labrie Y, Simard J, Belvedere P, Simontacchi C, Labrie F, Colombo L (1995) Occurrence of cytochrome P450c17 mRNA and dehydroepiandrosterone biosynthesis in the rat gastrointestinal tract. Mol Cell Endocrinol 111:83–92

de Galarreta CMR, Fanju LF, Meidan R, Hsueh A (1983) Regulation of 3β-hydroxysteroid dehydrogenase activity by human chorionic gonadotropin androgens and anti-androgens in cultures testicular cells. J Biol Chem 258:10988–10996

de Launoit Y, Simard J, Durocher F, Labrie F (1992a) Androgenic 17 β-hydroxysteroid dehydrogenase activity of expressed rat type I 3β-hydroxysteroid dehydrogenase/delta 5-delta 4 isomerase. Endocrinology 130:553–555

de Launoit Y, Zhao HF, Bélanger A, Labrie F, Simard J (1992b) Expression of liver-specific member of the 3β-hydroxysteroid dehydrogenase family an isoform possessing an almost exclusive 3-ketosteroid reductase activity. J Biol Chem 267:4513–4517

de Peretti E, Forest MG, Feit JP, David M (1980) Endocrine studies in two chidren with male pseudohermaphroditism due to 3β-hydroxysteroid (3β-HSD) dehydrogenase defect. In: Genazzani AR, Thijssen JHH, Siiteri PK (eds) Adrenal androgens. Raven, New York, pp 141–145

Doody KM, Carr BR, Rainey WE, Byrd W, Murry BA, Strickler RC, Thomas JL, Mason JI (1990) 3β-hydroxysteroid dehydrogenase/isomerase in the fetal zone and neocortex of the human fetal adrenal gland. Endocrinology 126:2487–2492

Dumont M, Van LT, Dupont E, Pelletier G, Labrie F (1992) Characterization, expression, and immunohistochemical localization of 3β-hydroxysteroid dehydrogenase/Δ5-Δ4 isomerase in human skin. J Invest Dermatol 99:415–421

Dupont E, Luu-The V, Labrie F, Pelletier G (1990a) Ontogeny of 3β-hydroxysteroid dehydrogenase/delta 5-delta 4 isomerase (3β-HSD) in human adrenal gland performed by immunocytochemistry. Mol Cell Endocrinol 74:R7-10

Dupont E, Zhao HF, Rheaume E, Simard J, Luu TV, Labrie F, Pelletier G (1990b) Localization of 3β-hydroxysteroid dehydrogenase/Δ5-Δ4-isomerase in rat gonads and adrenal glands by immunocytochemistry and in situ hybridization. Endocrinology 127:1394–1403

Dupont E, Luu TV, Labrie F, Pelletier G (1991) Ontogeny of 3β-hydroxysteroid dehydrogenase/Δ5-Δ4 isomerase (3β-HSD) in human testis as studied by immunocytochemistry. J Androl 12:161–164

Dupont E, Labrie F, Luu TV, Pelletier G (1992) Immunocytochemical localization of 3 β-hydroxysteroid dehydrogenase/Δ5-Δ4-isomerase in human ovary. J Clin Endocrinol Metab 74:994–998

Dupont E, Labrie F, Luu TV, Pelletier G (1993) Ontogeny of 3β-hydroxysteroid dehydrogenase/Δ5-Δ4 isomerase (3 β-HSD) in rat testis as studied by immunocytochemistry. Anat Embryol (Berl) 187:583–589

Dupont E, Simard J, Luu TV, Labrie F, Pelletier G (1994) Localization of 3 β-hydroxysteroid dehydrogenase in rat brain as studied by in situ hybridization. Mol Cell Neurosci 5:119–23

Durocher F, Sanchez R, Laudet V, Labrie Y, Samson C, Tremblay Y, Labrie F, Simard J (1994) Structural and functional characterization of the guinea pig 3β-hydroxysteroid dehydrogenase/Δ5-Δ4isomerase expressed in the adrenal gland and gonads. Program, 76th annual meeting of the Endocrinological Society, abstr 1192, p 498

Forest MG, Cathiard AM (1975) Pattern of plasma testosterone and Δ4-androstenedione in normal newborns: evidence for testicular activity at birth. J Clin Endocrinol Metab 41:977–984

Frasier SD, Gafford F, Horton R (1969) Plasma androgens in childhood and adolescence. J Clin Endocrinol Metab 29:1404–1408

Gosh D, Pletnev V, Zhu D-W, Wawrzak Z, Duax W, Pangborn W, Labrie F, Lin S-X (1995) Structure of human estrogenic 17β-hydroxysteroid dehydrogenase at 220A resolution. Structure 3:503–513

Griffin JE, Wilson JD (1988) The testis. In: Browdy PK Rosenberg LE (eds) Metabolic control and disease, 8th edn. Saunders, Philadelphia, pp 1535–1578

Guérin SL, Leclerc S, Verrault H, Labrie F, Luu-The V (1995) Overlapping cis-acting elements located in the first intron of the gene for type I 3β-hydroxysteroid dehydrogenase modulate its transcriptional activity. Mol Endocrinol 9:1583–1597

Heinrich UE, Bettendorf M, Vecsei P (1993) Male pseudohermaphroditism caused by nonsalt-losing congenital adrenal hyperplasia due to 3β-hydroxysteroid dehydrogenase (3β-HSD) deficiency. J Steroid Biochem Mol Biol 45:83–85

Katsumata N, Tanae A, Yasunaga T, Horikawa R, Tanaka T, Hibi I (1995) A novel missense mutation in the type II 3β-hydroxysteroid dehydrogenase in a family with classical salt-wasting congenital adrenal hyperplasia due to 3β-hydroxysteroid dehydrogenase deficiency. Hum Mol Genet 4:745–746

Keeney DS, Mason JI (1992a) Expression of testicular 3β-hydroxysteroid dehydrogenase/Δ5-Δ4-isomerase: regulation by luteinizing hormone and forskolin in Leydig cells of adult rats. Endocrinology 130:2007–2015

Keeney DS, Mason JI (1992b) Regulation of expression of 3β-hydroxysteroid dehydrogenase is mediated by cAMP in rat leydig cells and H540-rat Leydig tumor cells. J Steroid Biochem Mol Biol 43:915–922

Keeney DS, Naville D, Milewich L, Bartke A, Mason JI (1993) Multiple isoforms of 3β-hydroxysteroid dehydrogenase/Δ5-Δ4-isomerase in mouse tissues – male-specific isoforms are expressed in the gonads and liver. Endocrinology 133:39–45

Kenny FM, Reynolds JW, Green OC (1971) Partial 3β-hydroxysteroid dehydrogenase (3β-HSD) deficiency in a family with congenital adrenal hyperplasia: evidence for increasing 3β-HSD activity with age. Pediatrics 48:756–765

Krosowski Z (1992) 11β-Hydroxysteroid dehydrogenase and the short-chain alcohol dehydrogenase (SCAD) superfamily. Mol Cell Endocrinol 84:C25-C31

Labrie C, Bélanger A, Labrie F (1988) Androgenic activity of dehydroepiandrosterone and androstenedione in the rat ventral prostate. Endocrinology 123:1412–1417

Labrie C, Simard J, Zhao HF, Bélanger A, Pelletier G, Labrie F (1989) Stimulation of androgen-dependent gene expression by the adrenal precursors dehydroepiandrosterone and androstenedione in the rat ventral prostate. Endocrinology 124:2745–2754

Labrie F (1991) Intracrinology. Mol Cell Endocrinol 78:C113–C118

Labrie F, Dupont A, Bélanger A (1985) Complete androgen blockade for the treatment of prostate cancer. In: de Vita VT Hellman S, Rosenberg SA (eds) Important advances in oncology. Lippincott, Philadelphia, pp 193–217

Labrie F, Simard J, Luu-The V, Pelletier G (1994a) Molecular genetics struc-
ture-function relationships and tissue-specific expression and regulation of
the 3β-HSD gene family. In: Bartke A (ed) Function of somatic cells in the
testis Serono symposia. Springer, Berlin Heidelberg New York, pp 26–150
Labrie F, Simard J, Luu-The V, Pelletier G, Belghmi K, Bélanger A (1994b)
Structure, regulation and role of 3β-hydroxysteroid dehydrogenase 17β-hy-
droxysteroid dehydrogenase and aromatase enzymes in formation of sex
steroids in classical and peripheral intracrine tissues. In: Sheppard MC, Stewart PM (eds) Hormone-nuclear receptors interactions in health and disease. Baillière Tindall, London, pp 451–474
Lachance Y, Luu-The V, Labrie C, Simard J, Dumont M, de Launoit Y,
Guérin S, Leblanc G, Labrie F (1990) Characterization of human 3β-hy-
droxysteroid dehydrogenase/Δ5-Δ4-isomerase gene and its expression in
mammalian cells. J Biol Chem 265:20469–20475
Lachance Y, Luu-The V, Verreault H, Dumont M, Rhéaume E, Leblanc G, Labrie F (1991) Structure of the human type II 3β-hydroxysteroid dehydroge-
nase/Δ5-Δ4 isomerase (3β-HSD) gene: adrenal and gonadal specificity.
DNA Cell Biol 10:701–711
Lachance Y, Luu-The V, Labrie C, Simard J, Dumont M, de Launoit Y,
Guérin S, Leblanc G, Labrie F (1992) Characterization of human 3β-hy-
droxysteroid dehydrogenase/Δ5-Δ4-isomerase gene and its expression in
mammalian cells (additions and corrections). J Biol Chem 267:3551
Lebrethon MC, Jaillard C, Defayes G, Begeot M, Saez JM (1994a) Human
cultured adrenal fasciculata-reticularis cells are targets for angiotensin-II:
effects on cytochrome P450 cholesterol side-chain cleavage cytochrome
P450 17α-hydroxylase and 3β-hydroxysteroid-dehydrogenase messenger
ribonucleic acid and proteins and on steroidogenic responsiveness to corticotropin and angiotensin-II. J Clin Endocrinol Metab 78:1212–1219
Lebrethon MC, Jaillard C, Naville D, Begeot M, Saez JM (1994b) Regulation
of corticotropin and steroidogenic enzyme mRNAs in human fetal adrenal
cells by corticotropin angiotensin-II and transforming growth factor β 1.
Mol Cell Endocrinol 106:137–143
Lorence MC, Corbin CJ, Kamimura N, Mahendroo MS, Mason JI (1990a)
Structural analysis of the gene encoding human 3β-hydroxysteroid dehy-
drogenase/Δ5-Δ4 isomerase. Mol Endocrinol 4:1850–1855
Lorence MC, Murry BA, Trant JM, Mason JI (1990b) Human 3 β-hydroxysteroid dehydrogenase/Δ5-Δ4 isomerase from placenta: expression in nonsteroidogenic cells of a protein that catalyzes the dehydrogenation/isomeriza-
tion of C21 and C19 steroids. Endocrinology 126:2493–2498
Luu-The V, Coté J, Labrie F (1988) Purification and characterization of human
placental 3β-hydroxysteroid dehydrogenase Δ5-Δ4 isomerase. Clin Invest
Med 11:C32

Luu-The V, Lachance Y, Labrie C, Leblanc G, Thomas JL, Strickler RC, Labrie F (1989) Full length cDNA structure and deduced amino acid sequence of human 3β-hydroxy-5-ene steroid dehydrogenase. Mol Endocrinol 3:1310–1312

Luu-The V, Coté J, Labrie F (1990) Purification of microsomal and mitochondrial 3β-hydroxysteroid dehydrogenase/Δ5-Δ4 isomerase from human placent. Ann N Y Acad Sci 595:386–388

Luu-The V, Lachance Y, Leblanc G, Labrie F (1992) Human 3β-hydroxysteroid dehydrogenase/Δ5-Δ4 isomerase: characterization of three additional related genes. Proceedings of the 74th annual meeting of the Endocrinological Society, abstr 1499

Martel C, Melner MH, Gagne D, Simard J, Labrie F (1994) Widespread tissue distribution of steroid sulfatase 3β-hydroxysteroid dehydrogenase/Δ5-Δ4 isomerase (3β-HSD), 17β-HSD 5α-reductase and aromatase activities in the rhesus monkey. Mol Cell Endocrinol 104:103–111

Mason JI (1993) The 3β-hydroxysteroid dehydrogenase gene family of enzymes. Trends Endocrinol Metab 4:199–203

Mébarki F, Sanchez R, Rhéaume E, Laflamme N, Simard J, Forest M, Bey-Omar F, David M, Labrie F, Morel Y (1995) Nonsalt-losing male pseudohermaphrodite due to novel homozygous N100S mutation in the type II 3β-hydroxysteroid dehydrogenase (HSD3B2) gene. J Clin Endocrinol Metab 80:2127–2134

Mendonca BB, Russell AJ, Vasconcelos Leite M, Arnhold IJ, Bloise W, Wajchenberg BL, Nicolau W, Sutcliffe RG, Wallace AM (1994) Mutation in 3β-hydroxysteroid dehydrogenase type II associated with pseudohermaphroditism in males and premature pubarche or cryptic expression in females. J Mol Endocrinol 12:119–122

Mesiano S, Coulter CL, Jaffe RB (1993) Localization of cytochrome P450 cholesterol side-chain cleavage cytochrome P450 17α-hydroxylase/17 20-lyase and 3β-hydroxysteroid dehydrogenase isomerase steroidogenic enzymes in human and rhesus monkey fetal adrenal glands: reappraisal of functional zonation. J Clin Endocrinol Metab 77:1184–1189

Milewich L, Shaw CE, Doody KM, Rainey WE, Mason JI, Carr BR (1991) 3β-Hydroxysteroid dehydrogenase activity in glandular and extraglandular human fetal tissues. J Clin Endocrinol Metab 73:1134–1140

Milewich L, Shaw CE, Mason JI, Carr BR, Blomquist CH, Thomas JL (1993) 3β-Hydroxysteroid dehydrogenase activity in tissues of the human fetus determined with 5α-androstane-3β17β-diol and dehydroepiandrosterone as substrates. J Steroid Biochem Mol Biol 45:525–537

Moghissi E, Ablan F, Horton R (1984) Origin of plasma androstanediol glucuronide in men. J Clin Endocrinol Metab 59:417–421

Moore JB, Smith GL (1992) Steroid hormone synthesis by a vaccinia enzyme: a new type of virus virulence factor [published erratum appears in EMBO J (1992) 11(9):3490]. EMBO J 11:1973–1980

Morissette J, Rheaume E, Leblanc JF, Luu TV, Labrie F, Simard J (1995) Genetic linkage mapping of HSD3B1 and HSD3B2 encoding human types I and II 3β-hydroxysteroid dehydrogenase/delta 5-delta 4-isomerase close to D1S514 and the centromeric D1Z5 locus. Cytogenet Cell Genet 69:59–62

Morrison N, Nickson DA, McBride MW, Mueller UW, Boyd E, Sutcliffe RG (1991) Regional chromosomal assignment of human 3β-hydroxy-5-ene steroid dehydrogenase to 1p131 by non-isotopic in situ hybridisation. Hum Genet 87:223–235

Murono EP, Washburn AL (1990) Platelet derived growth factor inhibits 5α-reductase and Δ5-3 β-hydroxysteroid dehydrogenase activities in cultured immature Leydig cells. Biochem Biophys Res Commun 169:1229–1234

Murono EP, Goforth DP, Washburn AL, Wu N (1993a) Evidence that biphasic effects of basic fibroblast growth factor on 5-ene-3β-hydroxysteroid dehydrogenase-isomerase activity in cultured immature Leydig cells are mediated by binding to heparan sulfate proteoglycans. J Steroid Biochem Mol Biol 46:557–563

Murono EP, Washburn AL, Goforth DP, Wu N (1993b) Effects of acidic fibroblast growth factor on 5-ene-3β-hydroxysteroid dehydrogenase-isomerase and 5 α-reductase activities and [125I]human chorionic gonadotrophin binding in cultured immature Leydig cells. J Steroid Biochem Mol Biol 45:477–483

Nahoul K, Perrin C, Leymarie P, Job JC (1989) Elevated levels of plasma 4-ene steroids in a case of congenital deficiency of 3β-hydroxysteroid dehydrogenase – Taux élevés des 4-ène stéroïdes plasmatiques dans un cas de déficit congénital en 3β-hydroxystéroïde déshydrogénase. Ann Endocrinol (Paris) 50:58–63

Naville D, Rainey WE, Mason JI (1991a) Corticotropin regulation of 3β-hydroxysteroid dehydrogenase/Δ5-Δ4-isomerase in ovine adrenocortical cells: inhibition by transforming growth factor β. Mol Cell Endocrinol 75:257–263

Naville D, Rainey WE, Milewich L, Mason JI (1991b) Regulation of 3β-hydroxysteroid dehydrogenase/Δ5-Δ4-isomerase expression by adrenocorticotropin in bovine adrenocortical cells. Endocrinology 128:139–145

New MI, White P, Pang S, Dupont B, Speiser PW (1989) The adrenal hyperplasias. In: Scriver CR, Beaudet A, Sly WS, Valle D (eds) The metabolic basis of inherited diseases. McGraw-Hill, New York, pp 1881–1917

Nickson DA, McBride MW, Zeinali S, Hawes CS, Petropoulos A, Mueller UW, Sutcliffe RG (1991) Molecular cloning and expression of human trophoblast antigen FDO161G and its identification as 3β-hydroxy-5-ene steroid dehydrogenase. J Reprod Fertil 93:149–156

Pang S, Levine LS, Stoner E, Opitz JM, Pollack MS, Dupont B, New MI (1983) Nonsalt-losing congenital adrenal hyperplasia due to 3β-hydroxysteroid dehydrogenase deficiency with normal glomerulosa function. J Clin Endocrinol Metab 56:808–818

Payne AH, Sha LL (1991) Multiple mechanisms for regulation of 3β-hydroxysteroid dehydrogenase/Δ5-Δ4-isomerase 17 alpha-hydroxylase/C17-20 lyase cytochrome P450 and cholesterol side-chain cleavage cytochrome P450 messenger ribonucleic acid levels in primary cultures of mouse Leydig cells. Endocrinology 129:1429–1435

Rainey WE, Naville D, Mason JI (1991) Regulation of 3β-hydroxysteroid dehydrogenase in adrenocortical cells: effects of angiotensin-II and transforming growth factor β. Endocr Res 17:281–296

Rheaume E, Lachance Y, Zhao HF, Breton N, Dumont M, de Launoit Y, Trudel C, Luu TV, Simard J, Labrie F (1991) Structure and expression of a new complementary DNA encoding the almost exclusive 3β-hydroxysteroid dehydrogenase/Δ5-Δ4-isomerase in human adrenals and gonads. Mol Endocrinol 5:1147–1157

Rheaume E, Simard J, Morel Y, Mebarki F, Zachmann M, Forest MG, New MI, Labrie F (1992) Congenital adrenal hyperplasia due to point mutations in the type II 3β-hydroxysteroid dehydrogenase gene. Nat Genet 1:239–245

Rheaume E, Sanchez R, Simard J, Chang YT, Wang J, Pang S, Labrie F (1994) Molecular basis of congenital adrenal hyperplasia in two siblings with classical nonsalt-losing 3β-hydroxysteroid dehydrogenase deficiency. J Clin Endocrinol Metab 79:1012–1018

Rheaume E, Sanchez R, Mebarki F, Gagnon E, Carel JC, Chaussain JL, Morel Y, Labrie F, Simard J (1995) Identification and characterization of the G15D mutation found in a male patient with 3β-hydroxysteroid dehydrogenase (3β-HSD) deficiency: alteration of the putative NAD-binding domain of type II 3β-HSD. Biochemistry 34:2893–2900

Riley SC, Dupont E, Walton JC, Luu-The V, Labrie F, Pelletier G, Challis JR (1992) Immunohistochemical localization of 3β-hydroxy-5-ene-steroid dehydroge-nase/Δ5-Δ4 isomerase in human placenta and fetal membranes throughout gestation. J Clin Endocrinol Metab 75:956–961

Riley SC, Bassett NS, Berdusco E, Yang K, Leystralantz C, Luu-The V, Labrie F, Challis G Jr (1993) Changes in the abundance of messenger RNA for type-I 3β-hydroxy-steroid dehydrogenase/Δ5-Δ4 isomerase in the human placenta and fetal membranes during pregnancy and labor. Gynecol Obstet Invest 35:199–203

Rogerson FM, Lehoux JG, Mason JI (1995) Expression and characterization of isoforms of 3β-hydroxysteroid dehydrogenase /Δ5-Δ4 isomerase in the hamster. J Steroid Biochem Mol Biol (in press)

Rosenfield RL, Rich BH, Wolfsdorf JI, Cassorla F, Parks JS, Bongiovanni AM, Wu CH, Shackleton CH (1980) Pubertal presentation of congenital Δ5-3β-hydroxysteroid dehydrogenase deficiency. J Clin Endocrinol Metab 51:345–353

Russell AJ, Wallace AM, Forest MG, Donaldson MD, Edwards CR, Sutcliffe RG (1994) Mutation in the human gene for 3β-hydroxysteroid dehydrogenase type II leading to male pseudohermaphroditism without salt loss. J Mol Endocrinol 12:225–237

Sakai N, Tanaka M, Takahashi M, Fukada S, Mason JI, Nagahama Y (1994) Ovarian 3β-hydroxysteroid dehydrogenase/delta 5-4-isomerase of rainbow trout: its cDNA cloning and properties of the enzyme expressed in a mammalian cell. FEBS Lett 350:309–313

Sanchez R, de Launoit Y, Durocher F, Belanger A, Labrie F, Simard J (1994a) Formation and degradation of dihydrotestosterone by recombinant members of the rat 3β-hydroxysteroid dehydrogenase/Δ5-Δ4 isomerase family. Mol Cell Endocrinol 103:29–38

Sanchez R, Mebarki F, Rheaume E, Laflamme N, Forest MG, Bey Omard F, David M, Morel Y, Labrie F, Simard J (1994b) Functional characterization of the novel L108 W and P186L mutations detected in the type II 3 b-hydroxysteroid dehydrogenase gene of a male pseudohermaphrodite with congenital adrenal hyperplasia. Hum Mol Genet 3:1639–1645

Sanchez R, Rhéaume E, Laflamme N, Rosenfield RL, Labrie F, Simard J (1994c) Detection and functional characterization of the novel missense mutation Y254D in type II 3β-hydroxysteroid dehydrogenase (3β-HSD) gene of a female patient with nonsalt-losing 3β-HSD deficiency. J Clin Endocrinol Metab 78:561–578

Sasano H, Mason JI, Sasaki E, Yajima A, Kimura N, Namiki T, Sasano N, Nagura H (1990a) Immunohistochemical study of 3β-hydroxysteroid dehydrogenase in sex cord-stromal tumors of the ovary. Int J Gynecol Pathol 9:352–362

Sasano H, Mori T, Sasano N, Nagura H, Mason JI (1990b) Immunolocalization of 3β-hydroxysteroid dehydrogenase in human ovary. J Reprod Fertil 89:743–751

Sasano H, Nagura H, Harada N, Goukon Y, Kimura M (1994) Immunolocalization of aromatase and other steroidogenic enzymes in human breast disorders. Hum Pathol 25:530–535

Sauer LA, Chapman JC, Dauchy RT (1994) Topology of 3β-hydroxy-5-ene-steroid dehydrogenase/Δ5-Δ4-isomerase in adrenal cortex mitochondria and microsomes. Endocrinology 134:751–759

Scrutton NS, Berry A, Perham RN (1990) Redesign of the coenzyme specificity of a dehydrogenase by protein engineering. Nature 343:38–43

Simard J, de Launoit Y, Labrie F (1991a) Characterization of the structure-activity relationships of rat types I and II 3β-hydroxysteroid dehydrogenase/Δ5-Δ4 isomerase by site-directed mutagenesis and expression in HeLa cells. J Biol Chem 266:14842–14845

Simard J, Melner MH, Breton N, Low KG, Zhao HF, Periman LM, Labrie F (1991b) Characterization of macaque 3β-hydroxy-5-ene steroid dehydrogenase/Δ5-Δ4 isomerase: structure and expression in steroidogenic and peripheral tissues in primate. Mol Cell Endocrinol 75:101–110

Simard J, Couët J, Durocher F, Labrie Y, Sanchez R, Breton N, Turgeon C, Labrie F (1993a) Structure and tissue-specific expression of a novel member of the rat 3β-hydroxysteroid dehydrogenase/Δ5-Δ4 isomerase (3β-HSD) family – the exclusive 3β-HSD gene expressed in the skin. J Biol Chem 268:19659–19668

Simard J, Rhéaume E, Sanchez R, Laflamme N, de Launoit Y, Luu-The V, van Seters AP, Gordon RD, Bettendorf M, Heinrich U, Moshang T, New MI, Labrie F (1993b) Molecular basis of congenital adrenal hyperplasia due to 3β-hydroxysteroid dehydrogenase deficiency. Mol Endocrinol 7:716–728

Simard J, Rhéaume E, Leblanc JF, Wallis SC, Joplin JF, Gilbey S, Allanson J, Mettler G, Bettendorf M, Heinrich UE, Labrie F (1994) Congenital adrenal hyperplasia caused by a novel homozygous frameshift mutation 273deltaAA in type II 3β-hydroxysteroid dehydrogenase gene (HSD3B2) in three male patients of Afghan/Pakistani origin. Hum Mol Genet 3:327–334

Simard J, Rheaume E, Mebarki F, Sanchez R, New M, Morel Y, Labrie F (1995) Molecular basis of 3β-hydroxysteroid dehydrogenase deficiency. J Steroid Biochem Mol Biol 53:127–138

Sordoillet C, Chauvin MA, de PE, Morera AM, Benahmed M (1991) Epidermal growth factor directly stimulates steroidogenesis in primary cultures of porcine Leydig cells: actions and sites of action. Endocrinology 128:2160–2168

Tajima T, Fujieda K, Nakae J, Shinohara N, Yoshimoto M, Baba T, Ei-ichi K, Igarashi Y, Oomura T (1995) Molecular analysis of type II 3β-hydoxysteroid dehydrogenase deficiency. Hum Mol Genet 4:969–971

Thomas JL, Myers RP, Strickler RC (1989) Human placental 3β-hydroxy-5-ene-steroid dehydrogenase and steroid 5→4-ene-isomerase: purification from mitochondria and kinetic profiles biophysical characterization of the purified mitochondrial and microsomal enzymes. J Steroid Biochem 33:209–217

Thomas JL, Myers RP, Rosik LO, Strickler RC (1990) Affinity alkylation of human placental 3 β-hydroxy-5-ene-steroid dehydrogenase and steroid 5-4-ene-isomerase by 2 alpha-bromoacetoxyprogesterone: evidence for separate dehydrogenase and isomerase sites on one protein. J Steroid Biochem 36:117–123

Thomas JL, Strickler RC, Myers RP, Covey DF (1992) Affinity labeling of human placental 3β-hydroxy-Δ5-steroid dehydrogenase and steroid delta-isomerase: evidence for bifunctional catalysis by a different conformation of the same protein for each enzyme activity. Biochemistry 31:5522–5527

Thomas JL, Nash WE, Myers RP, Crankshaw MW, Strickler RC (1993) Affinity radiolabeling identifies peptides and amino acids associated with substrate binding in human placental 3β-hydroxy-Δ5-steroid dehydrogenase. J Biol Chem 268:18507–18512

Trudel C, Couet J, Martel C, Labrie C, Labrie F (1991) Regulation of adrenal 3β-hydroxysteroid dehydrogenase/Δ5-Δ4-isomerase expression and activity by adrenocorticotropin and corticosterone in the rat. Endocrinology 129:2077–2084

Tusie-Luna MT, Traktman P, White PC (1990) Determination of functional effects of mutations in the steroid 21-hydroxylase gene (CYP21) using recombinant vaccinia virus. J Biol Chem 265:20916–20922

Turgeon C, Sanchez R, Rhéaume E, Labrie F, Simard J (1995) Characterization of the unique cofactor specificity of liver-specific rat 3β-hydroxysteroid dehydrogenase by side-rected mutagenesis. Proceedings of the 77th annual meeting of the Endocrinological Society, abstr P-3–633, p 619

Voutilainen R, Ilvesmaki V, Miettinen PJ (1991) Low expression of 3β-hydroxy-5-ene steroid dehydrogenase gene in human fetal adrenals in vivo; adrenocorticotropin and protein kinase C-dependent regulation in adrenocortical cultures. J Clin Endocrinol Metab 72:761–767

Winter JSD Hughes IA Reyes FI (1976) Pituitary-gonadal relations in infancy 2. Patterns of serum gonadal steroid concentrations in man from birth to two years of age. J Clin Endocrinol Metab 42:679–686

Zachmann M, Vsllmin JA, Mürset G, Curtius HC, Prader A (1970) Unusual type of congenital adrenal hyperplasia probably due to deficiency of 3β-hydroxysteroid dehydrogenase. Case report of a surviving girl and steroid studies. J Clin Endocrinol Metab 30:719–726

Zhao HF, Simard J, Labrie C, Breton N, Rhéaume E, Luu-The V, Labrie F (1989) Molecular cloning cDNA structure and predicted amino acid sequence of bovine 3β-hydroxy-5-ene steroid dehydrogenase/delta5-delta4 isomerase. FEBS Lett 259:153–157

Zhao HF, Rhéaume E, Trudel C, Couet J, Labrie F, Simard J (1990) Structure and sexual dimorphic expression of a liver-specific rat 3β-hydroxysteroid dehydrogenase/isomerase. Endocrinology 127:3237–3239

Zhao HF, Labrie C, Simard J, de Launoit Y, Trudel C, Martel C, Rhéaume E, Dupont E, Luu-The V, Pelletier G, Labrie F (1991) Characterization of rat 3β-hydroxysteroid dehydrogenase/Δ5-Δ4 isomerase cDNAs and differential tissue-specific expression of the corresponding mRNAs in steroidogenic and peripheral tissues. J Biol Chem 266:583–593

11 The Src Family of Protein Tyrosine Kinases

C. Couture and T. Mustelin

11.1   Introduction 219
11.2   Protein Tyrosine Kinases 220
11.3   The Src Family of Protooncogenes 222
11.3.1 Evolution of the Src Gene Family 223
11.3.2 Overall Structure of Src-like PTKs 224
11.3.3 The Nine Family Members 228
11.4   Regulation and Regulators of Src-like PTKs 233
11.4.1 Autophosphorylation 234
11.4.2 Suppression by C-terminal Phosphorylation 235
11.4.3 Positive Regulation by N-terminal Tyrosine Phosphorylation ... 239
11.5   Future Directions and Concluding Remarks 243
References 244

11.1 Introduction

The protein tyrosine kinases (PTKs) of the Src family play a central role in regulating cellular development, proliferation, and function in a variety of tissues (reviewed in Mustelin 1994a). Their activity is tightly regulated and constitutive activity of these PTKs results in uncontrolled proliferation and even transformation. It has therefore been a major objective to understand how these enzymes are regulated. For many reasons, T lymphocytes have provided a very useful model system to address the mechanisms of Src-related PTK regulation (reviewed in Couture and Mustelin 1995; Mustelin and Burn 1993; Mustelin 1994b) both during development and antigen receptor-mediated activation. The function of a T lymphocyte is induced when it encounters its specific antigen bound to a major histocompatibility (MHC) molecule on the surface of an antigen-presenting cell. This ligand is specifically recognized by the lymphocyte's multicomponent T-cell antigen receptor (TCR), which contains both polymorphic subunits that are used for antigen/MHC binding, and nonpolymorphic subunits that are used to generate a cascade of events which signal the occupancy of the receptor and lead to modulation of gene expression and of the activity of gene products that are crucial to cell function. If appropriate secondary signals are present, these changes also result in progression through the cell cycle and clonal expansion (Altman et al. 1990; Zenner et al. 1995). A few years ago, the importance of tyrosine phosphorylation in these events was recognized (Mustelin et al. 1990; Mustelin and Altman 1991), and much work has been devoted to the identification of the PTKs involved in T-cell activation, including a few members of the Src family, and the mechanisms by which these enzymes are regulated. In this chapter, we will first describe all nine members of the Src family of PTKs and discuss the molecular mechanisms by which Src family members expressed in T cells are regulated and participate in TCR-mediated T-cell activation.

11.2 Protein Tyrosine Kinases

The majority of cellular proteins are covalently modified with phosphate through ester bonds with the side chains of a number of different amino acid residues. Best known is the acid-stable phosphorylation of serine, threonine, and tyrosine residues by serine/threonine-specific proteins kinases (E.C. 2.7.10) or tyrosine-specific protein kinases (E.C. 2.7.11), respectively. Of all protein-bound, acid-stable phosphate in intact cells, ~ 95% is present as phosphoserine (PSer), ~5% as phosphothreonine (PThr) and only 0.01%–0.1% as phosphotyrosine (PTyr). Nevertheless, phosphorylation of proteins on tyrosine residues plays a crucial role in the regulation of cell proliferation and differentiation, cell cycle control, and in the transmission of various signals. To date, over 200 different mammalian protein kinases or putative kinases have been identified and the vast majority of them are structurally related. Of these

Table 1. The ten currently known families of nonreceptor PTKs

Families	Members	Size of PTKs (kDa)
Src	c-Src, c-Yes, Fyn, Yrk, c-Fgr, Lyn, Lck, Hck, Blk	55–62
Brk	Brk, Frk (=Rak), Sik, Srm	50–55
Abl	c-Abl, Arg	150
Fes	c-Fes/Fps, Fer	92–98
Syk	Syk, Zap, HTK16	70–72
Tec	Tec, Itk, Btk, Bmx	62–80
Jak	Jak1, Jak2, Jak3, Tyk2	130
Fak	Fak	125
Ack	Ack	120
Csk	Csk, Ctk (=Lsk,Ntk), Matk	50–60

PTK, protein tyrosine kinase.

kinases, more than half phosphorylate serine and threonine residues, somewhat fewer are specific for tyrosine residues, and a few are bifunctional, i.e., they phosphorylate both tyrosine and serine/threonine residues.

PTKs can be divided into two main categories: the receptor-type transmembrane PTKs and the nonreceptor PTKs. While most members of the former class function as receptors for growth or differentiation factors, or are suspected to do so, the physiological function of the nonreceptor class of PTKs is not understood nearly as well. Recent findings suggest that some nonreceptor PTKs function as parts of receptor complexes (e.g., the Jak family PTKs with lymphokine receptors, Lck with CD4 and CD8 etc.), making the name "nonreceptor" more historical than accurate. The main difference between receptor and nonreceptor PTKs is the presence or absence of a transmembrane region in the PTK molecule itself. Based on structural similarities and sequence homology, the nonreceptor PTKs can be further subdivided into ten families (Table 1), namely, the Src, Brk, Abl, Fes, Syk, Tec, Jak, Fak, Ack, and Csk families. This chapter will focus on one family of nonreceptor PTKs, the Src family (reviewed in Mustelin 1994a).

11.3 The Src Family of Protooncogenes

There are currently nine known members of the Src family of nonreceptor PTKs: c-Src, c-Yes, Fyn, Yrk, c-Fgr, Lck, Hck, Lyn, and Blk
(Table 2). The genes for three of these (Src, Yes, and Fgr) were initially
discovered as viral oncogenes carried by the Rous sarcoma virus, Yamaguchi 73/Esh avian sarcoma virus, and Gardner-Rasheed feline sarcoma
virus, respectively. These retroviruses have the capacity to acutely
transform host cells by virtue of the v-*src*, v-*yes,* and v-*fgr* oncogenes,
which encode highly active and transforming versions of these PTKs.
Of these three oncogenes, v-*src* was the first to be cloned and the
encoded protein, v-Src, was the first oncogene product found to possess
PTK activity. The cellular counterparts of the three viral oncogenes
were subsequently identified and found to be quite similar genes encoding closely related, but distinct, proteins. The high degree of homology
between the viral (collectively termed v-*onc*) and the cellular (c-*onc*)
genes raised the now widely accepted notion that the viral genes originate from the cellular ones. Originally quite harmless viruses apparently
incorporated the c-*onc* genes and, in the process, modified them to better
serve the viral life cycle. These modifications caused a deregulation of
the encoded PTKs and thereby malignant transformation of the host cell.
The advantage of this event to the virus is evident.

The main mechanism by which the retroviruses transformed the
borrowed Src family genes was by deleting or replacing the nucleotide

Table 2. The Src family of PTKs

PTK	Protein (kDa)	Expression
c-Src	60	Ubiquitous, brain, platelets
c-Yes	59/62	Ubiquitous, T cells
Yrk	60	Monocytes
Fyn	59	Ubiquitous, brain, T cells, B cells
c-Fgr	59	Macrophages, granulocytes
Lck	56 (60/62)	T cells, NK cells
Hck	56/59	Granulocytes, monocytes
Lyn	53/56	B cells, granulocytes
Blk	55	B cells

PTK, protein tyrosine kinase; NK, natural killer.

sequences encoding the extreme C-terminal tail of the PTKs, which contains a normally phosphorylated tyrosine residue crucial for the repression of the catalytic activity. The v-*onc*-encoded PTKs invariably lack this critical tyrosine and therefore cannot be regulated by this mechanism. Indeed, transformed cells contain very high levels of PTyr in a number of cellular substrate proteins, some of which apparently cause the altered morphology and unrestricted growth behavior characteristic of malignant cells. The c-*onc* genes do not transform the host cell even when expressed at high levels, but can be made oncogenic by point mutations or deletions at the C-terminal tyrosine residue or other alterations disrupting their phosphorylation or proper function.

11.3.1 Evolution of the Src Gene Family

Src family genes have been cloned from many organisms, including such diverse species as *Drosophila melonogaster* and the simple metazoan *Hydra attenuata* , indicating that an ancestral Src family PTK was present at, or evolved shortly after, the emergence of multicellular organisms and has been conserved in both arthropods and vertebrates. Since only a single Src-like gene seems to be present in lower organisms, it can be assumed that the ancestral Src-like PTK diversified into a family in parallel with the evolution of multicellular organisms and the specialization of cell types within these more complex organisms. The notion that the family arose by gene duplication events is supported by the finding that they share a highly conserved exon/intron structure. They span up to 60 kb of DNA and usually have one untranslated exon (exon 1), sometimes located a long distance from exon 2, which usually contains the translation initiation codon. Different members of the family have a variable number of alternatively used exons, but generally only exons 1–2 (encoding the unique N-terminus) differ significantly in sequence between the family members. This suggests that the various family members were generated from the duplicated ancestral gene by exon shuffling, where novel 5' sequences containing tissue-specific promoter regions and encoding unique N-termini were recombined with the 3' sequences of one copy of the duplicated ancestral *src*-like gene. More members then evolved by a repetition of the duplication and exon-shuffling events.

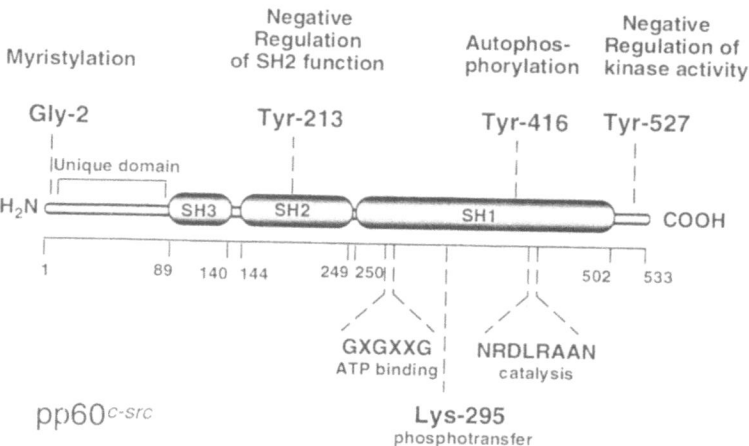

Fig. 1. Schematic presentation of the overall structure of Src family protein tyrosine kinases

That the individual genes are important and ideally adapted to their unique functions is shown by the strong pressure to maintain their amino acid sequence unchanged through more recent evolution. For example, the human and murine Lyn are 96% homologous, murine and human Lck are 96.7% homologous, and the C-terminal two-thirds of avian and human c-Src are 98.5% homologous. Thus, the Src family is very old and its members well conserved, indicating that these enzymes participate in very fundamental cellular processes.

11.3.2 Overall Structure of Src-like PTKs

The structure of all Src-like PTKs is based on a common multidomain architecture (Fig. 1). They all have a unique 80–100 amino acid N-terminus, in which only a glycine residue in position 2, required for membrane localization of the PTKs, is fully conserved. This member-specific N-terminus is followed by a ~50 amino acid Src-homology 3 (SH3) domain, a ~100 residue Src-homology 2 (SH2) domain, a 250 amino acid catalytic domain (also termed SH1 domain) and, finally, a highly conserved short C-terminal regulatory tail. The SH3, SH2 and

SH1 regions were initially identified based on homology between Src family PTKs, other PTKs and some other non-kinase signaling molecules, such as phospholipase Cγ1, Ras-GTPase activating protein, and cytoskeletal proteins (Pawson 1995; Cohen et al. 1995). The SH3 and SH2 regions are found independently of each other in one or several copies at any location in a multitude of proteins involved in signal transduction. Today, these regions are known to form separate nodular domains that may not influence the folding of the rest of the protein.

11.3.2.1 Myristylation and Palmitylation: The SH4 Domain

All Src family PTKs, as well as a multitude of other viral and cellular proteins, are modified with a myristic acid residue in an amide linkage to the glycine at position 2. All examined myristylated proteins contain the consensus sequence M-G-X-X-X-S/T, now termed the SH4 domain (Resh 1994). The 14-carbone saturated fatty acid is added during translation and seems to be important for localization of the Src family PTKs to the inside of the plasma membrane. Mutations designed to block myristylation of Src-like PTKs (for example the glycine residue at +2) prevent their efficiently binding to the plasma membrane as well as their participation in cell signaling. In addition, at least some Src family members (e.g., Lck and Fyn) have a pair of cysteine residues adjacent to G2 (e.g., C3 and C5 in Lck) which serve as acceptors for palmitic acid. These extra fatty acids may serve to anchor the proteins to the membrane more tightly.

11.3.2.2 The Member-Specific N-terminus

The remainder of the N-terminus is very different between various family members, raising the possibility that it confers unique properties to each member. There is some support for the notion that some Src family members associate via this domain with specific transmembrane or substrate proteins. Lck, for example, binds the intracellular tail of the CD4 and CD8 glycoproteins via a unique cysteine-containing motif within its first 30 amino acids. The capacity of Fyn to associate with the TCR/CD3 complex also resides within the first ten amino acids of its unique N-terminus.

11.3.2.3 The SH3 Domain

The SH3 domain is a hemispherical domain consisting of approximately 50 amino acids involved in protein–protein interaction. SH3 domains are found in a variety of proteins, such as signaling molecules, cytoskeletal proteins, and many nonreceptor PTKs. The function of the SH3 domain of Src family PTKs (as well as SH3 domains in other molecules) is to bind specific proline-rich sequences of ~10 amino acids in other cellular proteins. The minimum consensus sequence for SH3 binding is X-P-p-X-P, where X represents mostly aliphatic residues and p is usually a proline. It is currently believed that each SH3 domain prefers a unique type of ligand defined by the positions of the prolines and the nature of the other amino acids between the prolines. A number of ligands for the SH3 domains of Src family PTKs have been reported, including the 85-kDa subunit of phosphatidylinositol 3-kinase, Lck-BP, YAP65, and c-Cbl, but their relevance in intact cells remains unclear. Interestingly, the SH3 domain of the Src family PTK Lck binds a proline residue located within the SH2 domain of the same molecule. This SH2/SH3 dimer is thought to be involved in intramolecular repression of the PTK activity by binding to the phosphorylated C-terminal tail of the enzyme.

11.3.2.4 The SH2 Domain

SH2 domains are found in a variety of proteins, many of which are involved in signal transduction, and can mediate PTyr-dependent, sequence-specific interactions with other molecules. Within the Src family, the SH2 domain is highly conserved, and it seems that they all prefer the same type of ligand: PTyr followed by two acidic residues followed by isoleucine or leucine, Y*-E-E-I/L (Y*=PTyr). The crystal structure of the SH2 domains of c-Src and Lck revealed that they form a slightly depressed hemisphere with a deep pocket lined with basic residues into which the ligand PTyr residue fits and binds to a conserved arginine residue. A second, mostly hydrophobic pocket makes contact with all three amino acids following the PTyr residue and is largely responsible for the sequence specificity of the SH2 domain. Despite this preference of Src-related PTK SH2 domains, it is generally believed that the negative regulatory tyrosine residue in the C-terminal tail of Src family PTKs binds to the SH2 domain within the same kinase molecule and thereby forces the kinase domain into an inactive conformation. The sequence of this site (Y*-Q-X-G/Q) differs quite extensively from the preferred Y*-E-E-I/L sequence and, accordingly, binding occurs with considerably lower affinity (at least in vitro). In fact, this lower affinity might be crucial for the regulation of Src family PTKs in the intact cell, where competing ligands may activate these PTKs locally by sequestering their SH2 domains. This will be discussed in more detail later.

11.3.2.5 The Catalytic or SH1 Domain

The catalytic domain of Src-like PTKs occupies most of the C-terminal half of the molecules. A number of conserved residues are found in the catalytic region, and significant homology to other protein kinases can be observed. Although the catalytic domain of a Src family PTK has not yet been crystallized, the high degree of conservation and the reported crystal structure of other protein kinases, including the insulin receptor kinase, enables us to model the SH1 domain with a relatively high degree of accuracy. All kinase domains consist of a smaller upper lobe and a larger substrate-binding lower lobe kept together by a flexible hinge region. During catalysis the upper lobe, which contains the conserved G-X-G-X-X-G loop as part of the ATP-binding pocket, moves in relation to the lower lobe, which contains most of the catalytic residues facing the upper lobe, including a conserved lysine residue involved in transfer of the γ-phosphate from ATP to the substrate. Mutation of this lysine (e.g., to arginine) results in total loss of kinase activity. The site of autophosphorylation in Src family PTKs is located on the lower lobe close to the catalytic cleft between the lobes. In the unphosphorylated state this tyrosine residue fits into the substrate binding cleft and thereby blocks substrate phosphorylation (and ATP binding). Following phosphorylation, however, this tyrosine residue moves out of the pocket and the phosphate group forms a salt bridge to a conserved arginine and thereby stabilizes the active conformation. A nearby arginine interacts with the γ-phosphate of ATP and extracts the proton from the acceptor tyrosine residue. This residue replaces a lysine found in all serine/threonine-specific protein kinases, a difference that apparently can be explained by the much higher pKa for the hydroxyl group in serine and threonine compared to that in tyrosine.

It is not clear which amino acids are directly responsible for substrate recognition. The three-dimensional models predict that the substrate polypeptide interacts with a rather large surface surrounding the catalytic cleft of the catalytic domain. A glutamic acid residue in protein kinase A is known to interact with a basic residue in the substrate, and in PTKs this acidic residue is replaced by a basic residue (R389), suggesting that this arginine may interact with an acidic residue upstream of the acceptor tyrosine in the substrate. Indeed, many PTKs prefer substrates with acidic residues upstream of the acceptor tyrosine. In the case of the Src family PTKs, the optimal substrate has the sequence E-E-E-I-Y-E-E-I-E. Notably, the three amino acids following the tyrosine residue are exactly the same as those prefered by the SH2 domain. This raises the interesting possibility that Src family PTKs phosphorylate sites in cellular substrate proteins that their own SH2 domain subsequently will bind to. In fact, some identified substrates have multiple tyrosines followed by suitable acidic amino acids and isoleucines, suggesting that initial phosphorylation of a single site may result in physical association through the SH2 domain, resulting in recruitment of Src-related PTKs and enhanced phosphorylation of more sites.

11.3.2.6 The C-Terminal Regulatory Tail

A hallmark of the Src family PTKs is the highly conserved C-terminal tail, which contains a tyrosine residue known to be important for the regulation of kinase activity. When phosphorylated, this residue is believed to bind the SH2 domain of the same kinase molecule, thereby forcing the catalytic domain into an inactive conformation incapable of phosphorylating substrate proteins. It seems likely that this suppression involves a restriction in the movement of the upper lobe of the SH1 domain.

11.3.3 The Nine Family Members

The following is a short presentation of each of the currently known nine members of the Src family in order of their discovery. Expression patterns and features unique to each member are discussed.

11.3.3.1 c-Src, the Prototypic Nonreceptor PTK

The c-*src* gene is widely expressed, with particularly high levels found in neurons and platelets. Since both these cell types represent terminally differentiated cells without proliferative capacity, the physiological function of c-Src in these cells must be unrelated to the regulation of cell growth. This conclusion is in striking contrast to the well established fact that v-*src* and certain c-*src* mutants can acutely transform cells, and that c-Src is transiently activated during mitosis of normal cells, suggesting that it plays a role in cell division (e.g., by regulating the cytoskeletal reorganizations that occur before and during mitosis). Despite the tremendous efforts spent on this topic, our understanding of the function of both normal and activated Src proteins is still very limited. Additional disappointment came recently from the description of c-*src* null mice generated by homologous recombination ("knockout"), in which the only recognizable defect was a marked osteopetrosis, probably reflecting impaired osteoclast function. This result suggests that other Src family PTKs can take over and compensate for the loss of c-Src, and/or that the physiological function of c-Src is limited to a few specialized cellular functions, many of which may have been overlooked in the c-*src* null animals. In platelets, c-Src has been suggested to participate in signal transduction from the thrombin receptor together with c-Yes and perhaps Hck.

11.3.3.2 c-Yes, Yamaguchi's Kinase

The cellular homologue of the transforming v-*yes* gene of the Yamaguchi 73 virus, c-*yes*, is also widely expressed in adult tissues. The expression of c-*yes* seems to be very low or absent in most leukocytes. Detectable levels are found only in platelets and T cells, including freshly isolated blood T lymphocytes (our unpublished observation). c-Yes can respond by enzymatic activation to triggering of some surface receptors on leukocytes, such as CD36 on platelets and the FcεRI on some mast cell lines. Overall, the physiological function of c-Yes is largely unknown.

11.3.3.3 c-Fgr, the Third Member

The third family member, c-*fgr*, originally identified as a viral oncogene, is expressed in many types of leukocytes, notably granulocytes, eosinophils, macrophages, and natural killer (NK) cells. The expression to c-*fgr* also increases during differentiation of HL-60 promyelocytic cells towards a granulocytic or monocytic phenotype and following infection of B cells with Epstein-Barr virus. Although c-Fgr is activated following receptor triggering in phagocytic cells, particularly by simultaneous co-crosslinking of both Fc receptors and complement receptors, the role of c-Fgr in leukocyte biology remains unclear. The activation of c-Fgr in response to crosslinking of these surface structures suggests that it may be involved in the response of these cells to opsonized invading microorganisms. However, since mice lacking c-*fgr* do not show any overt phenotype or sensitivity to bacterial infections, c-Fgr is likely dispensable for this response.

11.3.3.4 Lck, the T-Cell-Specific Src Family PTK

Lck was the first PTK suggested to participate in signal transmission from the TCR. This kinase is unique in its T lymphocyte-restricted expression. It is expressed in all subsets of T lymphocytes and is detected very early during T-cell ontogeny in the thymus, with double negative (CD4-8-) thymocytes having particularly high levels. A few B cell lines and some colonic carcinomas also express Lck.

An important advance in our understanding of the biology of Lck was the finding that Lck is physically associated with the cytoplasmic domain of the CD4 and CD8 glycoproteins in T cells. This observation opened up new perspectives on the potential role and regulation of Lck in T-cell activation and maturation (Mustelin and Altman 1989), particularly since these two surface molecules were known to play an important role in T-cell interactions with antigen-presenting cells and in T-cell-receptor repertoire selection in the thymus. Lck has also been found to associate with many other transmembrane or surface glycoproteins. In many cases, the stoichiometry and affinity of the interactions seem to be much lower than that with CD4 and the domain of Lck that is involved remains undetermined. The reported association with the TCR, CD5, and CD2 may be indirect, and perhaps partly due to the formation of multimeric complexes containing several of these molecules and CD4 or CD8.

Lck seems to have multiple roles in T-cell physiology. First, Lck is crucial for thymic development and maturation. This role is partly due to very early effects on TCR gene rearrangements, allelic exclusion, and surface expression. Lck is also involved in TCR-dependent positive and negative selection in the thymus and in the progression to the mature CD4$^-$8$^+$ or CD4$^+$8$^-$ phenotype. Second, Lck is involved in TCR-driven activation of mature, resting T cells during an immune response. This function of Lck seems to be redundant with other Src family PTKs (Fyn and c-Yes) and consists of phosphorylating subunits of the TCR-CD3 and receptor-associated molecules. Exactly how Lck participates in TCR signaling is not clear, but association with CD4 and CD8 plays some role (even if Lck can participate in the absence of CD4 or CD8). Quite surprisingly, it has been recently reported that the SH1 function of Lck may not be required for its participation in T-cell signaling (Collins and Burakoff 1993; Xu and Littman 1993). The interaction of proteins with the SH2 or SH3 domains of Lck might therefore be crucial (Caron et al. 1992), and among the proteins that associate with Lck this way are two PTKs, the Syk and Zap kinases (see below).

11.3.3.5 Fyn, a Src Family PTK Involved in TCR Signaling

Another Src family PTK, Fyn, is found in two distinct isoforms arising by alternative splicing of two exons 7 (7A and 7B). The *fyn*(B) isoform, expressed predominantly in the brain, contains exon 7A, while the hematopoietic form of Fyn, *fyn*(T), contains exon 7B. In T cells, Fyn can be co-immunoprecipitated with the TCR complex and co-caps with the TCR in intact T cells, suggesting that this kinase may also be important for TCR signaling. This notion was supported by the observation that Fyn is activated up to fourfold after receptor triggering, and that single-positive thymocytes from mice expressing a *fyn* transgene were more readily triggered by TCR stimulation and produced higher levels of interleukin-2 than controls. Conversely, single-positive thymocytes from mutant mice lacking Fyn displayed greatly diminished responses. Mature T lymphocytes from *fyn*$^{-/-}$ mice, however, responded at substantial, albeit reduced, levels, suggesting that, while Fyn may be crucial for TCR signaling in immature thymocytes, other PTKs (presumably Lck and perhaps c-Yes) can substitute for Fyn in mature T cells. Thus, it seems that Lck and Fyn have distinct and unique functions in the thymus, while being more redundant in the periphery. To complicate the picture, it has been shown that Fyn also associates with CD2, CD5, and Thy-1 in T lymphocytes. How these associations occur and if they differ from the associations of Lck with the same molecules remains unclear.

11.3.3.6 Lyn, the B-Cell and Granulocyte Kinase

Lyn is expressed in B cells, granulocytes, macrophages, and platelets, and in T lymphocytes infected with the human T-cell leukemia virus type I. Lyn exists in two M_r forms of 53 and 56 kDa, respectively, due to alternative mRNA splicing. The smaller protein lacks 21 amino acids in the second half of the unique N-terminus and may associate with different regulators and/or targets and may have different physiological functions.

Lyn associates physically and functionally with the B-cell antigen receptor (BCR) in B lymphocytes. Thus, it seems that the physiological role of Lyn, at least partly, is connected to the signaling of the BCR complex in B cells. However, Lyn is also activated by interleukin 3 in a myeloid cell line and by interleukin 2 in a pre-B cell line.

11.3.3.7 Hck, the Granulocyte and Macrophage-Specific PTK

The Hck kinase also comes in two sizes, 56–57 and 59 kDa, respectively, but in this case this is due to alternative initiation of translation. The kinase is abundant only in platelets, granulocytes, monocytes, and macrophages, and its expression increases during macrophage activation and differentiation of promyelocytic cells towards a more mature granulocyte phenotype. Hck seems to participate in the regulation of signal transduction and specialized functions unique to mature granulocytes, monocytes and macrophages, such as secretion, phagocytosis, chemotaxis, or the induction of a respiratory burst. Indeed, elimination of the *hck* gene by homologous recombination ("knockout") leads to impaired phagocytosis. Interestingly, in Hck-negative mice the PTK activity of Lyn was increased, suggesting that this kinase may compensate for the loss of Hck. Mice lacking both Hck and c-Fgr were more susceptible to infection by *Listeria monocytogenes*, a pathogen normally raising a macrophage and monocyte-centered immune response. Macrophages from the *hck-/-, c-fgr-/-* animals nevertheless displayed many other normal functional properties. An attractive possibility would be that Hck, c-Fgr and Lyn are coupled to multiple surface receptors on these cells, e.g., receptors for immunoglobulins, bacterial peptides, complement proteins, or chemotactic factors, and that they have largely overlapping functions in the induction of cellular responses. So far, however, no specific receptor associations have been identified and the biology of Hck awaits further investigation.

11.3.3.8 Blk, the B Cell-Specific Kinase

The eighth Src family member to be cloned was Blk in 1991. This kinase is also bound to the BCR and is activated by receptor crosslinking. During B-cell maturation the expression of the *blk* gene gradually increases and is highest in mature cells. The available data suggest that Blk participates in BCR signaling, but details are still lacking.

11.3.3.9 Yrk, the Monocyte-Specific Kinase

The newest member of the Src family was cloned in New York and was appropriately named Yrk ("york") for Yes-related kinase. Little is presently known about this PTK except that it is ~60 kDa and is expressed at highest levels in spleen and cerebellum. In the spleen, it is the monocytes that express Yrk, suggesting that Yrk may be involved in some monocyte-specific function, perhaps signal transduction from a receptor mainly expressed on these cells.

11.4 Regulation and Regulators of Src-like PTKs

The function of the Src family PTKs is under tight regulation at all available levels: transcriptional, translational, and posttranslational. Little is known about the often highly tissue-specific transcription factors that regulate Src family gene expression and factors that determine translational efficiency. There are many indications that there are negative feedback loops from the PTKs to their production, and that the amount of these enzymes in a cell is critical for responsiveness to extracellular stimuli. Posttranslational mechanisms for regulation of catalytic activity and interaction with other proteins are potentially responsible for more rapid (seconds to minutes) changes in the function of Src family PTKs in T cells, for example, in response to triggering of the TCR. The best characterized posttranslational mechanisms include autophosphorylation, suppression by reversible phosphorylation of the C-terminal negative regulatory site, phosphorylation at other tyrosine residues, N-terminal serine/threonine phosphorylation, association with transmembrane receptors and other potential regulators or substrates, and binding to cytoskeletal elements. These have all been extensively reviewed recently (Mustelin 1994a), and only those mechanisms potentially involved in TCR signaling will be discussed here.

11.4.1 Autophosphorylation

The catalytic activity of Src family PTKs correlates with autophospho-rylation at a conserved tyrosine residue within the catalytic domain (Y394 in Lck, Y417 in Fyn), and it seems that this autophosphorylation is required for activity towards other polypeptide substrates. In the intact cells, normal cellular Src family PTKs contain very little (usually unde-tectable) phosphate at this site, suggesting that the kinases are mostly inactive or, alternatively, that the autophosphorylation site is the target for very efficient dephosphorylation. Increased autophosphorylation of normal Src-like PTKs in intact cells has only been reported for Lck following CD4-mediated crosslinking. This forced oligomerization ap-parently juxtaposes Lck molecules and increases the accessibility of Y394 residues to the PTK domains, resulting in increased phosphoryla-tion at this site. As a consequence of this increased autophosphorylation, the catalytic activity towards an exogenous substrate (enolase) increased severalfold.

Although there is no definitive evidence, and despite the fact that the autophosphorylation site is located close to the active center of the catalytic domain and the γ-phosphate of the bound ATP, there are some indications that autophosphorylation of Src family PTKs may occur as an intermolecular event, as is the case with growth factor receptor PTKs and perhaps all other PTKs as well. This notion is supported by the finding that autophosphorylation of Lck in vitro is exponentially de-pendent on the concentration of enzyme in the reactions (unpublished observation). If autophosphorylation of Src family PTKs really occurs only in trans, it implies that these kinases have the capacity to dimerize at least transiently. Since the kinase domain is highly conserved among the members of the family, there is no reason to assume that this transient dimerization is only homotypic; heterotypic interaction and "transphosphorylation" at the autophosphorylation site probably also take place.

11.4.2 Suppression by C-terminal Phosphorylation

The suppression (or repression) of Src family PTKs by phosphorylation of a highly conserved tyrosine residue in their C-terminal tail is perhaps the most important mechanism of posttranslational regulation. In all the examined cases, this tyrosine residue in normal Src family PTKs is phosphorylated in vivo. In most cells, the stoichiometry is thought to be very high, perhaps approaching 100%. Leukocytes, however, seem to differ from other cell types in that significant fractions of C-terminally unphosphorylated Src family PTKs (at least Lck) exist in the cells, suggesting a constant need for Src-family kinase activity in those cells.

The importance of C-terminal phosphorylation was initially suggested by the deletion of this portion of the enzyme in the transforming retroviral forms, and by subsequent studies showing that point mutations of the conserved tyrosine residue (e.g., Y-to-F) resulted in high (de-repressed) kinase activity and usually malignant transformation of transfected NIH 3T3 fibroblasts. The transfected cells displayed high levels of tyrosine phosphorylation of cellular proteins, indicating that the mutated kinases were highly active also in vivo.

It is important to note, however, that experiments demonstrating these striking effects of activated Src family PTKs were not performed in T cells. The fact that some C-terminally unphosphorylated Src family PTKs can be detected in lymphoid cells (and probably other leukocytes as well) indicates that suppression by C-terminal phosphorylation may not be as crucial in T cells as in other cell types. For example, transfection of Y505-to-F505 mutated Lck into a CD4$^-$8$^-$ T-cell line did not alter its level of basal tyrosine phosphorylation, but nevertheless augmented TCR-induced tyrosine phosphorylation and interleukin-2 production. This indicates that the level of tyrosine phosphorylation in T cells does not simply reflect the catalytic activity of PTKs. This response was also seen in a T-cell hybridoma transfected with v-Src (which lacks the codon for a C-terminal regulatory tyrosine). Finally, both the brain form and the T-cell form of Fyn mutated at their C-terminal regulatory tyrosine (Y531 and Y528, respectively) caused some elevation in basal tyrosine phosphorylation, and both augmented TCR-induced tyrosine phosphorylation. Curiously, only cells transfected with Fyn(T)F528 displayed increased interleukin-2 production upon TCR triggering.

The mechanism by which phosphorylation of the C-terminal tyrosine causes suppression of the catalytic activity of Src family PTKs is thought to involve an intramolecular binding of the phosphorylated tyrosine to the SH2 domain of the same kinase molecule, thereby forcing it into an inactive conformation. This PTyr-dependent interaction is of low affinity, but is probably stabilized by the participation of the SH3 domain. Hence, inactivation or deletion of either the SH2 or SH3 domain results in a de-repression of the enzyme.

Even if the C-terminal phosphorylation of Lck and Fyn in T cells seems to contribute to the suppression of these kinases, there is no evidence for acute changes in this phosphorylation after TCR triggering. Instead, the PTyr content of Lck increases after T-cell activation. This suggests that Lck is recruited and/or activated primarily through some mechanism other than sudden dephosphorylation of Y505.

11.4.2.1 Csk, the Suppressor of Src-like PTKs

The PTK apparently responsible for the suppressive phosphorylation of Lck at Y505 and Fyn at Y528 has been identified as the C-terminal Src kinase (Csk) (Bergman et al. 1992), a ubiquitously expressed 50-kDa cytosolic enzyme. The finding that disruption of the csk gene is lethal and that cells recovered from the early embryos contain greatly activated Src family PTKs, suggest that Csk is truly important for suppression of Src family PTKs in intact cells (at least during embryogenesis). At present, no other PTK seems to have this specificity, although other recently discovered tissue-restricted Csk family members might substitute for Csk in certain tissues or cell types, such as in T cells.

Very little is presently known about Csk. Its structure offers only a few clues to its regulation and properties; it contains single SH3 and SH2 domains and a catalytic domain as a Src family PTK, but lacks a glycine residue at position 2 for myristylation, the long N-terminal unique region of these kinases, the tyrosine autophosphorylation site, and the typical C-terminal Src family tail. Indeed, Csk appears to be predominantly cytosolic with only a minor fraction localized at the plasma membrane or in adhesion plaques in fibroblastic cells. The membrane-associated Csk (10%–20%) could be bound to Src family PTKs, but this has been difficult to verify by co-immunoprecipitation experiments (unpublished observations). The SH2 and SH3 domains of Csk presumably direct it to interact with other cellular proteins.

Instead of a tyrosine residue, Csk contains an S-S-T motif in the usual autophosphorylation site of PTKs, raising the possibility that it could be regulated by a serine/threonine-specific kinase. Presently, there is no evidence for this. Surprisingly, however, in vitro-translated Csk contains PTyr, and isolated Csk can autophosphorylate on a single tyrosine residue in vitro (our unpublished observation). So far, however, we and others have been unable to detect any tyrosine phosphorylation of Csk in intact T cells. It remains nonetheless possible that such autophosphorylation occurs to low stoichiometry in vivo and/or might be under the tight control of an unidentified tyrosine phosphatase.

An active role of Csk in TCR-induced signal transduction was suggested by a recent study (Oetken et al. 1994), showing that Csk is transiently activated within 1 min after TCR stimulation in Jurkat T cells. Concomitantly with this activation, Csk associated with a PTyr-containing 72-kDa protein, probably via its SH2 domain. Identification of this protein is in progress and will presumably clarify the significance of this association. Such engagement of Csk via its SH2 domain could serve to change the subcellular location of Csk and either bring it to the vicinity of Src family PTKs at the TCR or, conversely, keep it from interacting with these kinases.

Another recent study indicated that the role of Csk in TCR signaling is mainly suppressive by showing that overexpression of Csk in T cells caused a marked reduction of TCR-induced tyrosine phosphorylation and interleukin-2 production (Chow et al. 1993). Surprisingly, however, no elevation in the phosphorylation of the C-terminal negative regulatory site of Lck or Fyn could be detected, raising the possibility that Csk reduced the response to TCR stimulation by some other mechanism than repressing Lck and/or Fyn. Our observation that Csk also phosphorylates the leukocyte common antigen, CD45, and stimulates its PTPase activity (Autero et al. 1994) might be relevant to this phenomenon. Since tyrosine phosphorylation of CD45 has been reported to occur upon triggering of T cells via the TCR and the same sites were phosphorylated in vivo, it seems likely that this regulation of CD45 occurs in intact T cells.

11.4.2.2 CD45 Dephosphorylates the C-terminus of Lck and Fyn
In late 1988, we observed that the overall tyrosine kinase activity in T-cell membranes was spontaneously activated within 1–3 min when

the membranes were kept at 30°C (Mustelin et al. 1989). This effect was also seen in membranes isolated from LSTRA cells which contain 50–60 times more Lck than normal blood T lymphocytes, and it was partially blocked by 1 mM O-phosphotyrosine and completely blocked by Na_3VO_4, a known inhibitor of PTyr phosphatases (PTPases). Based on the simultaneously published observation that CD45 displayed extensive homology to the first cloned PTPase and was directly shown to have PTPase activity, we tested the possibility that this membrane-bound enzyme might be the PTPase responsible for the rapid activation of Lck. Indeed, no activation of Lck was seen in the isolated membrane fraction of a CD45-negative mutant of a murine lymphoma cell line, indicating that CD45 is involved in this process in normal cells. We then found that isolated Lck was activated in vitro by co-incubation with immunoprecipitated CD45, and that the C-terminal negative regulatory site of Lck, Y505, was indeed dephosphorylated by CD45 (Mustelin and Altman 1990). Our conclusion that CD45 can positively regulate Lck by dephosphorylating Y505 was supported by another paper (Ostergaard et al. 1989), which showed that Y505 was hyperphosphorylated in lymphoid cells lacking CD45. From these results it was calculated that ~50% of Y505 is unphosphorylated in the CD45-positive cells.

Numerous papers have later confirmed these findings and extended them to Fyn (Mustelin et al. 1992) and c-Yes in T cells. Curiously, however, phosphorylation of transfected c-Src at Y527 was not altered in the CD45-negative cells. In addition, the preference of CD45 for specific Src family members is not entirely clear: data from some laboratories suggest that CD45 primarily acts on Fyn, while others see more effects on Lck. Nevertheless, dephosphorylation of these two kinases by CD45 seems to correlate with increased responsiveness of the T cells to TCR stimulation, suggesting that CD45-mediated dephosphorylation and activation of Src family PTKs is important for TCR signal transmission. Findings with CD45-negative B lymphocytes and NK cells suggest that Src family kinases specific to these cells are similarly regulated by CD45. Since CD45 is expressed at high levels on all leukocytes and since all Src family PTKs have a highly conserved C-terminus including the negative regulatory site, we believe that all Src family PTKs present in leukocytes are positively regulated by CD45 via similar mechanisms.

The interaction of CD45 with Src family PTKs in intact cells can also be seen as co-immunoprecipitation of Lck with CD45 and a third 31- to 34-kDa protein, and by co-localization of both Lck and Fyn with CD45 during antibody-induced redistribution of CD45 in the membrane. Anti-PTyr immunofluorescence staining further suggested that the CD45-associated pool of Lck and Fyn is unphosphorylated.

Although it is now widely accepted that the C-terminal tyrosine of Src family PTKs in T cells is a physiological substrate for CD45, other PTPases can also regulate Src family PTKs. For example, expression of the CD45-related receptor-like PTPase, PTPα, in fibroblasts activated the transforming potential of c-Src by dephosphorylating its negative regulatory Y527. In vitro, c-Src can also be activated by dephosphorylation at Y527 by potato acid phosphatase. In addition, it is not known whether CD45 is truly specific for the C-terminal tyrosine or mostly dephosphorylates it because it contains most of the phosphate in Src family PTKs in vivo. Autophosphorylated ^{32}P-labeled recombinant Lck is also dephosphorylated by immunoprecipitated CD45 in vitro (our unpublished observation), and, during antibody-mediated co-crosslinking of CD4 and CD45, the phosphorylation of Lck at Y394 decreased, suggesting that CD45 can also dephosphorylate this site in vivo. Nevertheless, it seems that this PTPase dephosphorylates the C-terminus of Src kinases more readily.

11.4.3 Positive Regulation by N-terminal Tyrosine Phosphorylation

There are several reports on additional sites of tyrosine phosphorylation in Src family PTKs. The transforming v-Src protein encoded by the Prague strain of Rous sarcoma virus contains phosphate at Y205 or Y208 in its SH2 domain, and, during treatment of intact cells with Na_3VO_4, an inhibitor of PTPases, there is an increase in tyrosine phosphorylation of c-Src at undefined N-terminal sites. This increase is accompanied by activation of the kinase. Amino-terminal tyrosine phosphorylation and an increase in relative molecular weight on sodium dodecyl sulfate (SDS) gels of c-Src molecules associated with polyoma virus middle T antigen has also been reported. Treatment of T cells with Na_3VO_4 or phenylarsine oxide, another potent inhibitor of PTPases, causes hyperphosphorylation of Lck on tyrosine and an increase in its apparent molecular weight on SDS gels. Some of this hyperphosphorylation occurs at Y192 in the SH2 domain of Lck. Finally, incubation of purified recombinant Lck with ATP leads not only to autophosphorylation at Y394, but also incorporation of phosphate at one or several N-terminal tyrosine residues.

Phosphorylation of Src family PTKs on N-terminal tyrosine residues has also been observed in the platelet-derived growth factor receptor system. This receptor PTK is a transmembrane molecule with an extracellular ligand-binding domain and an intracellular PTK domain. Ligand-induced dimerization of the platelet-derived growth factor receptor induces autophosphorylation in trans of a number of tyrosine residues. When phosphorylated, these residues act as high-affinity ligands for the SH2 domains of a number of signal transduction molecules, including the Src family PTKs c-Src, Fyn, and c-Yes. Following this binding, the Src family PTKs are phosphorylated at an N-terminal tyrosine residue, increase in apparent molecular weight on SDS gels, and are enzymatically activated two- to fourfold. The mechanism of this activation is unknown, but one could imagine that phosphorylation in the SH3 or SH2 domains could alter the interaction between these domains and the phosphorylated C-terminus, and thereby destabilize the inactive conformation. It has not been determined whether the Src family PTKs that bind the platelet-derived growth factor receptor via their SH2 domains are C-terminally dephosphorylated, or if they are phosphorylated but bind with higher affinity for the PTyr residue on the receptor PTK. In the latter case the Src family PTKs would be expected to be activated already by the binding event.

T cells do not express platelet-derived growth factor receptor, but during T-cell activation Lck becomes phosphorylated at an N-terminal tyrosine, Y192, located in the SH2 domain (Couture et al. 1996). Presently, the best candidate for the PTK responsible for this event is the Syk family nonreceptor PTKs, Syk and Zap. Both these kinases have recently been found to participate in TCR signaling in T cells (Couture et al. 1994a) and we have found that Syk activates Lck in vitro or in co-transfected COS-1 cells and phosphorylates Lck at Y192 in the SH2 domain (Couture et al. 1994b). A Y192-to-F192 mutation abrogated both phosphorylation and activation of Lck by Syk in co-transfected COS-1 cells as measured by enolase phosphorylation assays in vitro. Since Syk also synergizes with Fyn in co-transfected COS-1 cells, it is likely that Syk also phosphorylates Fyn at Y205, the equivalent tyrosine residue which is present in all Src family PTKs.

11.4.3.1 The Syk Family of Nonreceptor PTKs

Unlike the Src family PTKs, the two mammalian Syk-family PTKs, Syk and Zap, as well as the closely related PTK encoded by the *Hydra attenuata* gene HTK16, lack an SH3 domain and instead have two SH2 domains. These kinases also lack myristylation signals or other recognized membrane localization motifs. Despite the overall similarity in domain organization between Syk and Zap, they are not as closely related as Src family members are to each other. The greatest divergence between Syk and Zap is located in the region between the second SH2 domain and the SH1 domain (only ~30% homology), and in the C-terminal tail, which is considerably longer in Zap. There also seem to be functional differences between the two kinases: First, the association of Syk with the TCR (as well as other receptors on leukocytes) seems to be independent of activation and tyrosine phosphorylation (Couture et al. 1994a), while association of Zap with TCR-ζ or CD3ε requires phosphorylation of two tyrosine residues located within a signaling motif and is cooperatively mediated by the two SH2 domains of the PTK. Whether this difference between Syk and Zap reflects a true difference in their biology or simply stem from insufficient comparative experimental data remains uncertain. In fact, it is likely that Syk also binds tyrosine-phosphorylated signaling motifs in ligated TCR complexes (and other receptors), particularly since the second SH2 domain of Syk is known to prefer the Y*-Q/E-X-L motif present in the smaller CD3 subunits. Thus, the constitutively TCR-bound Syk does not need to be recruited, but may nevertheless change its mode of receptor binding upon receptor ligation and tyrosine phosphorylation.

Second, when *syk* alone was transfected into COS cells, the resulting kinase was found to be highly phosphorylated on tyrosine residues and a number of cellular proteins also became tyrosine phosphorylated. This effect of Syk was critically dependent on its autophosphorylation site, Y518/519 (Couture et al. 1994b). Although Zap reportedly requires co-transfection of Src family PTKs to be active in COS cells, we find Zap to be tyrosine phosphorylated when expressed alone (unpublished). Nevertheless, Syk, but not Zap, becomes tyrosine phosphorylated upon

TCR triggering of the Lck-negative JCaM1 cells. Interestingly, Zap phosphorylation is also under the control of CD45 (Mustelin et al. 1995), but in contrast to the regulation of Src family PTKs by CD45, the effects are probably indirect.

TCR triggering induces a rapid tyrosine phosphorylation of both Syk and Zap, but the mechanism of this response is not entirely clear. The catalytic activity of Syk correlates positively with its degree of tyrosine phosphorylation, and a Y-to-F mutation of the conserved autophosphorylation site in Syk (Y518/Y519) reduces its tyrosine phosphorylation by >90% and abolishes its enzymatic activity in vitro and in intact transfected COS cells and T cells (unpublished). Together with the finding that Lck is not required for the activation of Syk in Jurkat T cells, these findings raise the possibility that Syk can activate itself by autophosphorylation. In the case of Zap, it is now known that autophosphorylation occurs on nonactivating tyrosine residues, such as Tyr-492. The observation that the Tyr-493 residue, recently shown to be critical for enzymatic activation, cannot be phosphorylated by Zap itself, but instead is a good substrate for Lck, confirms the requirement of Src-family PTKs for Zap activation. Syk can also be phosphorylated by Lck, but in this case there was no effect on its catalytic activity.

The possibility that Syk and Zap are important in T-cell activation was first suggested by the finding that transmembrane chimeric molecules having Syk or Zap as intracellular parts could induce Ca^{2+} mobilization, tyrosine phosphorylation, and targeted cytotoxicity upon antibody-mediated crosslinking. Interestingly, Syk was more effective while Zap required co-crosslinking with a Fyn-containing chimera to induce equivalent downstream effects, suggesting that Zap is more dependent on Src family PTKs for activation. Furthermore, patients with a mutation in the *zap* gene suffer from a severe immunodeficiency syndrome characterized by defective thymic maturation of CD8[+] T cells and deficient TCR signaling in the mature CD4[+] T cells. T cells lacking Syk have not yet been described, but B cells devoid of Syk respond to receptor triggering with a very limited tyrosine phosphorylation of cellular substrates and they fail to mobilize calcium.

11.4.3.2 Synergism Between Src and Syk Family PTKs

Co-expression of Zap or Syk with Lck or Fyn in COS cells gives rise to a synergistic increase in tyrosine phosphorylation of cellular substrates (Couture et al. 1994a, b). This effect is seen also in the absence of a co-expressed TCR-ζ construct, indicating that although TCR-ζ may act as a meeting place for the two classes of PTKs, there is also functional interaction at a more direct level. In our hands, the catalytic activity of Syk did not change by co-expression of Lck, while the catalytic activity of Lck was elevated severalfold by co-expression of Syk (Couture et al. 1994b, 1996). Since the activity of Lck towards the TCR-ζ construct in transfected COS cells reportedly depended on the presence of Zap, it seems that Zap also activates Src family PTKs. One mechanism by which this activation may occur is by the SH2 domain-dependent binding of Lck to tyrosine-phoshorylated Zap and Syk. Since the SH2 domain of Src family PTKs is involved in the maintenance of the inactive conformation of these kinases by binding to the C-terminal tail, one must assume that binding of the SH2 domain to another ligand (e.g., Zap or Syk) prevents or reverses this intramolecular suppression. Thus, the Lck molecules that bind Syk or Zap must either be preactivated (i.e., C-terminally dephosphorylated) or, alternatively, they become activated by the binding event. The former possibility seems unlikely since the stoichiometry of C-terminal phosphorylation of Src family PTKs in COS cells is very high and since a co-transfected Csk did not affect the synergism between Syk and Lck (our unpublished observation). Thus, a Src family PTK bound to Syk or Zap presumably is in the open conformation and, therefore, fully active. The phosphorylation of Lck at Y192 (and Fyn at Y205?) may serve to stabilize this activation.

11.5 Future Directions and Concluding Remarks

Up to now, the consensus model for the regulation of Src family PTKs and the basis for their participation during T-cell signaling was centered on the phosphorylation of conserved regulatory tyrosine residues, namely, the autophosphorylation site and the C-terminal tyrosine residue. These events were thought to initiate and regulate the functional participation of these kinases following antigen receptor stimulation. However, recent evidence suggests that the kinase domain of Lck is not required for potentiating antigen-specific activation of CD4-dependent T lymphocytes. Importantly, mutations affecting the function of either the SH2 or SH3 domains were each partly detrimental to antigenic stimulation. In a different system, our laboratory has examined the ability of SH2 domain mutants of Lck to restore TCR-mediated signaling in Lck-deficient JCaM1 cells. Although all constructs had a functional catalytic domain, a Y192E mutant known to be deficient in its SH2 domain function was totally unable to mediate TCR-mediated Erk2 activation, whereas a wild-type Lck construct or a Y192F mutant were fully active. These findings strongly suggest that the role of Src-family PTKs in antigen-receptor signaling depends on the regulated function of several independent domains, such as the SH2 and SH3 domains, which are involved in specific intermolecular interactions as well as the kinase domain. Until we achieve a better understanding of the regulation of the functional domains of Src family PTKs, our views and models on how these enzymes participate in lymphocyte activation are likely to represent oversimplifications of a much more sophisticated reality.

Acknowledgments. Work from our laboratory cited herein was supported by Le Fonds de la Recherche en Santé du Québec, and NIH grants GM48960 and AI35603. This is publication # 135 from the La Jolla Institute for Allergy and Immunology.

References

Altman A, Coggeshall KM, Mustelin T (1990) Molecular events mediating T cell activation. Adv Immunol 48:227–360

Autero M, Saharinen J, Pessa-Morikawa T, Soula-Rothhut M, Oetken C, Gassmann M, Bergman M, Alitalo K, Burn P, Gahmberg CG, Mustelin T (1994) Tyrosine phosphorylation of CD45 phosphotyrosine phosphatase by p50[csk] kinase creates a binding site for p56[lck] tyrosine kinase and activates the phosphatase. Mol Cell Biol 14:1308–1321

Bergman M, Mustelin T, Oetken C, Partanen J, Flint NA, Amrein KE, Autero M, Burn P, Alitalo K (1992) The human p50[csk] tyrosine kinase phosphorylates p56[lck] at Tyr-505 and down regulates its catalytic activity. EMBO J 11:2919–2924

Caron L, Abraham N, Pawson T, Veillette A (1992) Structural requirements for enhancement of T-cell responsiveness by the lymphocyte-specific tyrosine protein kinase p56[lck]. Mol Cell Biol 12:2720–2729

Chow LML, Fournel M, Davidson D, Veillette A (1993) Negative regulation of T-cell receptor signalling by the tyrosine kinase p50^{csk}. Nature 365:156–160

Cohen GB, Ren R, Baltimore D (1995) Modular binding domains in signal transduction proteins. Cell 80:237–248

Collins TL, Burakoff SJ (1993) Tyrosine kinase activity of CD4-associated p56^{lck} may not be required for CD4-dependent T-cell activation. Proc Natl Acad Sci USA 90:11885–11889

Couture C, Mustelin T (1995) Regulation of Src family PTKs during T cell activation. In: Lad PM, Kaptein JS, Lin C-KE (eds) Signal transduction in leukocytes, G protein-related and other pathway. CRC Press, Boca Raton

Couture C, Baier G, Altman A, Mustelin T (1994a) p56^{lck}-independent activation and tyrosine phosphorylation of p72^{syk} by T-Cell antigen receptor/CD3 stimulation. Proc Natl Acad Sci USA 91:5301–5305

Couture C, Baier G, Oetken C, Williams S, Telford D, Marie-Cardine A, Baier-Bitterlich G, Fischer S, Burn P, Altman A, Mustelin T (1994b) Activation of p56^{lck} by p72^{syk} through physical association and N-terminal tyrosine phosphorylation. Mol Cell Biol 14:5249–5258

Couture C, Songyang Z, Williams S, Tailor P, Cantley LC, Mustelin T (1996) Regulation of an SH2 domain by tyrosine phosphorylation (submitted for publication)

Mustelin T (1994a) Src family tyrosine kinases in leukocytes. Landes, Austin

Mustelin T (1994b) T cell antigen receptor signaling: three families of tyrosine kinases and a phosphatase. Immunity 1:351–356

Mustelin T, Altman A (1989) Do CD4 and CD8 control T-cell activation via a specific tyrosine protein kinase? Immunol Today 10:189–192

Mustelin T, Altman A (1990) Dephosphorylation and activation of the T cell tyrosine kinase pp56^{lck} by the leukocyte common antigen (CD45). Oncogene 5:809–813

Mustelin T, Altman A (1991) Tyrosine phosphorylation in T-cell activation. Scand J Immunol 34:259–264

Mustelin T, Burn P (1993) Regulation of src family tyrosine kinases in lymphocytes. Trends Biochem Sci 18:215–220

Mustelin T, Coggeshall KM, Altman A (1989) Rapid activation of the T-cell tyrosine protein kinase pp56^{lck} by the CD45 phosphotyrosine phosphatase. Proc Natl Acad Sci USA 86:6302–6306

Mustelin T, Coggeshall KM, Isakov N, Altman A (1990) T-cell antigen receptor-mediated activation of phospholipase C requires tyrosine phosphorylation. Science 247:1584–1587

Mustelin T, Pessa-Morikawa T, Autero M, Gassman M, Andersson LC, Gahmberg CG, Burn P (1992) Regulation of the p59^{fyn} protein tyrosine kinase by the CD45 phosphotyrosine phosphatase. Eur J Immunol 22:1173–1178

Mustelin T, Williams S, Tailor P, Couture C, Zenner G, Burn P, Ashwell JD, Altman A (1995) Regulation of the p70zap tyrosine protein kinase in T cells by the CD45 phosphotyrosine phosphatase. Eur J Immunol 25:942–946

Oetken C, Couture C, Bergman M, Bonnefoy-Berard N, Williams S, Alitalo K, Burn P, Mustelin T (1994) TCR/CD3-triggering causes increased activity of the p50^{csk} tyrosine kinase and engagement of its SH2 domain. Oncogene 9:1625–1631

Ostergaard HL, Shackelford DA, Hurley TR, Johnson P, Hyman R, Sefton BM, Trowbridge IS (1989) Expression of CD45 alters phosphorylation of the lck-encoded tyrosine protein kinase in murine lymphoma T-cell lines. Proc Natl Acad Sci USA 86:8959–8963

Pawson T (1995) Protein modules and signalling networks. Nature 373:573–580

Resh MD (1994) Myristylation and palmitylation of Src family members: the fats of the matter. Cell 76:411–413

Xu H, Littman DR (1993) A kinase-independent function of Lck in potentiating antigen-specific T cell activation. Cell 74:633–643

Zenner G, Zur Hausen JO, Burn P, Mustelin T (1995) Towards unraveling the complexity of T cell signal transduction. Bioessays 17:967-975

12 Sperm–Zona Pellucida Interaction: A Model for Zona Receptor Kinase-Mediated Signaling

P.M. Saling, D.J. Burks, and C.N. Tomes

12.1	Introduction	247
12.2	Identification of Zona Receptor Kinase (ZRK)	250
12.3	A Working Hypothesis for the Role of ZRK	252
12.3.1	Receptor PTKs and Signaling Pathways in Somatic Cells	252
12.3.2	ZRK and Signaling in Sperm: A Model	253
12.4	Structural Features of the ZRK Intracellular Domain	256
12.5	ZRK Interaction with PLCγ	256
12.5.1	PLCγ1 Is Phosphorylated on Tyrosine in Capacitated Sperm	259
12.5.2	ZP3 Activates PLC Activity in Capacitated Sperm via Tyrosine Phosphorylation	261
12.5.3	PLCγ1 Coprecipitates with ZRK in Capacitated Sperm	262
12.6	ZRK Interaction with PI 3-K	263
12.7	Summary and Perspectives	265
References		267

12.1 Introduction

Successful mammalian fertilization requires the precise recognition and interaction of specific molecules on the sperm with complementary molecules of the egg. Over the last decade, the identification of many of the proteins involved in these events has significantly advanced our understanding of the molecular basis of gamete interaction. In addition to permitting focused attention on each of the individual gamete compo-

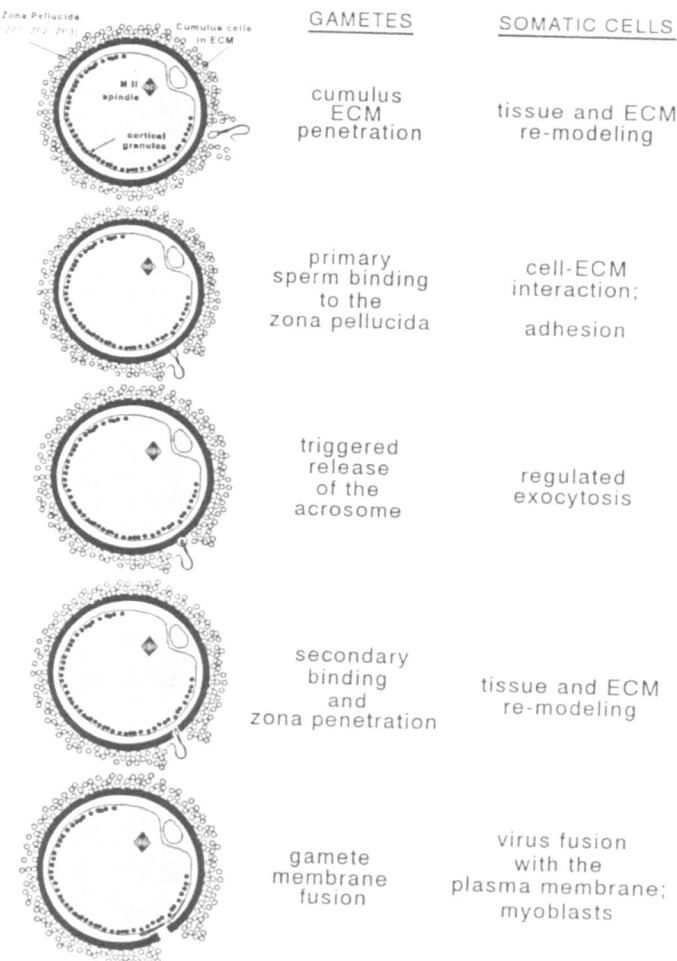

Fig. 1. Steps of gamete interactions leading to fertilization paired with parallel processes in somatic cells. *ECM*, extracellular matrix

nents identified, this analysis has re-enforced the concept that the intercellular interactions between sperm and eggs that lead to fertilization are similar to many aspects of somatic cell interactions.

A brief summary of the major interactions between mammalian gametes that lead to fertilization illustrates the parallels among gamete and somatic cellular interactions (Fig. 1). Upon reaching the egg in the oviduct, the sperm must initially pass through an extracellular matrix (ECM) secreted by the follicular cumulus cells that accompany the egg at ovulation. Sperm progress through this matrix appears to be facilitated by the hyaluronidase activity of PH-20 (Gmachl et al. 1993; Lin et al. 1994), similar to the migration of a somatic cell through a glycosaminoglycan-rich ECM. Sperm must then pass through a second ECM, the zona pellucida (zp), secreted in this case by the egg. Initial work in the mouse demonstrated that the zp has a rather simple composition, consisting largely of the three glycoproteins ZP1, ZP2, and ZP3 (Wassarman 1994, 1995). The genes that encode these proteins are well conserved across mammalian species (Epifano and Dean 1994), suggesting functional relationships. Primary binding occurs between ZP3 and proteins of the sperm plasma membrane. It is likely that several different sperm proteins are involved in primary binding; some may act as adhesins whereas others may be predicted to have transmembrane signaling potential. The ZP3-binding proteins galactosyltransferase (Miller et al. 1992) and sp56 (Bookbinder et al. 1995; Cheng et al. 1994) might fall into the former category, with zona receptor kinase (ZRK) (Burks et al. 1995a) in the latter category. As a consequence of binding to ZP3, the sperm cell is stimulated to discharge the contents of the acrosomal vesicle, an event known as the acrosome reaction (AR). This phenomenon is an example of regulated exocytosis, akin to the processes that, for example, mast cells or neurons undergo when stimulated appropriately. It is reasonable to expect that conserved pathways and components utilized by somatic cells for these processes will operate in gametes as well (Bennett and Scheller 1993). In keeping with this notion, ZP3 activates two highly conserved pathways in sperm, those that are protein-tyrosine kinase (PTK) and G_i protein mediated (Ning et al. 1995; Saling et al. 1995; Ward and Kopf 1993). These may operate either in series or in parallel to open calcium channels that elevate intracellular levels of Ca^{2+} and trigger exocytosis. The exposed contents of the acrosomal vesicle, in particular proacrosin (Lo Leggio et al. 1994;

Topfer-Petersen and Cechova 1990; Williams and Jones 1993) and PH-20 (Myles and Primakoff 1991) participate in secondary binding to the zp matrix; the likely ligand in this interaction is ZP2. PH-20 appears to be responsible for maintenance of binding whereas proacrosin is involved in binding as well as limited proteolysis of the zp matrix after autoactivation to the active enzyme acrosin. Like sperm interaction with the cumulus ECM, the mechanisms used here are similar to those used by somatic cells during tissue remodeling. Following penetration through the zp matrix, the acrosome-reacted sperm adheres to the egg plasma membrane and then fuses with it. The molecular characteristics of fertilin (Blobel et al. 1992), with a disintegrin domain for binding to presumptive integrin receptors in the egg plasma membrane (Almeida et al. 1995) and a viral fusion peptide for fusion, make it a good candidate for a sperm protein involved in fusion with the egg. Whereas the fusion of intracellular membranes with the plasma membrane, for instance, during exocytosis, is a process in which all cells engage, the fusion of two plasma membranes is less common. Gametes are one of the few cell types that exhibit this behavior. The differentiation of myoblasts into myotubes is another example; recently, a fusion protein with characteristics similar to fertilin was identified in this system (Yagamihiromasa et al. 1995). Perhaps the most studied form of membrane fusion is that catalyzed by viral fusion proteins; structural similarities to fertilin have also been found in this group of proteins (Wolfsberg et al. 1995).

Undoubtedly, new proteins that are not considered here will be identified to further our understanding of the processes by which fertilization occurs. It seems fully apparent, however, that fundamental paradigms of cellular interaction extend to gametes, and our analysis of this topic is likely to be facilitated by considering ongoing developments in the relevant fields.

12.2 Identification of Zona Receptor Kinase (ZRK)

Cells modulate their behavior in response to signals from their environment. These signals may be soluble or insoluble components of an adjacent cell or ECM. In all cases, the external signals must be transduced across the membrane to generate an effect. We identified a 95-kDa mouse sperm protein with characteristics of a PTK as a receptor for ZP3 (Leyton and Saling 1989a) and suggested that this protein may be responsible for transducing the signal of binding to ZP3 to the sperm cell's interior. Several lines of evidence indicate that this 95-kDa ZP3-receptor in mouse sperm is a member of the PTK receptor family: (1) it contains phosphotyrosine (PY), the level of which increases upon exposure to zp proteins (Leyton and Saling 1989a); (2) PTK activity is stimulated by direct exposure of the isolated receptor to ligand (Leyton et al. 1992); and (3) ZP3 receptor aggregation is an initiating signal in the cascade leading to acrosomal exocytosis (Leyton and Saling 1989b). Given these characteristics, we refer to this 95-kDa protein as ZRK.

Consistent with these observations in mice, we found that a 95-kDa protein is the major PY-containing protein in human sperm, and its level of PY increases both with capacitation (Burks et al. 1995a) and with exposure to human ZP3 (Burks et al. 1995b). Moore and colleagues reported some years ago on the monoclonal antibody (mAb) 97.25, which blocks human sperm interaction with the human zp and recognizes a 95-kDa human sperm membrane protein (Moore et al. 1987). We found that the protein recognized by mAb 97.25 is tyrosine phosphorylated and is located on the sperm surface in the acrosomal region (Burks et al. 1995a). Since these findings suggested that mAb 97.25 recognizes a human ZRK homolog, we screened a human testis cDNA expression library sequentially with anti-PY Ab and with mAb 97.25 probes predicted to identify the intracellular and extracellular domains, respectively, of human ZRK. A cDNA, *hu9*, that encodes a novel PTK with the predicted structure of a transmembrane receptor was isolated with this approach (Burks et al. 1995a).

When Northern blots containing RNA from various human tissues are probed with the *hu9* cDNA, a single transcript of approximately 2.2 kb is detected in human testis, suggesting the cloned insert represents the complete mRNA encoding the Hu9 protein (Burks et al. 1995a). *Hu9* does not hybridize with RNA from the other human tissues surveyed, suggesting that *hu9* expression is testis specific; in situ hybridization indicates that the *hu9* transcript is confined to postmeiotic germ cells (Burks et al. 1995a).

12.3 A Working Hypothesis for the Role of ZRK

Several lines of evidence indicate that *hu9* encodes human ZRK. First, we have raised an antibody in rabbits (K16) against a synthetic peptide that corresponds to residues 539–553 of the deduced amino acid sequence of *hu9*. Immunoblot analysis indicates that K16 recognizes a tyrosine-phosphorylated, 95-kDa human sperm protein (Burks et al. 1995a). Human ZP3 stimulates acrosomal exocytosis in human sperm, and this effect is blocked by tyrphostin RG50864, a specific tyrosine kinase inhibitor (Burks et al. 1995b). K16 immunoprecipitates display kinase activity that is stimulated by human ZP3 (Burks et al. 1995a) and human ZP3 increases the tyrosine phosphorylation of ZRK (Burks et al. 1995b). Finally, synthetic peptides corresponding to sequences in the predicted extracellular domain of Hu9 inhibit human sperm zp binding in hemi-zona assays (Burks et al. 1995a).

Of the various zp receptors identified so far, only ZRK has intrinsic signaling function, with the structure and activity of a receptor PTK. Recent work on galactosyltransferase suggests that the 13-residue, sperm-specific portion of its cytoplasmic domain interacts with a G_i protein (Gong et al. 1995); however, the validity of an assay that is fundamental to those findings has recently been challenged (Cardullo and Wolf 1995).

12.3.1 Receptor PTKs and Signaling Pathways in Somatic Cells

With respect to signaling pathways initiated in response to receptor PTK binding of their ligands, an enormous amount of information has been learned during the last decade (Van der Geer et al. 1994). Upon liganding, receptor PTKs undergo changes in conformation that promote oligomerization and intermolecular autophosphorylation, which, in turn, stimulates the kinase activity of the oligomerized receptor PTKs for phosphorylation of cytosolic substrates. Many receptor PTKs contain multiple autophosphorylation sites that serve to recruit specific substrates and binding proteins. Commonly, *src* homology 2 (SH2)-domains of specific signaling components, such as phospholipase Cγ (PLCγ) or phosphatidylinositol 3-kinase (PI 3-K), recognize and bind to these new PY residues. In many cases, these enzymes themselves serve as substrates and become tyrosine phosphorylated, causing their activation. Alternatively, several SH2-containing proteins (Grb-2, Shc, Crk) that associate with tyrosine-phosphorylated receptors lack enzymatic activity but act as adaptors, linking other components or signaling pathways to the receptors; in several cases, an adaptor links the activated PTK to the Ras family of low-molecular-weight G proteins via GTPase-activating proteins (RasGap) or guanine nucleotide exchange factors (Sos). In turn, activated Ras stimulates the Raf kinase which activates additional kinase pathways that affect the growth and differentiation characteristics of cells. Critical regulation of signaling pathways involving tyrosine phosphorylation is also mediated by protein tyrosine phosphatases (PTPases). In addition to modulating signaling pathways by removing tyrosine phosphates from the substrates of PTKs, PTPases have also been shown to exhibit complex interactions with PTKs themselves, either activating or inhibiting them. In another related paradigm, a PTPase has also been identified that links a receptor PTK to Grb-2, thus serving an adapter function (Li et al. 1994).

12.3.2 ZRK and Signaling in Sperm: A Model

With respect to the function of ZRK in acrosomal exocytosis, we have developed a working model (Fig. 2). From our previous work as well as by analogy with other ligand-induced cellular responses, we suggest that acrosomal exocytosis is triggered by the aggregation of receptors for ZP3 in the sperm's plasma membrane. We have identified ZRK as one ZP3 receptor. However, based on numerous results in the literature concerning sperm–zp interaction as well as results concerning somatic cell interactions, we suggest that ZRK is but one of several proteins in the sperm plasma membrane that forms a multimeric adhesion and signaling complex resulting in acrosomal exocytosis. At present, ZRK is the only candidate protein with intrinsic signaling potential and becomes a focal point of our model.

Capacitation is known to be associated with increased fluidity of the membrane (Yanagimachi 1994). Thus, if not pre-existing, this process might allow the formation of multimeric complexes consisting of adhesion components (e.g., sp56, galactosyltransferase) and signaling components (e.g., ZRK), all of which may be necessary for proper position-

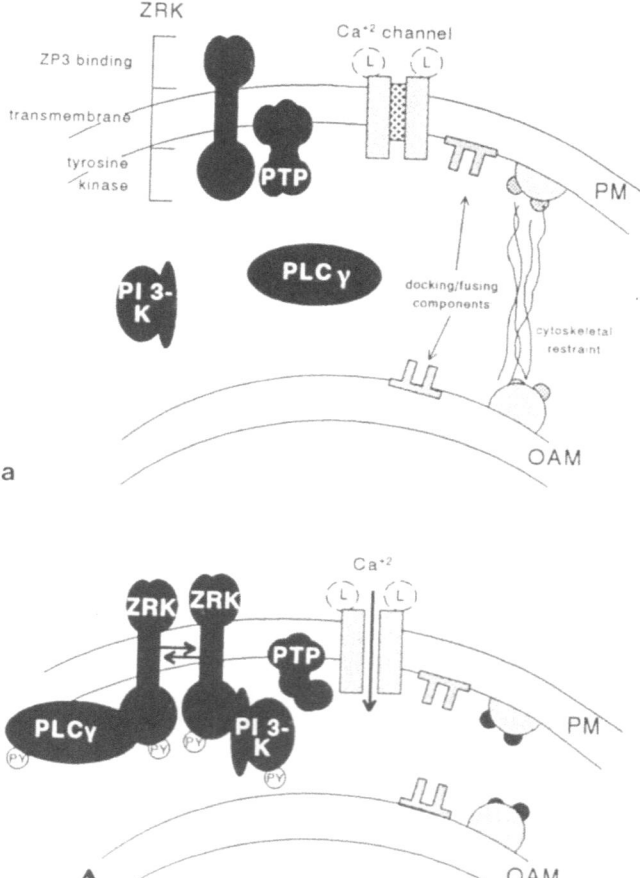

Fig. 2. Legend see p. 255

◀ **Fig. 2a,b.** A hypothetical model for sperm activation and triggering of acrosomal exocytosis. As a protein with signaling potential, zona receptor kinase (*ZRK*) forms a focus of the model shown. Other ZP3-binding proteins (not depicted due to spatial limits) also participate in assembling an active multimeric signaling complex at the plasma membrane (*PM*). G_i proteins are also involved in ZP3-triggered acrosome reactions (ARs), but are not depicted here. **a** Several components of the plasma and outer acrosomal membranes (*OAM*), as well as components in the intervening cytosolic space between these membranes, for a nonactivated sperm cell. ZRK is suggested to remain inactivated (nontyrosine-phosphorylated) via an active hypothetical tyrosine phosphatase (*PTP*). Other signaling components thought to participate in ARs, such as phospholipase Cγ (*PLCγ*) and phosphatidylinositol 3-kinase (*PI 3-K*), are shown with a cytosolic distribution in nonactivated sperm. Ca^{2+} channels (probably *L* type-like) in the plasma membrane are suggested to be inactive in nonactivated sperm and are drawn here as *closed*. Other machinery of exocytosis, although not yet identified in sperm, is predicted; this includes vesicle docking and fusing proteins (akin to syntaxin, synaptotagmin, and cellubrevin, for instance) as well as cytoskeletal restraints that will prevent the target and vesicle membranes from approaching too closely. These latter components can be predicted to be critical for maintaining sperm in an acrosome-intact state during transit through the male and female reproductive tracts to the site of fertilization. **b** Activated sperm. The putative PTPase(s) has been inactivated, permitting expression of phosphorylated tyrosine residues due to basal activity of the ZRK tyrosine kinase. These phosphorylated tyrosine residues provide coupling sites for SH2-containing proteins, such as PLCγ and PI 3-K. Liganding of ZRK by ZP3 increases the activation of these, and perhaps other, coupled proteins and initiates a signaling cascade. Activation of downstream signaling components could provide for coupling to the G_i protein(s), and leads to opening of Ca^{2+} channels and increased intracellular Ca^{2+}. As a consequence of these, and perhaps other, events, cytoskeletal restraints disassemble, permitting docking and subsequent fusion of the vesicle and plasma membranes

ing of the sperm at the zp surface. Interaction of ZP3 and ZRK will result in PTK activation, with recruitment of intracellular signaling components that are required for the exocytotic stimulus. The machinery of acrosomal exocytosis (the docking and fusing components and cytoskeletal elements) is predicted to be similar to that used in other exocytotic systems and is modulated by the cascade set into motion by ZP3 activation of ZRK. Based on findings with receptor PTKs in somatic cells, it can be predicted that activated ZRK will recruit cytosolic substrates and activate them, if they bear enzymatic activity. Identification of these substrates is therefore fundamental to understanding the signaling pathways involved in acrosomal exocytosis.

12.4 Structural Features of the ZRK Intracellular Domain

Examination of the sequence of ZRK's intracellular domain reveals that many of the tyrosine residues are in consensus motifs for binding of SH2-containing proteins to activated receptor PTKs (Cunningham et al. 1995; Songyang et al. 1994) (Fig. 3). SH2-containing proteins that are involved directly in signaling, such as PLCγ and PI 3-K, as well as adapter proteins, such as Grb2, SHC, and 3BP2, that link receptor PTKs with G-protein signaling pathways, are thus predicted to potentially bind to ZRK.

As an initial test of this prediction, we have directly analyzed human and mouse sperm for the presence of two of these candidate signaling proteins and their possible involvement in the regulation of gamete interaction.

12.5 ZRK Interaction with PLCγ

The activation of the enzyme PLC by extracellular factors to generate intracellular second messengers is a ubiquitous mechanism involved in the stimulation of a number of cellular processes, including secretion, cell division, and differentiation. This step is the focal point for two major pathways, one initiated by G-protein-linked receptors (activating PLCβ) and the other initiated by tyrosine kinase-linked receptors (activating PLCγ) (Rhee and Choi 1992a). Both of these PLC isoforms

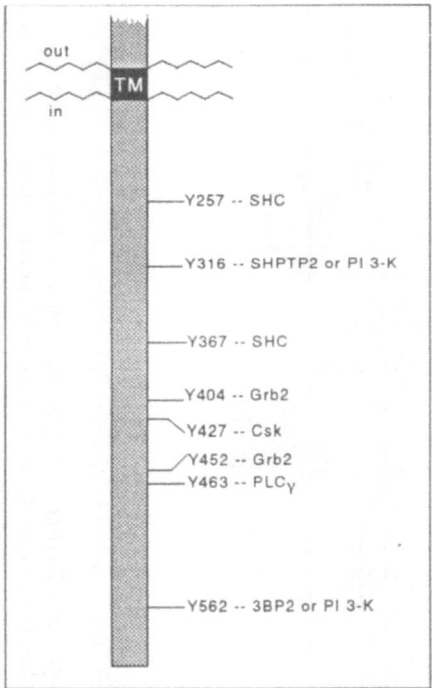

Fig. 3. Identification of consensus motifs in zona receptor kinase for potential binding of Src homology 2 (SH2) domain-containing signaling proteins. *TM*, transmembrane; *SHC*, SH2 domain-containing protein; *PLCγ*, phospholipase Cγ; *PI 3-K*, phosphatidylinositol 3-kinase

generate two second messengers in Ca^{2+}-dependent processes: 1,2-dia-cylglycerol (DAG) and inositol polyphosphates (in particular, I-1,4,5P$_3$) (Fig. 4). Association between PTKs and PLCγ is mediated largely by the SH2 region of PLC binding to PY of the activated PTK. Phosphorylation of PLCγ1 on tyrosine residues is sufficient to increase its catalytic activity (Nishibe et al. 1990; Rhee and Choi 1992a).

We examined sperm for the presence of PLCγ1 using a mixture of six mAbs raised against various PLCγ1 epitopes contained in bovine brain (Suh et al. 1988). Immunostaining studies indicate that PLCγ1 localizes

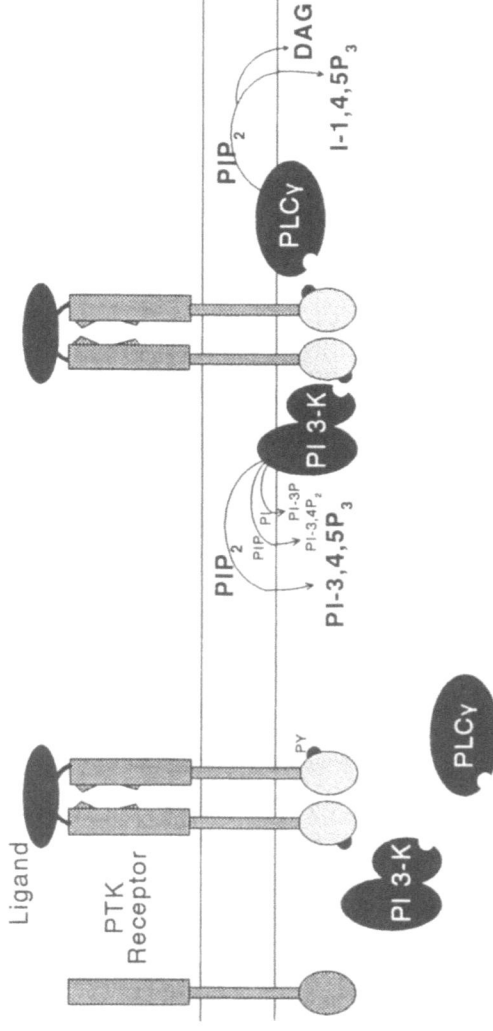

Fig. 4. A model for activation of phospholipase Cγ (*PLCγ*) and phosphatidylinositol 3-kinase (*PI 3-K*) signaling pathways downstream from coupling to a receptor tyrosine kinase. *PTK*, protein tyrosine kinase; *DAG*, diacylglycerol

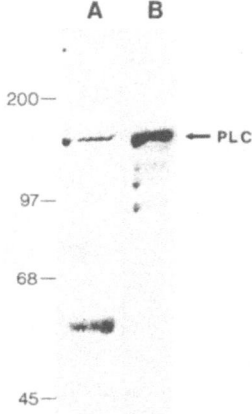

Fig. 5. Anti-phospholipase Cγl antibodies detect PLCγl (*PLC*) in mouse sperm (*lane A*) and brain (*lane B*). An anti-PLCγl monoclonal antibody cocktail was used to probe the samples indicated, and reactivity was detected using ECL (Amersham). The molecular weight standards (kDa×10^{-3}) are indicated to the *left* of lane A

to the acrosomal region (Tomes et al. 1995), a location consistent with a role in acrosomal exocytosis. Immunoblot analysis demonstrates the presence of a 145-kDa protein in mouse sperm that comigrates with mouse brain PLCγl (Fig. 5), suggesting that related, if not identical, forms are present in these tissues. However, the amount of enzyme from the two sources appears to differ significantly, since a substantially lower anti-PLCγl signal is observed in the sperm sample (lane A) despite a tenfold greater protein load.

12.5.1 PLCγl Is Phosphorylated on Tyrosine in Capacitated Sperm

To determine whether the PLCγl present in sperm is catalytically active, we measured PLC activity in immunoprecipitates. Phosphatidylinositol 4,5-bisphosphate (PIP$_2$)-PLC activity from capacitated sperm is recovered in immunoprecipitates with antibodies to PLCγl as well as to

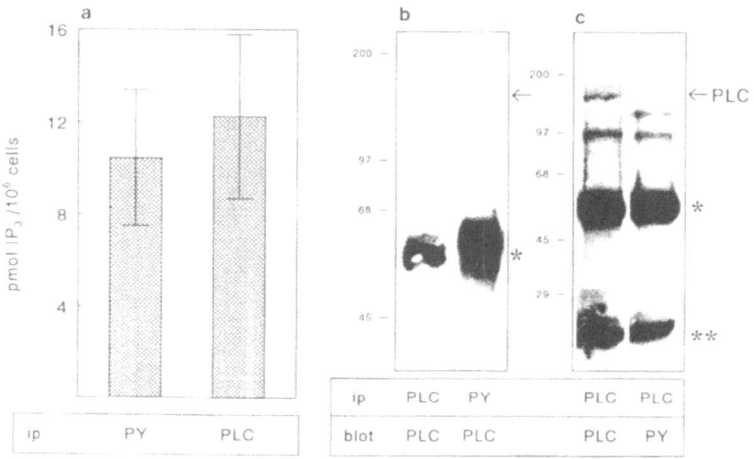

Fig. 6a–c. Phospholipase Cγ1 (*PLC*) is tyrosine phosphorylated in capacitated sperm. **a** Immunoprecipitation of PIP$_2$-PLC activity by antibodies to PLCγ1 and phosphotyrosine (*PY*). Sperm lysates were solubilized in NP40 lysis buffer and incubated with anti-PLCγ1 antibody for 2 h at room temperature followed by overnight incubation with anti-mouse IgG coupled to agarose at 4°C. Identical extracts were incubated with PY20-agarose overnight at 4°C. Immunoprecipitates were washed with cold lysis buffer and assayed for PLC activity using a modification of the method of Rhee et al. (1991). Generation of IP$_3$ in the PLC assay was confirmed by ion-exchange chromatography on Dowex AG 1-X8 (Sigma, St. Louis, MO, USA) (Berridge et al. 1983). Results are expressed as pmol IP$_3$ formed per million cells. The data represent the mean and SD of three independent experiments. **b** Triton X-100 extracts of capacitated cells were immunoprecipitated (*ip*) using anti-PLCγ1 or anti-PY antibodies. The immunoprecipitates were subjected to sodium dodecyl sulfate-polyacrylamide gel electrophoresis (SDS-PAGE), transferred, and probed with anti-PLCγ1 antibodies. Electrophoretic migration of PLCγ1 is indicated with an *arrow*. An *asterisk* indicates the position of immunoglobulin heavy chain. The molecular weight standards (kDa×10^{-3}) are indicated to the *left* of **b**. **c** Triton X-100 extracts of capacitated cells were immunoprecipitated (ip) using anti-PLCγ1 antibodies. The immunoprecipitates were subjected to SDS-PAGE, transferred, and probed with anti-PLCγ1 or anti-PY antibodies. Electrophoretic migration of PLCγ1 is indicated with an *arrow*. An *asterisk* indicates the heavy chain and a *double asterisk* indicates the light chain of immunoglobulin. The 97-kDa band present in **c** represents material that is precipitated with protein A-agarose purchased from Sigma; the corresponding product from Pierce (Rockford, IL, USA) (**b**) does not precipitate this protein. The molecular weight standards (kDa×10^{-3}) are indicated to the *left* of **c**

PY (Fig. 6a). Immunoblot analysis confirms the presence of PLCγ1 in both of these immunoprecipitates (Fig. 6b). While considerable PLC was measured in the anti-PY immunoprecipitates, no direct comparison between the levels of PLC activity recovered here can be attempted due to the use of unrelated primary antibodies, each with an independent efficiency of precipitation. Tyrosine phosphorylation of the γ class of PLC has been reported in a variety of cell types (Rhee and Choi 1992a, b). To determine whether PLCγ in capacitated mouse sperm is tyrosine phosphorylated, extracts from capacitated cells were immunoprecipitated with anti-PLCγ1 antibodies and probed on blots with anti-PY (Fig. 6c). A band at 145 kDa comigrating with PLCγ1 is observed, suggesting that a portion of the PLCγ1 present in capacitated mouse sperm is phosphorylated in vivo.

12.5.2 ZP3 Activates PLC Activity in Capacitated Sperm via Tyrosine Phosphorylation

Stimulation of cells with a variety of ligands, including growth factors, hormones, mitogens, and antigens, leads to an increased turnover in phosphoinositide metabolism through activation of tyrosine kinases and PLCγ1. We observe analogous results when mouse sperm are exposed to their stimulating ligand, zp proteins (Tomes et al. 1995). For these experiments, sperm were capacitated and then exposed to solubilized zp proteins. After treatment for 30 min, PIP_2-PLC activity was measured in cell lysates. We found that PLC activity was increased nearly twofold in zp-treated cells compared to nontreated controls. Recombinant mouse ZP3 substitutes for whole solubilized zp proteins in stimulating PIP_2-PLC activity. Pretreatment of capacitated sperm with tyrphostin, at doses similar to those that block zp-induced ARs (Leyton et al. 1992), prevents the zp-stimulated formation of I-1,4,5P_3. The inhibitory effect of tyrphostin did not result from drug toxicity since sperm motility was not affected significantly by culture in the presence of tyrphostin for 2 h. These results indicate that ZP3 binding to capacitated mouse sperm stimulates PLC activity, and that this stimulation relies on the functional operation of a sperm tyrosine kinase(s).

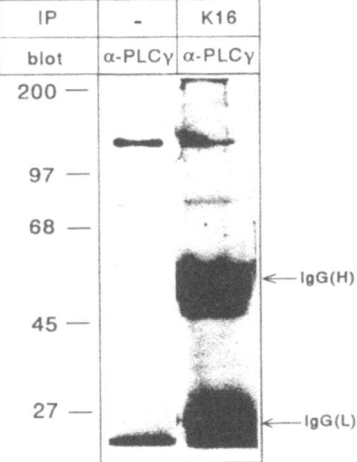

Fig. 7. Phospholipase Cγ1 (α-PLCγ) coprecipitates with zona receptor kinase (ZRK) in capacitated human sperm. *Left lane*: To ascertain the presence of PLCγ1, human sperm proteins were separated by sodium dodecyl sulfate-poly-acrylamide gel electrophoresis (SDS-PAGE), transferred to nitrocellulose, and probed with anti-PLCγ1 antibodies. *Right lane*: To determine whether PLCγ1 coprecipitates with ZRK, extracts of capacitated sperm were immunoprecipitated using K16, an anti-ZRK antibody (Burks et al. 1995a); precipitated proteins were analyzed by immunoblot using anti-PLCγ1 antibodies, as described. A band of approximately 145 kDa that comigrates with PLCγ1 is found. Due to the indirect method of detection, the heavy [*IgG (H)*] and light [*IgG (L)*] immunoglobulin G chains of the immunoprecipitating antibody are also apparent. The molecular weight standards (kDa×10^{-3}) are indicated on the *left*

12.5.3 PLCγ1 Coprecipitates with ZRK in Capacitated Sperm

Cell fractionation studies indicate that the majority of mouse sperm PLCγ1 is located in the cytosol when noncapacitated sperm are examined. In contrast, when capacitated sperm are analyzed, approximately half of the detectable PLCγ1 partitions with the membrane fraction. A coincident shift in electrophoretic mobility suggests phosphorylation of PLCγ1 in capacitated cells (see also Fig. 6) (Tomes et al. 1995). Immunoprecipitation studies using the K16 antibody with human sperm reveal that PLCγ1 coprecipitates with ZRK in capacitated sperm (Fig. 7); this association is not detected in noncapacitated sperm, consistent with our observation of PLCγ1 translocation to mouse sperm membranes during capacitation (Tomes et al. 1995). Collectively, these data suggest that PLCγ1 couples to ZRK as a consequence of capacitation, a process during which ZRK becomes tyrosine phosphorylated. Furthermore, our observations that ZP3 stimulates IP_3 production in a PTK-mediated pathway indicates that PLCγ1 may constitute a key element in the cascade that couples sperm binding to ZP3 with regulated acrosomal exocytosis.

12.6 ZRK Interaction with PI 3-K

PI 3-K associates with and is activated by a number of proteins containing PTK activity, including receptor PTKs (Varticovski et al. 1994). This enzyme, which exists as a heterodimer of a regulatory 85-kDa subunit (p85) and a catalytically active 110-kDa subunit (p110) (Fry and Waterfield 1993), catalyzes the formation of a family of phosphoinositides with phosphate at the D-3 position of the inositol ring (Auger et al. 1989). The production of PI-3,4,5P_3 in particular by PI 3-K correlates well with the activation of differentiated cellular functions, such as granule secretion in platelets (Stephens et al. 1993). The p85 subunit contains SH2 and SH3 domains, but no intrinsic PI 3-K activity; this subunit may be considered an adapter, using its SH2 domains to bind activated PTKs to the catalytically active p110 subunit (Fig. 4). Wortmannin has recently been described as a membrane-permeable inhibitor of PI 3-K, both in extracts and in whole cells, with an IC_{50} of ~2 nM; inhibition is due to wortmannin binding to p110 and inactivation of its catalytic activity (Yano et al. 1993). In the mast cell line RBL 2H3, wortmannin inhibition of PI 3-K blocks histamine secretion (Yano et al. 1993).

We have detected both the p85 and the p110 subunits of PI 3-K in sperm and found that, together with ZRK, p85 displays a capacitation-dependent increase in tyrosine phosphorylation (Burks et al. 1995c). We have also found that p85 translocates from a soluble (S) to a particulate (P) fraction of mouse sperm as a consequence of capacitation (Fig. 8). When p85 immunoprecipitates of human sperm are probed with anti-

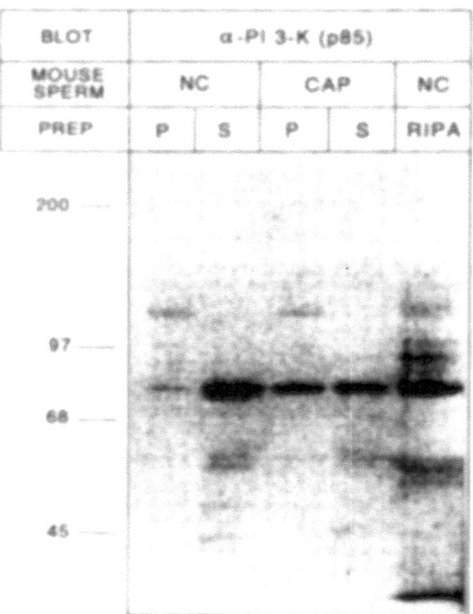

Fig. 8. Phosphatidylinositol 3-kinase *[α-PI 3-K (p85)]* translocates to the membrane in capacitated mouse sperm. Noncapacitated (*NC*) and capacitated (*CAP*) mouse sperm were separated into soluble (*S*) and particulate (*P*) fractions and probed on blots with anti-PI 3-K (p85α). An extract of NC unfractionated mouse sperm (*RIPA*) was analyzed similarly. The molecular weight standards (kDa×10⁻³) are indicated on the *left*. *PREP*, type of sperm preparation

PY, ZRK is also detected in capacitated, but not noncapacitated, sperm preparations. Reciprocally, anti-PY immunoprecipitates of capacitated sperm demonstrate the presence of p85 (Burks et al. 1995c). These experiments suggest that ZRK and p85 are associated physically and tyrosine-phosphorylated in capacitated, but not in noncapacitated, sperm. Consistent with models developed in somatic cells, p85 appears to serve as a substrate for activated ZRK. When the kinase activity of K16 immunoprecipitates is assessed, ^{32}P incorporation into an 85-kDa band that comigrates with p85 is increased significantly with ZP3 preincubation. Not unexpectedly, ZRK phosphorylation is also increased in this situation as is the phosphorylation of several other proteins (Burks et al. 1995a). To test whether PI 3-K activation is relevant to acrosomal exocytosis, we incubated human sperm with the PI 3-K inhibitor wortmannin (Burks et al. 1995c). Treatment of capacitated human sperm with 1 or 100 nM wortmannin resulted in inhibition of hZP3 stimulated ARs by 64% and 87%, respectively (Burks et al. 1995c). Since these same wortmannin treatments inhibited A23187-stimulated ARs four- to fivefold less effectively, it appears that PI 3-K acts predominantly prior to Ca^{2+} influx.

Given the presence of consensus motifs for binding both PI 3-K(p85) and for Grb-2 in ZRK, the interaction between PI 3-K and ZRK could be either direct or indirect (Fig. 3). There is precedence for both possibilities (Van der Geer et al. 1994) and it will be exciting to determine which mode(s) of interaction operates in sperm.

12.7 Summary and Perspectives

Our present results indicate that a 95-kDa protein with characteristics of a tyrosine kinase, named ZRK, serves as a ZP3 receptor in sperm. Since ZP3 binding triggers acrosomal exocytosis in sperm, we are eager to explore the potential role of ZRK in regulated exocytosis. Molecular cloning studies define a cDNA isolated from human testis, *hu9*, that is likely to encode human ZRK and predict that its structure is that of a receptor PTK. Expression of bioactive human ZP3 in COS cells (Burks et al. 1995b) has allowed us to examine ZP3–ZRK interaction and its consequences. We have found that human ZP3 stimulates acrosomal exocytosis as well as the tyrosine kinase activity of ZRK. Conversely, tyrphostin RG50864, a specific tyrosine kinase inhibitor, blocks both acrosomal exocytosis and tyrosine phosphorylation of ZRK. To investigate the signaling pathways that ZRK might exploit in the sperm cell to promote exocytosis, we noted that the primary structure of ZRK contains consensus motifs for the binding of a variety of SH2 domain-containing signaling proteins. Thus far, we have analyzed interaction of ZRK with two of these candidates: PLCγ and PI 3-K. We have found that PLCγ is present in the sperm head acrosomal region and associates with tyrosine-phosphorylated ZRK. A consequence of this interaction is tyrosine phosphorylation of PLCγ. Consistent with this association, we find that ZP3 stimulates IP_3 production in sperm via a tyrosine kinase-mediated pathway. Turning to PI 3-K, we have identified both the regulatory (p85) and catalytic (p110) subunits in sperm. The p85 subunit associates with tyrosine-phosphorylated ZRK and itself becomes tyrosine phosphorylated. The relevance of this interaction to sperm pathways is highlighted by the finding that wortmannin, a PI 3-K inhibitor, blocks ZP3-stimulated acrosomal exocytosis. Collectively, these findings suggest a crucial role for tyrosine phosphorylation in sperm fertilizing ability and initiate the delineation of signaling pathways activated by ZP3 binding.

However, many questions regarding ZRK-mediated signaling remain to be investigated. Regulation of the tyrosine kinase activity of ZRK demands the presence of a corresponding PTPase. A prime candidate PTPase is SHPTP2 (PTP1D, Syp), a widely distributed cytoplasmic PTPase that has been shown to interact via its SH2 domains with receptor PTKs such as epidermal growth factor (EGF)-R and platelet-derived growth factor (PDGF)-R. The ZRK sequence has revealed a SHPTP2 SH2 binding consensus site. Similarly, the presence of a consensus binding site in ZRK for the SH2 domain of Csk prompts curiosity about the potential role of Csk, or related tyrosine kinases, in ZRK signaling. Csk is a PTK that inactivates Src through phosphorylation of its C-terminal Tyr (Y527). These and related questions about ZRK will be facilitated by an examination of expressed ZRK in cultured cells, which is an approach that we would like to pursue to ultimately define individual residues in ZRK that are essential for its functions of ZP3 binding and signal transduction.

Acknowledgements. Work in the authors' laboratory was supported by grants from the NIH (HD18201 and HD29125) and the Andrew W. Mellon Foundation. CT is a Pew Latin American Fellow, supported by fellowships from The Pew Charitable Trusts, The Lalor Foundation, and the Fogarty International Center of the NIH.

References

Almeida EA, Huovila AP, Sutherland AE, Stephens LE, Calarco PG, Shaw LM, Mercurio AM, Sonnenberg A, Primakoff P, Myles DG (1995) Mouse egg integrin $\alpha6\beta1$ functions as a sperm receptor. Cell 81:1095–1104

Auger KR, Serunian LA, Soltoff SP, Libby P, Cantley LC (1989) PDGF-dependent tyrosine phosphorylation stimulates production of novel polyphosphoinositides in intact cells. Cell 57:167–175

Bennett MK, Scheller RH (1993) The molecular machinery for secretion is conserved from yeast to neurons. Proc Natl Acad Sci USA 90:2559–2563

Berridge MJ, Dawson M, Downes CP, Heslop JP, Irvine RF (1983) Changes in the levels of inositol phosphates after agonist-dependent hydrolysis of membrane phosphoinositides. Biochem J 212:473–482

Blobel CP, Wolfsberg TG, Turck CW, Myles DG, Primakoff P, White JM (1992) A potential fusion peptide and an integrin ligand domain in a protein active in sperm-egg fusion. Nature 356:248–252

Bookbinder LH, Cheng A, Bleil JD (1995) Tissue- and species-specific expression of sp56, a mouse sperm fertilization protein. Science 269:86–89

Burks DJ, Carballada R, Moore HDM, Saling PM (1995a) Interaction of a tyrosine kinase from human sperm with the zona pellucida at fertilization. Science 269:83–86

Burks DJ, McLeskey SB, Morales P, Saling PM (1995b) Activation of human sperm ZRK using recombinant human ZP3 (submitted)

Burks DJ, Tomes CN, Saling PM (1995c) PI 3-Kinase couples to ZRK and regulates acrosomal exocytosis in human sperm (submitted)

Cardullo RA, Wolf DE (1995) Distribution and dynamics of mouse sperm surface galactosyltransferase: implications for mammalian fertilization. Biochemistry 34:10027–10035

Cheng A, Le T, Palacios M, Bookbinder LH, Wassarman PM, Suzuki F, Bleil JD (1994) Sperm-egg recognition in the mouse: characterization of sp56, a sperm protein having specific affinity for ZP3. J Cell Biol 125:867–878

Cunningham SA, Waxham MN, Arrate PM, Brock TA (1995) Interaction of the Flt-1 tyrosine kinase receptor with the p85 subunit of phosphatidylinositol 3-kinase – mapping of a novel site involved in binding. J Biol Chem 270:20254–20257

Epifano O, Dean J (1994) Biology and structure of the zona pellucida: a target for immunocontraception. Reprod Fertil Dev 6:319–330

Fry MJ, Waterfield MD (1993) Structure and function of phosphatidylinositol 3-kinase: a potential second messenger system involved in growth control. Philos Trans R Soc Lond 340:337–344

Gmachl M, Sagan S, Ketter S, Kreil G (1993) The human sperm protein PH-20 has hyaluronidase activity. FEBS Lett 336:545–548

Gong XH, Dubois DH, Miller DJ, Shur BD (1995) Activation of a G protein complex by aggregation of β-1,4-galactosyltransferase on the surface of sperm. Science 269:1718–1721

Leyton L, Saling P (1989a) 95 kD sperm proteins bind ZP3 and serve as tyrosine kinase substrates in response to zona binding. Cell 57:1123–1130

Leyton L, Saling P (1989b) Evidence that aggregation of mouse sperm receptors by ZP3 triggers the acrosome reaction. J Cell Biol 108:2163–2168

Leyton L, LeGuen P, Bunch D, Saling PM (1992) Regulation of mouse gamete interaction by a sperm tyrosine kinase. Proc Natl Acad Sci USA 89:11692–11695

Li W, Nishimura R, Kashishian A, Batzer AG, Kim WJH, Cooper JA, Schlessinger J (1994) A new function for a phosphotyrosine phosphatase: linking GRB2-Sos to a receptor tyrosine kinase. Mol Cell Biol 14:509–517

Lin Y, Mahan K, Lathrop WF, Myles DG, Primakoff P (1994) A hyaluronidase activity of the sperm plasma membrane protein PH-20 enables sperm to penetrate the cumulus cell layer surrounding the egg. J Cell Biol 125:1157–1163

Lo Leggio L, Williams RM, Jones R (1994) Some effects of zona pellucida glycoproteins and sulfated polymers on the autoactivation of boar sperm proacrosin and activity of β-acrosin. J Reprod Fertil 100:177–185

Miller DJ, Macek MB, Shur BD (1992) Complementarity between sperm surface β-1,4-galactosyltransferase and egg-coat ZP3 mediates sperm-egg binding. Nature 357:589–593

Moore HDM, Hartman TD, Bye AP, Lutjen P, De Witt M, Trounson AO (1987) Monoclonal antibody against a sperm antigen Mr 95,000 inhibits attachment of human spermatozoa to the zona pellucida. J Reprod Immunol 11:157–166

Myles DG, Primakoff P (1991) Sperm proteins that serve as receptors for the zona pellucida and their post-testicular modification. Ann N Y Acad Sci 637:486–493

Ning X, Ward CR, Kopf GS (1995) Activation of a Gi protein in digitonin/cholate-solubilized membrane preparations of mouse sperm by the zona pellucida, an egg-specific extracellular matrix. Mol Reprod Dev 40:355–363

Nishibe S, Wahl MI, Hernandez-Sotomayor SM, Tonks NK, Rhee SG, Carpenter G (1990) Increase of the catalytic activity of phospholipase C-γ1 by tyrosine phosphorylation. Science 250:1253–1256

Rhee SG, Choi KD (1992a) Regulation of inositol phospholipid-specific phospholipase C isozymes. J Biol Chem 267:12393–12396

Rhee SG, Choi KD (1992b) Multiple forms of phospholipase C isozymes and their activation mechanisms. Adv Sec Messenger Phosphoprot Res 26:35–61

Rhee SG, Ryu SH, Lee KY, Cho KS (1991) Assays of phosphoinositide-specific phospholipase C and purification of isozymes from bovine brains. Methods Enzymol 197:502–511

Saling PM, Burks DJ, Carballada MR, Dowds CA, Leyton L, McLeskey SB, Robinson AG, Tomes CN (1995) Sperm interaction with the zona pellucida: the role of ZRK. In: Fenichel P, Parinaud J (eds) The human sperm acrosome reaction. Libbey Eurotext, Montrouge, France, pp 85–104

Songyang Z, Shoelson SE, McGlade J, Olivier P, Pawson T, Bustelo XR, Barbacid M, Sabe H, Hanafusa H, Yi T, Ren R, Baltimore D, Ratnofsky S, Feldman RA, Cantley LC (1994) Specific motifs recognized by the SH2 domains of Csk, 3BP2, fps/fes, GRB-2, HCP, SHC, Syk, and Vav. Mol Cell Biol 14:2777–2785

Stephens LR, Jackson TR, Hawkins PT (1993) Agonist-stimulated synthesis of phosphatidylinositol(3,4, 5)-trisphosphate: a new intracellular signalling system. Biochim Biophys Acta Mol Cell Res 1179:27–75

Suh PG, Ryu SH, Choi WC, Lee KY, Rhee SG (1988) Monoclonal antibodies to three phospholipase C isozymes from bovine brain. J Biol Chem 263:14497–14504

Tomes CN, McMaster C, Saling PM (1995) Activation of mouse PIP_2-PLC by zona pellucida is modulated by tyrosine phosphorylation. Mol Reprod Dev (in press)

Topfer-Petersen E, Cechova D (1990) Zona pellucida induces conversion of proacrosin to acrosin. Int J Androl 13:190–196

Van der Geer P, Hunter T, Lindberg RA (1994) Receptor protein-tyrosine kinases and their signal transduction pathways. Annu Rev Cell Biol 10:251–337

Varticovski L, Harrison-Findik D, Keeler ML, Susa M (1994) Role of PI 3-kinase in mitogenesis. Biochim Biophys Acta Mol Basis Dis 1226:1–11

Ward CR, Kopf GS (1993) Molecular events mediating sperm activation. Dev Biol 158:9–34

Wassarman PM (1994) Gamete interactions during mammalian fertilization. Theriogenology 41:31–44

Wassarman PM (1995) Mammalian fertilization – egg and sperm (glyco)proteins. Am J Reprod Immunol 33:253–258

Williams RM, Jones R (1993) Specificity of binding of zona pellucida glycoproteins to sperm proacrosin and related proteins. J Exp Zool 266:65–73

Wolfsberg TG, Primakoff P, Myles DG, White JM (1995) ADAM, a novel family of membrane proteins containing a disintegrin and metalloprotease domain – multipotential functions in cell-cell and cell-matrix interactions. J Cell Biol 131:275–278

Yagamihiromasa T, Sato T, Kurisaki T, Kamijo K, Nabeshima Y, Fujisawasehara A (1995) A metalloprotease-disintegrin participating in myoblast fusion. Nature 377:652–656

Yanagimachi R (1994) Mammalian fertilization. In: Knobil E, Neill JD (eds) The physiology of reproduction. Raven, New York, pp 189–317

Yano H, Nakanishi S, Kimura K, Hanai N, Saitoh Y, Fukui Y, Nonomura Y, Matsuda Y (1993) Inhibition of histamine secretion by wortmannin through the blockade of phosphatidylinositol 3-kinase in RBL-2H3 cells. J Biol Chem 268:25846–25856

13 The Use of Spermatids for Human Conception

I. Aslam and S. Fishel

13.1 Introduction 272
13.2 Abnormal Spermatogenesis and Infertility 273
13.2.1 Hypospermatogenesis 273
13.2.2 Maturation Arrest 273
13.2.3 Sertoli Cell Only Syndrome 274
13.3 Spermatid Microinjection: A New Approach in the Treatment
  of Male Infertility 275
13.4 Changes in DNA and Nucleoproteins During Spermatogenesis .. 276
13.5 The Stage of Cell Cycle and Its Effect on Success
  of Spermatid Microinjection 276
13.6 The Role of Genomic Imprinting 277
13.7 The Role of Oocyte Activation 280
13.8 The Role of Sperm Centrosome in Fertilisation 280
13.9 The Method of Separation, Culture and Cryopreservation
  of Spermatids 281
13.10 Conclusion 281
References 282

13.1 Introduction

Human conception is initiated by fertilisation, a process involving the interaction between the male and female gametes – the spermatozoon and ovum, respectively. Their interaction is complex and, for the spermatozoa this involves penetration of the cumulus oophorous and corona radiata cells, temporary and permanent binding to the zona pellucida, release of the acrosomal contents and a change in the state of motility to one of hyperactivation, penetration of the zona pellucida and fusion with the vitelline membrane. Once the spermatozoon is incorporated into the ooplasm of the activated oocyte, the latter being induced by a putative sperm cytosolic component (Swann 1990), the sperm nucleus is triggered to decondense in synchrony with the female nucleus to form two visible pronuclei. Fertilisation culminates in the fusion of the genetic material from both gametes (syngamy) following breakdown of the pronuclei membranes at this zygote stage. For an optimal chance of conception in vivo, a minimum number of sperm need to be ejaculated; this is estimated to be approximately 20 million per millilitre, or 40 million per ejaculate, with 50% or more having forward progression and 30% or more with normal morphology (WHO 1992).

In preparation for fertilisation, both male and female germ cells undergo a number of changes. Mature spermatozoa arise from the metamorphosis of precursor cells. Primordial prospermatogenic germ cells colonise the developing gonads early in fetal life, and, at puberty, the spermatogonia start a series of mitotic divisions (mitotic phase) resulting in an expansion of their number. These cells then undergo two reductional divisions (meiotic phase) resulting in the formation of spermatids. The early spermatids are rounded cells (round spermatids) which are remodelled through various elongating stages (elongated spermatids) to the fully formed spermatozoa (spermiogenic phase). During this phase, only pre-existing structures are reshaped. This sequence of cytological events that results in the formation of mature spermatozoa from precursor cells occurs in the seminiferous tubules of the adult male testes and is known as spermatogenesis (de Kretser and Kerr 1994).

In man, abnormalities can arise during any stage of spermatogenesis which result in a decrease in the number of developed spermatozoa (oligozoospermia) or affect the shape of mature spermatozoa (teratozoospermia) and/or the motility (asthenozoospermia). In many cases, all three conditions arise together. Furthermore, many men (perhaps 1%–2% of all cases of infertility) have such extreme dysfunction that spermatozoa do not develop at all (azoospermia); these men may ejaculate only immature cells – the spermatids, or these may be extracted from testicular material. It is the use of these immature cells for human conception that is considered in this chapter. Both approaches have resulted in normal human offspring (Fishel et al. 1995; Tesarik et al. 1995).

13.2 Abnormal Spermatogenesis and Infertility

The evaluation of testicular biopsy of the infertile male can be categorised within the following morphologic classification: hypospermatogenesis, maturation arrest and Sertoli cell only syndrome.

13.2.1 Hypospermatogenesis

Hypospermatogenesis is characterised by reduced spermatogenesis, affecting all stages of germinal cells in a uniform manner. This reduction can be mild, moderate or severe in degree (Colgan et al. 1980). For unknown reasons, many of these patients are azoospermic.

13.2.2 Maturation Arrest

In maturation arrest spermatogenesis is halted at either a late (spermatid) or early (spermatocyte) stage in the majority of tubules. In any particular patient, the level of the arrest is constant. Maturation of germinal cells is qualitatively and probably quantitatively determined by the genes. In some cases, the arrest of spermatogenesis at various stages can be brought about by gene mutations, the chromosomal pattern of the individual being either normal or abnormal (Skakkebaek et al. 1973). Probably not all cases of maturation arrest are due to genetic mutations. In some cases inadequate gonadotropic stimulation may be the cause of this condition. Franchimont et al. (1972) showed that azoospermic patients in whom spermatogenesis was arrested prior to the spermatid stage had elevated follicle-stimulating hormone (FSH) levels, while maturation arrest beyond the spermatid stage did not affect FSH levels. Another variant of maturation arrest is known as disorganised testis. Tubular walls are sometimes thickened, the tubular diameter is usually normal, and the Leydig cells are of normal appearance. Within the tubules, all stages of spermatogenesis can usually be observed, but immature cells are sloughed into the tubular lumen. Due to this premature separation of spermatogenic cells, the germinal epithelium may be depleted of distinct populations and appear arrested in its development prior to the stage presented by the sloughed cells. These may sometimes obstruct the tubular lumen, at least partially. The sloughing of immature germinal cells may be an expression of stress or injury exerted upon the testes. The ejaculates are mostly azoospermic or contain fragments of sloughed immature cells which are often misinterpreted as leucocytes (Glezerman 1982).

13.2.3 Sertoli Cell Only Syndrome

In Sertoli cell only syndrome the tubules demonstrate a total absence of germ cells, a decrease in size and the presence of Sertoli cells only. A variable degree of tubular fibrosis is present. The patients exhibit azoospermia (Glezerman 1982). This syndrome seems to occur rather frequently. In a series of 1294 cases of male infertility this condition was observed in 2.7% of patients (Dubin and Amelar 1971). Among azoospermic patients, this condition has been shown to account for approximately one third of cases (Chandley et al. 1976).

Quantitative analysis of testicular biopsy has proven that even when an extremely minute amount of sperm produced in a grossly deficient testicle results in absolute azoospermia in the ejaculate, there are a few spermatozoa being produced in the testicle (Silber and Rodriguez-Rigau 1981). For histological assessment of testicular cells fine needle aspiration can be used. Various seminiferous tubular cells can easily be identified in smears taken by fine needle aspiration (Rajwanshi et al. 1991).

In all cases, it is essential to appreciate the variations existing in the foci of seminiferous tubules. Does a single biopsy give an accurate picture of the above conditions? Definitions such as those described above may be erroneously recorded and patients denied an opportunity of treatment as a result.

13.3 Spermatid Microinjection:
A New Approach in the Treatment of Male Infertility

The development of intracytoplasmic sperm injection into oocytes (ICSI) has completely revolutionised the treatment of male infertility (Palermo et al. 1992). The combination of ICSI with percutaneous epididymal sperm aspiration (PESA), microscopic epididymal sperm aspiration (MESA), or testicular sperm extraction (TESE) requires only a few very weak, barely twitching sperm for normal fertilisation and pregnancy (Silber 1995). But even these may not be available in azoospermic patients due to incomplete spermatogenesis. This failure of spermatogenesis is seen clinically in Sertoli cell only syndrome, maturation arrest, postcryptorchidism tubular atrophy, postmumps orchitis and Klinefelters syndrome. There is no medical treatment for these conditions apart from the possibility of using the spermatids for conception to allow the man to have his own genetic offspring. The knowledge that the spermatids contain haploid DNA which is similar to that of the mature sperm led to this novel approach of injecting the spermatids into the oocytes for the treatment of such patients. The initial studies were done in mouse and hamster (Ogura and Yanagimachi 1993; Ogura et al. 1993) and live births have been reported in mouse (Ogura et al. 1994) and rabbit (Sofikitis et al. 1994). Since then there have been reports of fertilisation of the oocyte by spermatid injection in humans (Vanderzwalmen et al. 1995), ongoing pregnancy (Fishel et al. 1995) and live birth (Tesarik et al. 1995).

The success of these studies indicates that this option can help those azoospermic men who are capable of producing spermatids. There are a few aspects, however, which need careful consideration.

13.4 Changes in DNA and Nucleoproteins During Spermatogenesis

At the end of the mitotic phase, the germ cells undergo a phase of DNA replication which doubles the amount of DNA (S-phase resulting in 4n DNA) before progressing further into the meiotic phase (Tobias 1956). The first reductional division yields two daughter cells each with half the number of chromosomes (only one member of homologous pair), but each chromosome consisting of two chromatids and the 2n DNA. In the second meiotic division, chromatids separate to yield two haploid cells (spermatids), each containing only one complete set of chromosomes and 1n (half than somatic cell) DNA. The DNA is present in combination with nucleoproteins which are histones in the earlier stages of development. As the development of spermatids progresses, the histones of round spermatids are gradually replaced by protamines in elongated spermatids (Grimes 1986).

13.5 The Stage of Cell Cycle and Its Effect on Success of Spermatid Microinjection

The injected spermatid is at a different stage of the cell cycle and interacts with the cycle of the oocyte as they fuse together. The oocyte in metaphase II is in its M phase, whereas the spermatids are in the G2 phase (Edwards et al. 1994). This cell cycle imbalance is more pronounced if spermatids are injected into oocytes because the maturation factors that maintain oocytes in metaphase II drive the spermatid nuclei to M phase. There is a comparable situation when mature and immature oocytes are fused. When a mature metaphase II oocyte in M phase is fused with an immature oocyte with an intact germinal vesicle, the latter is forced to undergo premature chromosome condensation and enter meiosis (Balakier 1978). As the spermatids contain the haploid set of chromosomes, they behave like a cell in G1. G1 cells are compelled to form single chromatids, since their S phase has not begun and their chromatids have not divided. The problem of cell cycle imbalance between spermatid and metaphase II oocyte can be avoided by artificially activating the oocyte several hours before the injection. Non-physiological activation of the oocyte can be achieved by calcium ionophores or other stimuli. This drives the oocyte into its G2 phase. The cell cycle stages of spermatid and oocyte then coincide, and successful physiological activation is essential for clinical use.

An alternative approach is to inject the spermatid at the most advanced stage possible. In elongating spermatids, histone to protamine transition has begun and the presence of protamines might protect the sperm DNA from maturation factors of the oocyte (Edwards and Brody 1995). After fertilisation the sequence of events of formation of the male pronucleus are the breakdown of the sperm nuclear membrane, decondensation of the sperm chromatin, replacement of protamines with histones, formation of the pronuclear membrane and DNA synthesis (Wolgemuth 1983). Only activated oocytes between metaphase and telophase of the second meiosis are capable of dissociating the sperm nuclear membrane (Szollosi et al. 1988), and if the sperm nucleus is surrounded by its cytoplasm, this breakdown may not be instantaneous (Ogura et al. 1993).

Successful pregnancy and delivery after spermatid injection has proven that the sperm cytosolic factor required for oocyte activation is also present in the spermatid, and that spermatid injection can activate the oocyte (Tesarik et al. 1995). During the time interval in which the spermatid nuclear membrane is broken down (and it will be delayed if whole spermatid is injected), protamines are replaced by histones (if elongated spermatid is injected) and chromatin is decondensed, the oocyte passes from M to G2 and the cell cycle stages of spermatid and oocyte coincide. This results in the successful spermatid transfer. In the near future isolation and purification of the putative sperm cytosolic oscillogen (Swann 1990) may make this available for injection for oocyte activation.

13.6 The Role of Genomic Imprinting

Paternal and maternal genomes do not play an identical role during mammalian embryogenesis. The former appears to be preferentially needed for the development of extra-embryonic tissues and the latter for preimplantation development and embryogenesis (Barton et al. 1984). In addition, chromosomes of both parents are needed for development to proceed to term (McGrath and Solter 1984). While homologous chromosomes are spatially segregated during oogenesis and spermatogenesis, they are subjected to modifications that subsequently evoke different responses at later events throughout development. Hence, differential gene expression during development may be controlled in a major way by specific modifications of genes on homologous chromosomes prior to fertilisation (Surani 1986). DNA methylation has been postulated to play a role in this specific modification of the gene activity (Cedar 1984). DNA methylation renders the gene inactive (Keshet et al. 1986). So far, five imprinted genes have been found to be differentially methylated on the paternal and maternal alleles within somatic cells: mouse Igf2 (Brandeis et al. 1993), mouse Xist (Norris et al. 1994), and human SNRPN (Glenn et al. 1993) are paternally expressed and mouse Igf2r (Stoger et al. 1993) and mouse H19 (Bartolomei et al. 1993) are maternally expressed. A recent study proved that the methylation of DNA changes during development of sperm. Three genes were examined in mouse. All three genes were unmethylated in spermatogenic cells in the testis, but were remethylated in mature sperm. This shows that the remethylation is part of the process of sperm maturation which occurs in the epididymis (Ariel et al. 1994). If this proves to be similar in man, then, as the spermatid has not passed through the epididymal maturation process therefore, it can be suspected that spermatid injection into the oocyte may induce problems in embryo development. For example, the maternally inherited H19 allele is transcriptionally active, while the paternally inherited allele is silent (Bartolomei et al. 1991). The reactivation of the normally silent (paternal) allele has been reported in some Wilms tumor samples (Rainier et al. 1993).

As methylation is the basis of imprinting, by following the methylation changes of genes during gametogenesis and after fertilisation we can determine the role of genomic imprinting. While not all methylated sites in all genes behave identically, genes in sperm show more methylation than genes in eggs. The establishment of the methylation patterns of mature gametes is a gradual process. Both male and female fetal germ cells are unmethylated at embryonic day 12.5–13.5 and new methylation is not detected until day 15.5 (Howlett and Reik 1991; Kafri et al. 1992). It has been suggested that the ability of the fetal germ cells to avoid the wave of methylation which occurs at the late blastula/early gastrula stage is related to the migration of the fetal germ cell precursors from the epiblast into the yolk sac, where they remain before entering the fetal gonad. A combination of further methylations and new demethylations at specific sites occurs in both the male and female germ line, until the final gametic patterns are achieved postmeiotically during sperm and oocyte maturation. It should be noted that different sites within the same gene can be methylated in sperm alone or in both sperm and oocytes, i.e., differential parental methylation appears to occur at the level of individual sites and not necessarily entire genes (Kafri et al. 1992). The early embryo shows lower levels of methylation than do either mature sperm or oocytes, with indication of active demethylation during the first several cell divisions. The complete erasure of the methylation patterns of single-copy genes seems to be carried out by a two-step demethylation process. Sites methylated in sperm but not in oocytes are demethylated earlier and are completely unmethylated by the eight-cell stage of embryo development, whereas sites methylated in both gametes are demethylated between the eight- and sixteen-cell stage of development. Similarly, demethylation of multicopy genes appears to be a two-stage process. These waves of demethylation result in only 15% methylation at the blastocyst stage (Howlett and Reik 1991). A new wave of methylation occurs at about the time of implantation and increases at the time of gastrulation in embryonic lineages such that the patterns of methylation found in adult somatic tissues are established at about 6.5 days of gestation. The extra-embryonic lineages do not appear to undergo this wave of methylation (Monk et al. 1987). In imprinting genes, preferentially methylated sites maintain the methylation pattern even after fertilisation, and the pattern also persists in adult life (Razin and Kafri 1994).

It is known that paternal genome is needed for the development of the extra-embryonic tissue (Barton et al. 1984), therefore the risks involved are fairly low and in any case affect only the early viability of the zygote, not the fetus or the child. A recent study reported the increased success rate by changing the technique of spermatid transfer. When spermatids were electrofused with oocytes, the success rate was very low but by microinjection of spermatid into oocytes the success rate increased to 28.2% (Kimura and Yanagimachi 1995). These results suggest that changes in methylation pattern of certain genes after transport of testicular sperm through epididymis are not essential for embryonic development and perhaps the genomic imprinting is completed before the phase of spermiogenesis.

13.7 The Role of Oocyte Activation

Although it is generally agreed that intracellular calcium (Ca^{2+}) is the universal signal for triggering the oocyte activation (Vitullo and Ozil 1992; Homa et al. 1993; Tesarik et al. 1994), it is not clear how the sperm causes this Ca^{2+} change. Microinjection of cytosolic sperm extracts into unfertilised hamster eggs which stimulated a series of Ca^{2+} increases and mimicked fertilisation suggested that a cytosolic factor of sperm transferred into egg at the time of fertilisation causes the oocyte activation (Swann 1990). Later these findings were also confirmed in human oocytes (Tesarik et al. 1994; Dozortsev et al. 1995). Electron microscopic analysis of human oocytes that failed to display signs of fertilisation by ICSI suggested that this failure after ICSI is basically a failure of oocyte activation (Sousa and Tesarik 1994). This indicates that a suboptimal oocyte activation stimulus can arrest embryo development. The effect of oocyte activation on the success rate of spermatid miroinjection has been established by Kimura and Yanagimachi (1995). The highest rate (77%) of normal fertilisation of the oocytes with spermatid microinjection was obtained when the oocytes were first electrostimulated before injection. In human successful pregnancy and delivery after spermatid injection has indicated that the sperm cytosolic factor required for oocyte activation is probably present in the spermatid and spermatid injection can activate the oocyte (Fishel et al. 1995; Tesarik et al. 1995).

13.8 The Role of Sperm Centrosome in Fertilisation

In the process of fertilisation the sperm also contributes the centrosome, the microtubule-organising centre. The centrosome is composed of two centrioles: centriole duplication occurs at a specific stage in the cell cycle in order to produce two centrioles to regulate the two poles of the mitotic spindle (Edwards and Brody 1995). Their role is to organise the first and later cell divisions after fertilisation (Palermo et al. 1994). It was suggested very early that centriole is contributed by sperm (Boveri 1901), but the maternal inheritance observed in mice confused the picture (Schatten et al. 1991). It is now known that the centrosome has paternal inheritance (Simerly et al. 1995). Considering the critical role played by the centrosome in regulating first and later cell divisions of the embryo, by coupling cell growth with cell division (Maniotis and Schliwa 1991), a functionally imperfect centrosome, contributed by a spermatid, can induce problems both in early embryogenesis and at a later developmental stage. The microinjection of the whole spermatid will ensure the transfer of the centrosome.

13.9 The Method of Separation, Culture and Cryopreservation of Spermatids

In some patients suffering from azoospermia, spermatids are found in the ejaculate. Spermatids can be isolated from the semen or from testicular biopsies. Testicular material is digested with collagenase and trypsin and this results in the formation of the mixture of the germinal cells. This mixture of germinal cells is then separated into different fractions by sedimentation under unit gravity, with each fraction containing pure populations of a specific stage of germinal cells (Bellve 1993). For the separation of germinal cells from the human testicular material the same technique can be used (Shepherd et al. 1981), but the fraction which contains spermatids is contaminated with Leydig cells. Contaminating Leydig cells can be removed by density centrifugation in discontinuous Percoll gradients to yield 90%–95% pure, round spermatids (Narayan et al. 1983). The separated fractions of spermatids are viable as detected by the trypan blue exclusion test (I. Aslam and S. Fishel, unpublished). Spermatid fractions can be cultured for 48 h without much loss of the viability and even round spermatids show generation of flagella (Gerton and Millette 1984). Testicular sperms can be cryopreserved (Craft and Tsirigotis 1995). Therefore, it is hoped that spermatids can also be cryopreserved.

13.10 Conclusion

Some men produce spermatids as the only form of haploid genetic material for potential conception. These spermatids may be of testicular or ejaculate origin and may be in one of a varying number of stages between the round to elongated spermatid. It is known that there are subtle DNA-histone/protamine differences between the early- and late-stage spermatids and that genome imprinting may occur during this period. Whether the latter has any consequential bearing following conception using the spermatid is unclear, but this matter is currently under investigation. Some argue that the birth of three healthy offspring, two from ejaculated round spermatids (Tesarik et al. 1995) and one from a testicular elongated spermatid (Fishel et al. 1995), indicates that the concerns of genome imprinting are not an issue.

The fundamental processes required for successful conception after spermatid injection are oocyte activation, the presence of a centrosome and appropriately formed haploid DNA. Perhaps the future will see the microinjection "cocktail" as a mixture of paternal haploid DNA, reconstituted, purified oscillogen combined with a centrosome – ostensibly the only requirements from a spermatozoon for successful conception! With the advent of efficient methods for purification of specific stages of spermatids, especially from testicular material, and the addition of cryopreservation (Aslam I and Fishel S, unpublished), we will enter an era in which men will be given the option of producing their own genetic offspring by spermatid injection for hitherto intractable infertility.

References

Ariel M, Cedar H, McCarrey J (1994) Developmental changes in methylation of spermatogenesis-specific genes include reprogramming in the epididymis. Nature Genet 7:59–63

Balakier H (1978) Induction of maturation in small oocytes from sexually immature mice by fusion with meiotic or mitotic cells. Exp Cell Res 112:137–141

Bartolomei MS, Zemel S, Tilghman SM (1991) Parental imprinting of the mouse H19 gene. Nature 351:153–155

Bartolomei MS, Webber AL, Brunkov ME, Tilghman SM (1993) Epigenetic mechanisms underlying the imprinting of the mouse H19 gene. Genes Dev 7:1663–1673

Barton SC, Surani MAH, Norris ML (1984) Role of paternal and maternal genomes in mouse development. Nature 311:374–376

Bellve RA (1993) Purification, culture and fractionation of spermatogenic cells. Methods Enzymol 225:84–113

Boveri T (1901) Zellen-Studien: Über die Natur der Centrosomen IV. Fischer, Jena

Brandeis M, Kafri T, Ariel M, Chaillet JR, McCarrey JR, Razin J, Cedar H (1993) The ontogeny of allele-specific methylation associated with imprinted genes in the mouse. EMBO J 12:3669–3677

Cedar H (1984) DNA methylation and gene expression. In: Razin A, Cedar H, Riggs AD (eds) DNA methylation: biochemistry and biological significance. Springer, Berlin Heidelberg New York, pp 147–164

Chandley AC, Edmond P, Maclean N, Fletcher J, Watson ES (1976) Cytogenetics and infertility in man. II. Testicular histology and meiosis. Ann Hum Genet 40:165–176

Colgan TJ, Bedard YC, Strawbridge HTG, Buckspan MB, Klotz PG (1980) Reappraisal of the value of testicular biopsy in the investigation of infertility. Fertil Steril 33:56–60

Craft I, Tsirigotis M (1995) Simplified recovery, preparation and cryopreservation of testicular spermatzoa. Hum Reprod 10:1623–1627

de Kretser DM, Kerr JB (1994) The cytology of the testis. In: Knobil E, Neill JD (eds) The physiology of reproduction. Raven, New York, pp 1122–1290

Dozortsev D, Rybouchkin A, DeSutter P, Qian C, Dhont M (1995) Human oocyte activation following intracytoplasmic injection: the role of the sperm cell. Hum Reprod 10:403–407

Dubin L, Amelar RD (1971) Etiological factors in 1294 consecutive cases of male infertility. Fertil Steril 22:469–474

Edwards RG, Brody SA (1995) Principles and practice of assisted human reproduction. Saunders, Philadelphia

Edwards RG, Tarin JJ, Dean N, Hirsch A, Tan SL (1994) Are spermatid injections into human oocytes now mandatory? Hum Reprod 9:2217–2219

Fishel S, Green S, Bishop M, Thornton S, Hunter A, Fleming S, Al-Hassan S (1995) Pregnancy after intracytoplasmic injection of spermatid. Lancet 345:1641–1642

Franchimont P, Millet D, Vendrely E, Letawe J, Legros JJ, Netter A (1972) Relationship between spermatogenesis and serum gonadotrophin levels in azoospermia and oligospermia. J Clin Endocrinol Metab 34:1003–1008

Gerton GL, Millette CF (1984) Generation of flagella by cultured mouse spermatids. J Cell Biol 98:619–628

Glenn CC, Porter KA, Jong MTC, Nicholls RD, Driscoll DJ (1993) Functional imprinting and epigenetic modification of human SNRPN gene. Hum Mol Genet 2:2002–2005

Glezerman M (1982) Etiology of fertility disturbances in man. In: Bandhauer K, Frick J (eds) Disturbances in male fertility Springer, Berlin Heidelberg New York, pp 171–193 (Encyclopedia of urology, vol 16)

Grimes SR (1986) Nuclear proteins in spermatogenesis. Comp Biochem Physiol [B] 83:495–500

Homa ST, Carroll J, Swann K (1993) The role of calcium in mammalian oocyte maturation and egg activation. Hum Reprod 8:1274–1281

Howlett SK, Reik W (1991) Methylation levels of maternal and paternal genomes during preimplantation development. Development 113:119–127

Kafri T, Ariel M, Brandeis M, Shemer R, Urven L, McCarrey J, Cedar H, Razin A (1992) Developmental pattern of gene-specific DNA methylation in the mouse embryo and early germ lines. Genes Dev 6:705–714

Keshet I, Hurwitz JL, Cedar H (1986) DNA methylation affects the formation of active chromatin. Cell 44:535–543

Kimura Y, Yanagimachi R (1995) Mouse oocytes injected with testicular spermatozoa or round spermatids can develop into normal offspring. Development 121:2397–2405

Maniotis A, Schliwa M (1991) Microsurgical removal of centrosome blocks cell reproduction and centriole regeneration in BSC-1 cells. Cell 67:495–504

McGrath J, Solter D (1984) Completion of mouse embryogenesis requires both the maternal and paternal genomes. Cell 37:179–183

Monk M, Boubelik M, Lehnert S (1987) Temporal and regional changes in DNA methylation in the embryonic, extra-embryonic, and germ cell lineages during mouse embryo development. Development 99:371–382

Narayan P, Scott BK, Millette CF, DeWolf WC (1983) Human spermatogenic cell marker proteins detected by two-dimensional electrophoresis. Gemete Res 7:227–239

Norris DP, Patel D, Kay GF, Penny GD, Brockdorff N, Sheardown SA, Rastan S (1994) Evidence that random and imprinted Xist expression is controlled by preemptive methylation. Cell 77:41–51

Ogura A, Yanagimachi R (1993) Round spermatid nuclei injected into hamster oocytes form pronuclei and participate in syngamy. Biol Reprod 48:219–225

Ogura A, Yanagimachi R, Usui N (1993) Behaviour of hamster and mouse round spermatid nuclei incorporated into mature oocytes by electrofusion. Zygote 1:1–8

Ogura A, Matsuda J, Yanagimachi R (1994) Birth of normal young after electrofusion of mouse oocytes with round spermatid. Proc Natl Acad Sci USA 91:7460–7462

Palermo G, Joris H, Devroey P, Van Steirteghem AC (1992) Pregnancies after intracytoplasmic injection of single spermatozoon into an oocyte. Lancet 340:17–18

Palermo G, Munne S, Cohen J (1994) The human zygote inherits its mitotic potential from the male gamete. Hum Reprod 9:1220–1225

Rainier S, Johnson LA, Dobry CJ, Ping A, Grundy PA, and Feinberg AP (1993) Relaxation of imprinted genes in human cancer. Nature 362:747–749

Rajwanshi A, Indudhara R, Goswami AK, Radhika S, Das A, Sharma SK, Vaidyanathan S, Datta BN (1991) Fine needle aspiration cytology in azoospermic males. Diagn Cytopathol 7:3–6

Razin A, Kafri T (1994) DNA methylation from embryo to adult. Prog Nucleic Acid Res Mol Biol 48:53–81

Schatten G, Simerly C, Schatten H (1991) Maternal inheritance of centrosomes in mammals? Studies on parthenogenesis and polyspermy in mice. Proc Natl Acad Sci USA 88:6785–6789

Shepherd WR, Millette FC, DeWolf CW (1981) Enrichment of primary pachytene spermatocytes from the human testes. Gamete Res 4:487–498

Silber SJ (1995) What forms of male infertility are there left to cure. Hum Reprod 10:503–504

Silber SJ, Rodriguez-Rigau LJ (1981) Quantitative analysis of testicular biopsy: determination of partial obstruction and prediction of sperm count after surgery for obstruction. Fertil Steril 36:480–485

Simerly C, Wu G, Zoran S, Ord T, Rawlins R, Jones J, Navara C, Gerrity M, Rinehart J, Binor Z, Asch R, Schatten G (1995) The paternal inheritance of the centrosome, the cell's microtubule-organizing center, in humans and the implications for infertility. Nature Med 1:47–52

Skakkebaek N, Hulten M, Philip J (1973) Quantification of human seminiferous epithelium. IV. Histological studies in 17 men with numerical and structural autosomal aberrations. Acta Pathol Microbiol Scand [A] 81:112–124

Sofikitis N, Zavos P, Koutselinis A, Mourtzinis D, Loutradis D, Glanzounis G (1994) Achievement of pregnancy after injection of round spermatid (RS) nuclei into rabbit oocytes and embryo transfer:a possible mode of treatment for men with spermatogenic arrest at the spermatid stage. J Urol 5 [Suppl]:151

Sousa M, Tesarik J (1994) Ultrastructural analysis of fertilization failure after intracytoplasmic sperm injection. Hum Reprod 9:2374–2380

Stoger R, Kubicka P, Liu CC, Kafri T, Razin A, Cedar H, Barlow DP (1993) Maternal-specific methylation of the imprinted mouse Igf2r locus identifies the expressed locus as carrying the imprinting signal. Cell 73:61–71

Surani MZH (1986) Evidences and consequences of differences between maternal and paternal genomes during embryogenesis in the mouse. In: Rossant J, Pedersen RA (eds) Experimental approaches to mammalian embryonic development. Cambridge University Press, Cambridge, pp 401–435

Swann K (1990) A cytosolic sperm factor stimulates repetitive calcium increases and mimics fertilization in hamster eggs. Development 110:1295–1302

Szollosi D, Czolowska R, Szollosi M, Tarkowski AK (1988) Remodelling of mouse thymocyte nuclei depends on the time of their transfer into activated, homologous oocytes. J Cell Sci 91:603–613

Tesarik J, Sousa M, Testart J (1994) Human oocyte activation after intracytoplasmic sperm injection. Hum Reprod 9:511–518

Tesarik J, Mendoza C, Testart J (1995) Viable embryos from injection of round spermatids into oocytes. N Engl J Med 333:525

Tobias PV (1956) Chromosomes, sex cells and evolution in a mammal. Lund and Humphries, London

Vanderzwalmen P, Lejeune B, Nijs M, Bertin GS, Vandamme B, Schoysman R (1995) Fertilization of an oocyte microinseminated with a spermatid in an in vitro fertilization programme. Hum Reprod 10:502–503

Vitullo AD, Ozil JP (1992) Repetitive calcium stimuli derive meiotic resumption and pronuclei development during mouse oocyte activation. Dev Biol 151:128–136

WHO (1992) WHO laboratory manual for examination of human semen and sperm-cervical mucus interaction, 3rd edn. Cambridge University Press, Cambridge

Wolgemuth DJ (1983) Synthetic activities of the mammalian early embryo: molecular and genetic alterations following fertilisation. In: Hartmann JF (ed) Mechanism and control of animal fertilisation. Academic, New York, pp 415–452

14 Evidence-Based Andrology: The Importance of Controlled Clinical Trials

E. Leifke and E. Nieschlag

14.1   Introduction: Evidence-Based Medicine 287
14.2   Need for Controlled Clinical Trials 289
14.3   Considerations for the Design of Controlled Clinical Trials 290
14.4   Treatment Strategies in Andrology 292
14.4.1   Rational Therapy 294
14.4.2   Preventive Therapy 294
14.4.3   Empirical Therapy 296
14.4.4   Symptomatic Therapy with Assisted Fertilization 301
14.5   Conclusions 302
References 303

14.1 Introduction: Evidence-Based Medicine

The concept of *evidence-based medicine* has emerged over the past decades, and, by virtue of its pervasive influence, is becoming a "constitutional amendment" in all fields of clinical practice. Personal authority and skills born of experience are no longer the major determining factors when therapeutic decisions must be made. In addition to pathophysiological rationales and professional expertise, clinical practice should be based on properly designed studies and applied statistics, summarized under the term of *outcome research* (Evidence-Based Medicine Working Group 1992). While widely regarded as an oddity in

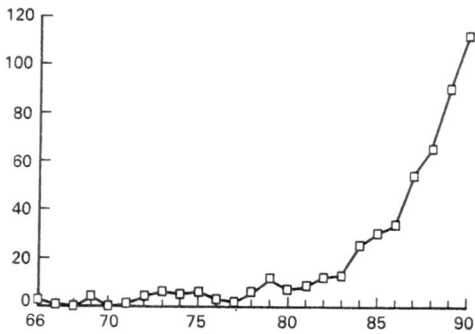

Fig. 1. The number of randomized, clinical trials displayed per year (*y-axis*) between 1966 and 1990 (*x-axis*) shows an exponential increase over the last decade (Vandekerckhove et al. 1993)

medicine up to the 1960s, today the controlled, prospective, randomized – and if possible – double-blind clinical trial is accepted as the most reliable method of proving the effectiveness of diagnostic and thera-peutic strategies. No drug, no surgical therapy, and not even a diagnostic test should enter or remain in clinical practice without evidence and outcome research-based confirmation of their benefits.

Compared to other fields of medicine, reproductive medicine and, in particular, andrology, was late in accepting the need for controlled clinical trials. Notwithstanding, the exponential increase in the number of published randomized, controlled clinical trials concerning infertility treatment over the last decade indicates the extent to which the paradigm of evidenced-based medicine has entered the field of reproductive medi-cine and andrology (Fig. 1) (Olive 1986; Vandekerckhove et al. 1993). The majority of these publications have focused on the newly intro-duced techniques of assisted reproduction as infertility treatment, while fewer concentrate on drug regimens. This proportion emphazises the need for more and intensified outcome research concerning empirical therapies widely used in andrology.

Approximately 10% of couples of reproductive age fail to conceive within 12 months of unprotected sexual intercourse and are considered infertile (Vessey et al. 1976). Male factors are responsible for about 30% of these cases (Hull et al. 1985). Relative to the high prevalence of male fertility disturbances in men of reproductive age, the therapeutic possibilities are rather limited. One reason is that the pathogenesis of many fertility disturbances has not yet been elucidated and therefore rational approaches to treatment are necessarily lacking in these cases. The question arises as to whether a profound biological understanding is always necessary to offer rational therapeutics in more or less unclear pathological conditions (Nieschlag 1994). In general, the less profound our basic understanding and laboratory models of therapeutic concepts are, the more necessary it is to perform clinical outcome research. Often it provides the only source for evidence-based clinical decisions. Furthermore, therapeutic concepts derived from laboratory results must be confirmed or challenged by clinical findings and require testing in controlled clinical trials.

14.2 Need for Controlled Clinical Trials

Ideally – but not very often – clinical trials prove what experimental studies and hypotheses have already suggested. For example, in conditions such as idiopathic hypogonadotropic hypogonadism (IHH) or its variant, Kallmann's syndrome, although pathogenetically not fully understood, specific substitution of what the endocrine system endogenously lacks will lead to reconstitution of male reproductive functioning. Here, the diagnostic entity as well as the outcome parameters for substitution therapy with pulsatile gonadotropin releasing hormone (GnRH) or gonadotropins are clearly definable (i.e., testosterone blood levels, testicular growth, appearance of sperm in the ejaculate). In this case, untreated control groups – ethical implications aside – would not reveal important information because there is good evidence that spontaneous recovery or reconstituition of reproductive functions cannot be expected without GnRH or gonadotropins (Schopohl et al. 1991; Kliesch et al. 1994). It is conceivable, however, that this situation may change, if in these cases of secondary hypogonadism a specific treatment regimen using certain hormone preparations has proved to be effective and a new treatment regimen with new hormone preparations should be tested. For example, it may seem appropriate to switch from intramuscular to subcutaneous gonadotropin application or to replace urinary by recombinant gonadotropin preparations. Such changes would require comparative controlled trials in order to establish which type of treatment is superior to the other.

The patients with secondary hypogonadism mentioned above comprise only a small portion of men attending an infertility clinic. About 30% of infertile patients suffer from nonspecific conditions generally summarized as "idiopathic infertility." In these cases the abnormalities found in semen parameters cannot be ascribed to a cause. In this condition, clinical outcome research applied to the varied and empirical therapies being offered is important to provide evidence for a nonstochastic cause-and-effect relationship. In addition to valid statistical methods, a clear-cut study design is necessary to minimize erroneous conclusions derived from possible selection bias and chance errors.

14.3 Considerations for the Design of Controlled Clinical Trials

Design and data analysis are the most important criteria for the quality of a fertility trial as well as in all other fields of clinical medicine (Olive 1986). Unlike laboratory research, clinical research is often less precise and more time-consuming. Prior to any high-quality study, much intellectual input is required if its design is to avoid bias and imprecision. Establishing cause-and-effect relationships is the essence of evaluating therapies in male infertility and the following points should be considered:

1. The study should be controlled to determine a baseline value for comparison and to exclude that effects seen are simply due to the change in time. When creating a control it should be taken into consideration that no medical intervention is without placebo effect (Kleijnen et al. 1994; Gotzsche 1994; Johnson 1994). Gotzsche introduced a pragmatic definition of what placebo is: *placebo is an intervention which is believed to lack a specific effect – i.e., an effect for which an empirically supported theory exists for its mechanism of action – on the condition in question, but which has been demonstrated to be better than no intervention.* That placebo does not exert a specific action for the condition being treated does, however, not mean that it is not evaluable or varying in magnitude. It

might be influenced itself by the physician's attitude and the expectations of patients. Patients, for example, who had good experience with certain drugs may react more favorably to placebos than those who had never used them or have had bad experience (Peck and Coleman 1991). In order to discriminate between intervention-associated specific and unspecific (placebo) effects it would be appropriate (although not always practicable) to include placebo-treated as well as untreated control groups in clinical studies.

2. Randomization is essential to ensure balance between known and unknown covariables in the control and the treatment groups, especially in poorly defined and therefore probably heterogenous conditions (such as idiopathic infertility).

3. In order to avoid the possibility that heterogeneity of patients masks or biases therapy effects, homogenization by inclusion or exclusion criteria, stratification, and a clear definition of the patients group is necessary.

4. Clear definition of outcome parameters such as semen concentration, motility or pregnancy rate, and sufficient follow-up investigations depending on the expected incidence of the parameter is necessary. Although cumulative pregnancies on the basis of life table calculation might be the best parameter for outcome research of male infertility treatment – because the induction of pregnancy and the birth of a healthy child is the goal of all infertility treatment – pregnancies may not always be a practical and, hence, reliable endpoint. Low pregnancy rates among infertile couples, small treatment effects with large sample sizes and long follow-ups are necessary as well, since additional female factors, previously not considered, may lead to interference. Despite these difficulties and because no sperm function test reliably predicting the fertility chances of a patient has yet been established, cumulative pregnancy rates will remain the most meaningful endpoint in infertility treatment studies.

5. Cross-over design should not be used. In particular the evaluation of drugs can be biased by carry-over effects of prolonged action. In addition, if pregnancy is the ultimate goal of therapy, responders in the first part of the trial would leave the study and thus bias the second part.

6. Statistics to estimate the power and the probability of false-positive (type I error) as well as false-negative (type II error) erroneous con-

clusions are necessary. The number of patients that has to be included in a trial on the basis of a power estimate is usually higher than the number of cases available in a given center at a certain period and the number of patients that can easily be handled by the investigators in a reasonable time.

7. Multicenter studies might provide larger sample sizes than single-center studies, but they may also have to deal with inhomogeneity between centers, and administrative problems may lead to difficulties and bias. In addition, the investigators may not be highly motivated since the most attractive reward in science (i.e., being first author of a good publication) is unlikely to be granted to them.

These points do not exclude, for example, that retrospective studies, observational surveys, or studies, in which a patient cohort is compared with historical control groups can also reveal meaningful information. However, they face a lot of potential problems and conclusions should be drawn with caution. Such studies must be reviewed critically by the authors, and placed or ranked appropriately in "a hierarchy of evidences" (Pocock 1983).

14.4 Treatment Strategies in Andrology

Male fertility disturbances may be classified according to pathophysiological concepts and therapeutic possibilities into

1. Those allowing rational treatment
2. Those requiring preventive treatment
3. Those for which no treatment is available
4. Those for which assisted fertilizing procedures offer symptomatic treatment
5. Those for which treatment is empirical or experimental

It is not the topic of the current paper to discuss the individual disorders and their therapies listed in Table 1 in detail. The reader is referred to more extensive reviews (e.g., Nieschlag 1993; Howards 1995) and here only a few examples will be highlighted. Especially group 5 will be discussed with regard to the considerations mentioned above.

Table 1. Classification of andrological therapies

Disorder	Therapy
1. Rational therapy	
Idiopathic hypogonadotropic hypogonadism and Kallman's syndrome	Pulsatile GnRH or hCG/hMG
Pituitary insufficiency	hCG/hMG
Prolactinoma/hyperprolactinemia	Dopamine agonists/surgery
Obstructive azoospermia	Reconstructive surgery
Retrograde ejaculation	Sympathomimetics
2. Preventive therapy	
Maldescended testes	Early hCG or GnRH or surgery
Infections	Antibiotics
Exogenous factors (toxins/drugs)	Elimination, avoidance of exposure
Chronic diseases, e.g., renal insufficiency, liver disease, diabetes mellitus	Therapy of basic disease
Malignant diseases	Cryopreservation of sperm
3. Currently no therapy available	
Anorchia	
Gonadal dysgenesis	
Klinefelter syndrome	
Sertoli-cell-only syndrome	
Azoospermia factor (on Y chromosome)	
Globozoospermia	
Androgen receptor disorder	
4. Symptomatic therapy	
Idiopathic oligoasthenoteratozoospermia	Insemination/IVF/ICSI
Hypospadia	Insemination
Ductal agenesis and inoperable obstructive azoospermia	Sperm aspiration – IVF/ICSI
Globozoospermia and axonemata defects	ICSI
5. Empirical therapy	
Varicocele	Surgical ligation, radiological embolization, counseling
Immunological infertility	Immunosuppression (glucocorticoids)
Idiopathic infertility	Kallikrein, hCG/hMG, GnRH, androgens, antiestrogens

GnRH, gonadotropin releasing hormone; hCG, human chorionic gonadotropin; hMG, human menopausal gonadotropin; ICSI, intracytoplasmic sperm injection; IVF, in vitro fertilization.

14.4.1 Rational Therapy

Although andrology is a multidisciplinary field with many contributing specialities and the emerging and powerful modern assisted fertilization techniques emphazise the need of strong collaboration between andrologists and gynecologists, endocrinology can be still considered as the backbone of andrology. Endocrinology has always provided clear pathophysiological concepts based on a close relationship between clinical and laboratory findings. It is therefore not surprising that infertility associated with endocrine defects are often considered treatable according to rationales derived from both experimentally and clinically proven concepts. Nevertheless, and as pointed out before, recent developments concerning, for example, the administration form or protocol of hormonal regimens should be evaluated by controlled clinical trials, where alternative regimens are compared with each other. However, it may be extremely difficult to perform such studies, as the example of IHH demonstrates, where to date it has not been possible to show convincingly whether GnRH or human chorionic gonadotropin/human menopausal gonadotropin (hCG/hMG) treatment may be more advantageous for the patient and his fertility (Liu et al. 1988; Schopohl et al. 1991; Kliesch et al. 1994). The number of available patients is so small and their clinical appearance so heterogenous that studies providing sufficient statistical power are almost impossible to perform. In such cases, prospective multicenter trials are preferred.

14.4.2 Preventive Therapy

Prospective clinical studies would also be necessary for the field of preventive therapies (Table 1). They may be regarded as a subgroup of rational therapy, because pathophysiological concepts constitute their backbone. Because of the great time span, however, between the original disease and its possible and harmful complications for male fertility, the benefit-risk ratios of therapeutic concepts are harder to evaluate and therefore more often subject to controversial discussion. This is the case, for example, in cases of classical venereal diseases (e.g., gonorrhea), in which acute inflammatory processes affect male fertility (e.g., by blocking the epididymides, so that obstructive azoospermia may occur). The preventive effect of early antibiotic treatment is evidenced by the low rate of obstructive azoospermia in developed countries where such treatment is readily available and the high rate in Africa where such treatment is often lacking. Clinical trials to prove the preventive effect of this treatment do not seem to be required and would be even unethical on the basis of already existing clinical data. Nowadays the spectrum of genital infection, however, has changed towards more chronic, almost asymptomatic forms, often with no signs of acute inflammation (Purvis and Christiansen 1993). The pathological significance of these infections for male fertility is not well established, and in this situation well-designed controlled clinical studies are mandatory to establish the necessity and effectiveness of antibiotic therapy which is widely applied in clinical practice. Indeed, a recently published large randomized controlled study could not show any beneficial effect of such treatment (Yanushpolski et al. 1995).

In other conditions where preventive therapy is recommended, such as in maldescended testes, the pathological significance for male fertility is mainly assumed on the basis of observational and retrospective data. For example, the incidence of maldescended testes is higher among infertile men than among the general male population, suggesting that there might be a causative relation (Schäfer et al. 1989). However, to our knowledge the incidence of infertility among patients with a past history of maldescended testes and different therapeutic regimens has not yet been evaluated in a prospective, comparative trial. Most studies addressing the long-term outcome and different therapeutic modalities are retrospective. Data concerning this issue are often drawn from a selected population of infertility patients and may therefore be biased. Here prospective studies are required. However, they will need long observational follow-up-periods of almost 30 years when the patients treated as young children wish to become fathers. We are not aware that such studies are being performed. Based on our current pathophysiological concept it would, however, be unethical to include an untreated control group. The variable parameter in such a study would be the time point for therapeutic intervention in groups of boys with maldescended testes.

14.4.3 Empirical Therapy

Controlled clinical trials are urgently needed for the vast number of patients with idiopathic male infertility. In this condition, no clear pathophysiological or pathogenetic concepts exist which could provide a basis for evidence-based therapeutics. No laboratory animal models exist for this condition, and it is uncertain whether treatment is better or worse than no treatment. Where concepts are highly speculative, prospective, randomized, controlled clinical studies offer the only chance to reveal evidence for therapeutic decisions. Empirical therapies have been widely used and represent a good example for the importance of clinical trials in andrology and reproductive medicine.

14.4.3.1 Varicocele

Varicoceles are the most frequent physical finding in infertile men (WHO 1992a; Nieschlag and Behre 1992). Based on these observational data and the speculative concept that varicocele may cause testicular and epididymal damage while elevating intrascrotal temperature, occlusion of the spermatic vein by ligation or embolization is generally accepted as the treatment of choice (Tulloch 1952; Takihara et al. 1991). However, most of the publications which have focused on this issue confirmed treatment benefits on merely "technical" grounds; i.e., whether the varicocele had disappeared after treatment or not. Purportive improvement of male fertility has hardly been assessed by controlled clinical trials aiming at pregnancy rates. In addition, in most studies female factors were not clearly defined by inclusion or exclusion criteria and results may be biased by undefined female covariables. It therefore remains unclear whether surgical treatment is superior to no treatment or to simple counseling. A properly randomized, controlled, and prospective trial recently showed no significant difference in the cumulative pregnancy rate over a 12-month period between the control and treatment group (Nieschlag et al. 1995) (Fig. 2), thus challenging the current concept of varicocele repair and emphasizing the need for further properly designed clinical studies. The study emphasizes the importance of placebo-controlled design. Although sham operation would be the best placebo in all cases concerning surgical therapies, it may be unethical to expose patients to the risk of anesthesia and surgery for nothing but the placebo effect (Johnson 1994). In order to evaluate the magni-

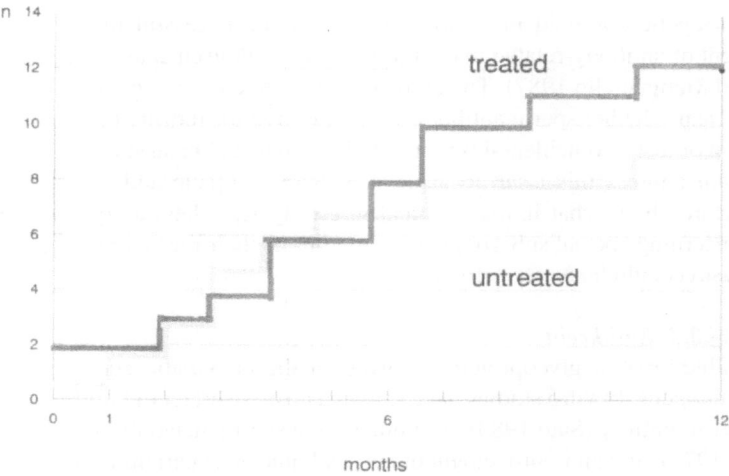

Fig. 2. Cumulative pregnancies of patients with varicocele after surgery (treated group) compared with counseling (untreated group) over a period of 12 months did not show any significant difference as results of a randomized, clinical trial (Nieschlag et al. 1995)

tude of the effect associated with counseling seen by the increase of cumulative pregnancies and to discriminate from the spontaneous course, it would be even more interesting to have an additional untreated – not only counseled – control group for comparison.

14.4.3.2 Immunological Male Infertility

The hypothesis of immunological infertility is yet not well established. The term refers mainly to the detection of sperm antibodies in the seminal fluid in infertile men whose infertility is otherwise unexplained. Its clinical significance, however, remains unclear. There are findings mostly based on laboratory tests supporting the relevance of IgG and IgA antibodies on the sperm surface for male fertility (Jager et al. 1979, 1980). Most studies concerning this issue are uncontrolled (e.g., Hendry et al 1981; Shulman and Shulman 1982). To our knowledge only one controlled clinical study has shown higher pregnancy rates in couples with prednisolone-treated men than in the placebo-controlled group (Hendry et al. 1990). Other controlled studies, however, have shown that cyclic corticoid immunosuppression is unsuccessful in the treatment of antibody-related male infertility (Bals-Pratsch et al. 1992; Haas and Manganiello 1987). The clinical results are conflicting and it is still unclear whether sperm antibodies are causative for fertility problems in men or just a coincidental finding. Well-designed clinical studies should again address this issue to achieve a more complete and convincing picture about what immunological infertility is, if laboratory findings concerning special subgroups of antibodies or their titer within seminal plasma could be better defined.

14.4.3.3 Kallikrein
Kallikrein is a glycoprotein involved in the enzymatic activation of kininogens. In vitro studies have shown a positive effect of kallikrein on sperm motility (Sato 1980), a stimulation in sperm metabolism (Leidl et al. 1975), and an improvement of cervical mucus penetration (Steiner et al. 1981). Following these observations orally administered kallikrein has been widely used in andrological practice for idiopathic male infertility. Most clinical studies claiming positive effects are methodologically inconclusive. Micic et al. (1985, 1990), for example, left the control group untreated, so that placebo effects in the treatment groups cannot be ruled out. Schill (1979) recorded pregnancies from retrospective questionnaires and covered a posttreatment period of 12 months, which seems too long to account for pregnancies to be ascribed only to kallikrein with its very short half-life. In contrast, more recent randomized, double-blind, placebo-controlled studies could not demonstrate any benefits of kallikrein given orally (600 IU/day) on sperm parameters or pregnancy rates in male idiopathic infertility (Glezerman et al. 1993; Keck et al. 1994). The implication of these studies for clinical andrology clearly highlights the importance of controlled studies.

14.4.3.4 Hormonal Treatment
Since GnRH, gonadotropins, and testosterone are required for normal testicular function (for review, see Weinbauer and Nieschlag 1993) and are effective in the treatment of hypogonadism, they were applied in the treatment of idiopathic male infertility as well, although no endocrine defect could be demonstrated as a cause of this type of infertility.

In the early 1960s gonadotropins became available for clinical use and were applied to idiopathic infertility on the hypothesis that elevation of gonadotropin levels may lead to stimulation of spermatogenesis. Surprisingly, they were used over many years without their effectiveness being properly assessed. A review in 1986 summarizing 39 studies, all uncontrolled and reporting pregnancy rates on average of 8%–14%, concluded that controlled, double-blind studies were urgently needed (Schill 1986). A randomized, double-blind, placebo-controlled study of hCG/hMG treatment for normogonadotropic oligoasthenoteratozoospermic men could not demonstrate any beneficial effect on sperm parameters or pregnancy rate (Knuth et al. 1987). If the hCG/hMG group is considered alone – as shown in Fig. 3. – a majority of patients would show an improvement in sperm parameters. However, each change in the verum group could be matched with a similiar change in the placebo group, emphasizing the risk of erroneous conclusion if the trial had not been placebo controlled.

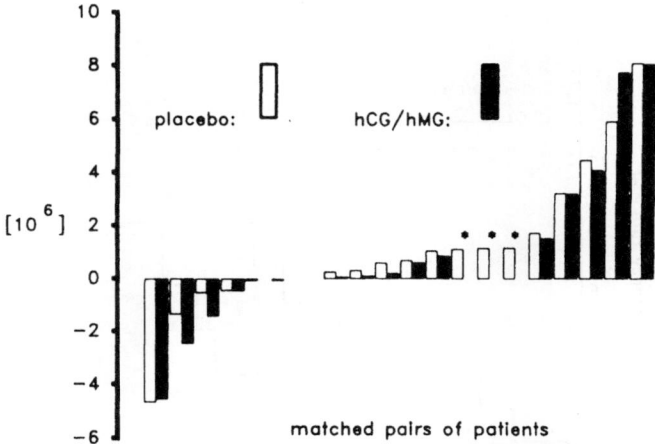

Fig. 3. Results of placebo-controlled, double-blind, randomized trial of human chorionic gonadotropin/human menopausal gonadotropin (*hCG/hMG*) treatment for normogonadotropic oligoasthenoteratozoospermia. The differences in the means of the total number of normally formed, motile sperm are shown. Individual values of patients are matched between groups according to the magnitude of differences. *Asterisks* indicate lack of appropriate counterpart (Knuth et al. 1987)

It was suggested that oligoasthenoteratozoospermia in patients with elevated follicle-stimulating hormone (FSH) levels might be caused by too infrequent GnRH pulses and thereby claimed that sperm parameters might be improved by pulsatile GnRH therapy (Wagner and Warsch 1984). This hypothesis could not be confirmed by a longitudinal study in which patients with oligoasthenoteratozoospermia and elevated FSH levels were treated with GnRH pulses every 90–120 min over a period of 12 and 24 weeks, respectively (Bals-Pratsch et al. 1989). This was an open, uncontrolled study, but since no change was observed compared with pretreatment semen values, a controlled study appeared superfluous.

The requirement of testosterone for normal spermatogenesis under physiological conditions led to the use of androgens in idiopathic male infertility, although abnormalities in serum testosterone or intratesticular testosterone could not be demonstrated in this condition (Nieschlag et al. 1979). Even without a clear pathophysiological rationale, androgens, especially mesterolone, were used over two decades in the

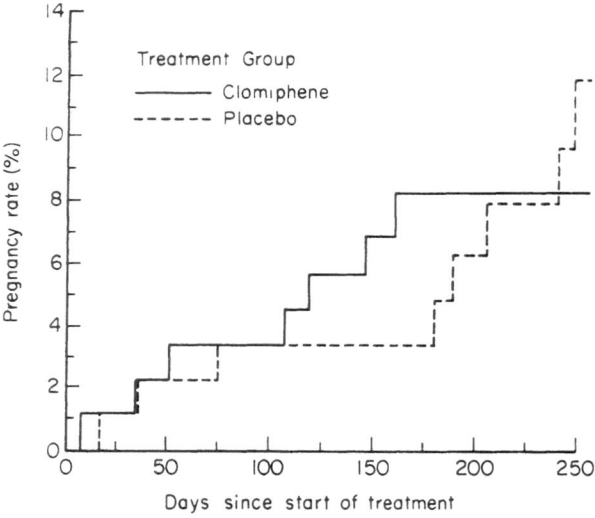

Fig. 4. Results of a randomized, double-blind, placebo-contolled multicenter study for clomiphene therapy in male idiopathic infertility. The cumulative pregnancies are shown for both groups. No significant difference can be observed over a period of 250 days (WHO 1992b)

treatment of idiopathic infertility until placebo-controlled, double-blind, randomized studies showed their ineffectiveness (Scottish Infertility Group 1984; WHO Task Force 1989).

It is well known that estrogens can have a negative feedback on the hypophyseal gonadotropin secretion. Antiestrogenic compounds competetively blocking estrogens at the receptor site might reduce the inhibitory feedback and lead to elevation of serum gonadotropin levels. Assuming that an increase in luteinizing hormone (LH) and FSH may improve sperm production, antiestrogens (in particular tamoxifen) have been widely used. To our knowledge, of 29 published studies concerning tamoxifen as a therapy in idiopathic male infertility, only eight were randomized and controlled (Rolf et al. 1996). None of these controlled studies have demonstrated any beneficial effect of tamoxifen therapy on fertility, neither could significant therapeutic effect be demonstrated for clomiphene, the other widely used antiestrogenic compund (Fig. 4; WHO 1992b).

14.4.4 Symptomatic Therapy with Assisted Fertilization

Because pharmacological therapies for idiopathic male infertility have been disappointing, attempts have been made to bring sperm and egg closer together. In addition to insemination, extracorporeal procedures like in vitro fertilization (IVF) and intracytoplasmic sperm injection (ICSI) have been developed. Especially the ICSI procedure, where a single sperm is injected into an oocyte by a micromanipulation, offers help in severe oligozooasthenozoospermia. For insemination and IVF procedures many controlled studies have been performed comparing different ovulation-stimulation protocols, sperm- and oocyte preparation techniques, embryo-transfer techniques, etc. (for review see Vandekerckhove et al. 1993).

If antibiotic therapy is not used in acute or chronic inflammation of the genital tract, obstruction of the efferent duct may occur, leading to azoospermia despite regular spermatogenesis. Reconstructive microsurgery can be applied in those cases to regain fertility. More recently, pregnancies were reported following IVF with sperm aspirated from the epididymis proximal to the occlusion (Hirsch et al. 1994). With improving fertilization techniques such as ICSI, this approach may provide an alternative if surgery fails to achieve reanastomosis. Furthermore, microsurgical aspiration of sperm from the epididymis followed by IVF or ICSI and pregnancy has become a treatment for patients with congenital absence of the ductuli deferentes, as in cystic fibrosis. Recently, pregnancies with sperm extracted from testicular tissue obtained by biopsy or aspiration have also been established from men with nonobstructive azoospermia (Tournaye et al. 1995).

It appears obvious that in men with azoospermia from whom single sperm may be obtained from epididymides or testes and which are used for microinjection into oocytes, clinical trials with the goal to establish pregnancy rates in untreated and treated groups are superfluous. However, comparative trials of various techniques will be required. Trials may also be required to establish a hierarchy of techniques of assisted fertilization in order to establish diagnostic criteria to decide which technique (intrauterine insemination, IUI, IVF, or ICSI) should be used at which degree of oligoasthenoteratozoospermia. Thus, controlled clinical trials also have a firm place in symptomatic treatment using assisted fertilization.

14.5 Conclusions

The treatment strategies mentioned above and discussed critically highlight the importance of controlled clinical studies in andrology. Often clinicians are confronted with situations of diagnostic and therapeutic uncertainty, or where evidence concerning risk-benefit ratios of competing therapeutic decisions is incomplete or contradictory. Obvious suffering as well as patients' expectations goad some doctors towards therapeutic action, i.e., doing something and providing hope is better than doing nothing. Other physicians tend towards therapeutic minimalism. Both attitudes may have their risks. In addition, anecdotal experience, the self-limiting or fluctuating course of some diseases, placebo-like effects of medical intervention or just physician's counseling may lead to overestimation of therapeutic intervention as being significant. The phenomenon of spontaneous change of parameters, also known in other fields as "regression towards the mean" may be especially obvious when patients with extreme values (in this case low sperm counts or low pregnancy rates) are selected for further consideration or treatment.

A genuine therapeutic effect can be considered to have taken place only when sample sizes are big enough for powerful statistical evaluation and changes in seminal parameters or pregnancies accumulated over a sufficient period of time differ significantly from those of a placebo-treated control group. Such studies are complex and time consuming, as has been discussed in detail in this chapter, and the standards demanded at times exceed available capacities. In addition, placebo treatment might be considered as unethical when verum, although unproven in its efficacy, can be given to patients. In our opinion it is, however, even more unethical to abandon clinicians as well as patients in a limbo of therapeutic uncertainty and to give ambiguous answers to patients' concerns about risk-benefit ratios of therapies being offered, i.e., that they may or may not help.

In this uneasy situation clinicians should be guided by the following principle in their decisions: *Any therapeutic procedures whose effectiveness has not been verified by placebo-controlled studies should be applied only in the context of clinical studies until their effectiveness is indeed proven.*

References

Bals-Pratsch M, Knuth UA, Hönigl W, Klein HM, Bergmann M, Nieschlag E (1989) Pulsatile GnRH-therapy in oligozoospermic men does not improve seminal parameters despite decreased FSH levels. Clin Endocrinol (Oxf) 30:549–560

Bals-Pratsch M, Dören M, Karbowski B, Schneider HPG, Nieschlag E (1992) Cyclic corticoid immunosuppression is unsuccessful in the treatment of sperm antibody-related male infertility: a controlled study. Hum Reprod 7:99–104

Evidence-based Medicine Working Group (1992) Evidence-based medicine: a new approach to teaching the practice of medicine. JAMA 268:2420–2425

Glezerman M, Lunenfeld E, Potashnik G, Huleihel M, Soffer Y, Segal S (1993) Efficacy of kallikrein in the treatment of oligozoospermia and asthenozoospermia: a double-blind trial. Fertil Steril 60:1052–1056

Gotzsche PC (1994) Is there logic in the placebo? Lancet 344:925–926

Haas G, Manganiello P (1987) A double-blind, placebo-controlled study of the use of methylprednisolone in infertile men with sperm-associated immunoglobulins. Fertil Steril 47:295–301

Hendry WF, Stedronska J, Parslow J, Hughes L (1981) The results of intermittent high dose steroid therapy for male infertility due to antisperm antibodies. Fertil Steril 36:351–355

Hendry W, Hughes L, Scammell G, Pryor J, Hargreave T (1990) Comparison of prednisolone and placebo in subfertile men with antibodies to spermatozoa. Lancet 335:85–88

Hirsch AV, Mills C, Bekir J, Dean N, Yovich JL, Tan SL (1994) Factors influencing the outcome of in vitro fertilization with epididymal spermatozoa in irreversible obstructive azoospermia. Hum Reprod 9:1710–1716

Howards SS (1995) Treatment of male infertility. N Engl J Med 2:312–317

Hull M, Glazener C, Kelley N, Conway D, Foster P, Hinton R, Coulson C, Lambert P, Watt E, Desai K (1985) Population studies of causes, treatment and outcome of infertility. Br Med J 291:1693–1697

Jager S, Kremer J, van Slochteren-Draaisma T (1979) Presence of sperm agglutination antibodies in infertile men and inhibition of in vitro sperm penetration into cervical mucus. Int J Androl 2:117–130

Jager S, Kremer J, Kuiken J, van Slochteren-Draaisma T (1980) Immunoglobulin class of antispermatozoal antibodies from infertile men and inhibition of in vitro sperm penetration into cervical mucus. Andrology 3:1–14

Johnson AG (1994) Surgery as a placebo. Lancet 344:1140–1142

Keck C, Behre HM, Jockenhövel F, Nieschlag E (1994) Ineffectiveness of kallikrein in treatment of idiopathic male infertility: a double-blind, randomized, placebo-controlled trial. Hum Reprod 9:325–329

Kleijnen J, de Craen AJM, van Everdingen J, Krol L (1994) Placebo effect in double-blind clinical trials: a review of interactions with medications. Lancet 344:1347–1351

Kliesch S, Behre HM, Nieschlag E (1994) High efficacy of gonadotropin or pulsatile GnRH treatment in hypogonadotropic hypogonadal men. Eur J Endocr 131:347–354

Knuth UA, Hönigl W, Bals-Pratsch M, Schleicher G, Nieschlag E (1987) Treatment of severe oligozoospermia with hCG/hMG. A placebo-controlled double blind trial. J Clin Endocrinol Metab 65:1081–1087

Leidl W, Prinzen R, Schill WB, Fritz H (1975) The effect of kallikrein on motility and metabolism of spermatozoa in vitro. In: Haberland GL, Rohen JW, Schirren C, Huber P (eds) Kininogenases. Kallikrein 2. Schattauer, Stuttgart, pp 33–40

Liu L, Banks SM, Barnes KM, Sherins RJ (1988) Two-year comparison of testicular responses to pulsatile gonadotropin-releasing hormone and exogenous gonadotropins from the inception of therapy in men with isolated .hypogonadotropic hypogonadism. J Clin Endoc Metabol 67:1140–1145

Micic S, Bila S, Nic V, Sulovic V (1985) Treatment of men with oligoasthenozoospermia and asthenozoospermia with kallikrein. Acta Eur Fertil 16:51–54

Micic S, Tulic C, Dotlic R (1990) Kallikrein therapy of infertile men with varicocele and impaired sperm motility. Andrologia 22:179–183

Nieschlag E (1993) Current therapy: care for the infertile male. Clin Endocrinol (Oxf) 38:123–133

Nieschlag E (1994) Clinical relevance and irrelevance of molecular and cellular research on the testis in molecular and cellular endocrinology of the testis. In: Verhoeven G, Habenicht UF (eds) Molecular and cellular endocrinology of the testis. Springer, Berlin Heidelberg New York, pp 273–292 (Ernst Schering Research Foundation Workshop, Suppl 1)

Nieschlag E, Behre HM (1992) Male Infertility due to testicular dysfunction. In: Drife JO, Templeton AA (eds) Infertility. Proceedings of the 25th study group of the Royal College of Obstetricians and Gynaecologists. Springer, Berlin Heidelberg New York, pp 65–80

Nieschlag E, Wickings EJ, Mauss J (1979) Endocrine testicular function in vivo and in vitro in infertile men. Acta Endocrinol (Copenh) 90:544–551

Nieschlag E, Hertle L, Fischedick A, Behre HM (1995) Treatment of varicocele: counselling as effective as occlusion of the vena spermatica. Hum Reprod 10 (2):347–353

Olive DL (1986) Analysis of clinical fertility trials: a methodologic review. Fertil Steril 45:157–171

Peck C, Coleman G (1991) Implications for placebo theory for clinical research and practice in pain management. Theor Med 12:247–270

Pocock SJ (1983) Clinical trials: a practical approach. Wiley, New York

Purvis K, Christiansen E (1993) Infection in the male reproductive tract. Impact, diagnosis and treatment in relation to male infertility. Int J Androl 16:1–13

Rolf C, Behre HM, Nieschlag E (1996) Tamoxifen bei männlicher Infertilität. Analyse einer fragwürdigen Therapie. Dtsch Med Wochenschr 121:33–39

Sato H (1980) Studies on the components of kallikrein-kinin system and treatment of male infertility. Keio J Med 29:19–38

Schäfer M, Brühl P, Jankowski (1989) Aktuelle Diagnostik und Therapie des Maldeszensus testis. Klin Padiatr 201:452–457

Schill WB (1979) Treatment of idiopathic oligozoospermia by kallikrein: results of a double-blind study. Arch Androl 2:163–170

Schill WB (1986) Medical treatment of male infertility. In: Insler V, Lunenfeld B (eds) Infertility: male and female. Churchill Livingstone, Edinburgh, pp 533--573

Schopohl J, Mehltretter G, von Zumbusch R, Eversman T, von Werder K (1991) Comparison of gonadotropin-releasing hormone and gonadotropin therapy in male patients with idiopathic hypothalamic hypogonadism. Fertil Steril 56:1143–1150

Scottish Infertility Group, Hargreave T, Kyle K, Baxby K, Rogers A, Scott R, Tolley D, Abel D, Orr T, Elton R (1984) Randomized trial of mesterolone versus vitamin C for male infertility Br J Urol 56:740–744

Shulman JF, Shulman S (1982) Methylprednisolone treatment of immunologic infertility in the male. Fertil Steril 38:591–599

Steiner R, Hofmann N, Hartmann R, Kaufmann R (1981) Kallikrein-enhanced human sperm motility in different media and cervical mucus measured with Laser-Doppler-spectroscopy. In: Haberland GL, Rohen J (eds) Kininogenases. Kallikrein 5. Schattauer, Stuttgart, pp 17–26

Takihara H, Sakatoku J, Cockett ATK (1991) The pathophysiology of varicocele in male infertility. Fertil Steril 55:861–868

Tournaye H, Camus M, Goosens A, Liu J, Nagy P, Silber S, Van Steirteghem AC, Devroey P (1995) Recent concepts in the management of infertility because of non-obstructive azoospermia. Hum Reprod 10 [Suppl 1]:115–119

Tulloch WS (1952) Consideration of sterility factors in light of subsequent pregnancies: subfertility in the male. Edinb Med J 59:29

Vandekerckhove P, O'Donavan PA, Lilford RJ, Harada TW (1993) Infertility treatment: from cookery to science. The epidemiology of randomized controlled trials. Br J Obstet Gynaecol 100:1005–1036

Vessey M, Doll R, Peto R, Johnson B, Wiggins P (1976) A long-term follow up study of women using different methods of contraception – an interim report. J Biosoc Sci 8:373–427

Wagner ROF, Warsch F (1984) Pulsatile LHRH therapy of "slow pulsing oligospermia": indirect evidence for a hypothalamic origin of the disorder. Acta Endocrinol (Copenh) 105 [Suppl 264]:142–145

Weinbauer GF, Nieschlag E (1993) Hormonal control of spermatogenesis. In: De Kretser D (ed) Molecular biology of the male reproductive system. Academic, New York, p 99

WHO Task Force on the Diagnosis and Treatment of Infertility (1989) Mesterolone and idiopathic male infertility: a double-blind study. Int J Androl 12:254–264

WHO (1992a) The influence of varicocele on parameters of fertility in a large group of men presenting to infertility clinics. Fertil Steril 57:1289–1293

WHO Special Programme of Research, Development and Research Training in Human Reproduction, Task Force on the Prevention and Management of Infertility (1992b) A double-blind trial of clomiphene citrate for the treatment of idiopathic male infertility. Int J Androl 15:299–307

Yanushpolski ET, Politch JA, HillJA, Anderson DJ (1995)Antibiotic therapy and leukocytospermia: a prospective randomized controlled study. Fertil Steril 63:142–147

15 Molecular Genetics and Neurobiology of Kallmann's Syndrome

P.-M.G. Bouloux, P. de Zoyza, V. Duke, and R. Quinton

15.1	Introduction	307
15.2	Developmental Biology of the Olfactory System and GnRH Cells	308
15.3	Neuroanatomical Abnormalities in Kallman's Syndrome	309
15.4	Characterization of the *KAL* Locus	310
15.5	Spatiotemporal *KAL* Expression in Chick and Human (and Relationship to Phenotype)	311
15.6	KAL Protein	313
15.7	Current Hypothesis of KAL Protein Function	314
15.8	Recent Work on KAL Protein	315
References		316

15.1 Introduction

Kallmann's syndrome (KS) is a human genetic disorder, occurring in both X-linked (XKS) and autosomal forms (less commonly). It is phenotypically characterized by the association of anosmia (lack of sense of smell) and hypogonadotrophic hypogonadism. The olfactory defect is due to defective development of the olfactory bulbs and tracts and the hypogonadotrophic hypogonadism results from hypothalamic deficiency of gonadotrophin-releasing hormone (GnRH).

Although the association of absent olfactory bulbs and hypogonadism was first recorded in 1856, the recognition of KS as a distinct genetic entity was only established by the seminal study of Kallmann and colleagues (1944). Since then, there have been several reports of the genetic heterogeneity of this condition which affects approximately 1 in 10 000 males and 1 in 50 000 females. Our own experience suggests that the X-linked recessive mode of inheritance is most frequently encountered, although in clinical practice, sporadic presentations are preponderant. The hypogonadism of KS is treatable. Puberty may be induced by the graded administration of sex steroids, and fertility achieved by the administration of either subcutaneous pulsatile GnRH or exogenous human menopausal (or, more recently, recombinant) gonadotrophins. The high incidence of cryptorchidism in male patients (50% in sporadic male KS and 85% in XKS) may be responsible for the disappointing results of spermatogenesis induction in these patients. In this review, we shall focus exclusively on the male with KS, highlighting some recent advances in the understanding of the pathogenesis of this condition and, in particular, the inter-relationship between sex and smell (reviewed in Bouloux et al. 1992).

15.2 Developmental Biology of the Olfactory System and GnRH Cells

Recent evidence has confirmed a common developmental origin for olfactory and GnRH neurones. Both originate in the olfactory placode, a discrete cranial ectodermal thickening destined to become olfactory epithelium (lateral olfactory placode) and to differentiate into GnRH cells (medial olfactory placode). From the lateral placode, olfactory neurones send axonal projections through the cribriform plate area to synapse with mitral cell dendrites in the developing olfactory bulb. During development, newly differentiated GnRH neurones migrate from the medial olfactory placode epithelium along a neural cell adhesion molecule (N-CAM)-rich scaffold along fascicles of the olfactory, terminal and vomeronasal nerves (the cranial nerve I complex) to the forebrain. During embryogenesis, immuno-histochemical evidence has accrued for differential distribution of two forms of N-CAM glycoproteins, differing in their sialic acid content. The N-CAM with low sialic acid content is present in the olfactory placode of the earliest embryos examined, and later throughout the migration route. The polysialated (PSA) N-CAM form is present only in nerve fibres streaming from the olfactory placode and along the caudal margin of the migration route below the forebrain, suggesting that the less adhesive PSA-N-CAM may be correlated with greater rates of GnRH cell movement, with the low sialic acid N-CAM required for stability of the migration route (Schwanzel-Fukuda et al. 1996).

GnRH cells traverse the forebrain to their final destination in the mediobasal hypothalamus (Schwanzel-Fukuda and Pfaff 1989). Synaptic contacts made by olfactory axons with mitral cell dendrites appear to play a key role in the induction of olfactory bulb development and also appear to play a role postnatally (Graziadei et al. 1978), vertebrate olfactory neurones which have a half-life of weeks being replaced by new neurones that differentiate from a neuronal stem cell population. The olfactory neuroepithelium in turn gains trophic support from the olfactory bulbs (Schwob et al. 1992), such that experimental bulbectomy, although not affecting the differentiation of olfactory sensory neurones, results in reduced cell lifespan.

15.3 Neuroanatomical Abnormalities in Kallman's Syndrome

Immunohistological analysis of a 19-week human male foetus with an Xpter chromosomal deletion (and hence complete *KAL* gene deletion) revealed that neurones of the cranial nerve I complex extended axonal projections rostrally but that these, instead of having penetrated the meninges and entered the forebrain, ended as neuronal tangles in the meninges overlying the cribriform plate (Schwanzel-Fukuda et al. 1989). GnRH neurones, whose most proximal sites lay in the upper nasal septum and cribriform plate areas, had clearly migrated along these axons to their furthest extension (but were unable to proceed to the hypothalamus). These observations led Schwanzel-Fukuda to hypothesize that the putative KAL protein (KALp) encoded a factor involved in olfactory axonal penetration of the meninges and, as a consequence, migration of GnRH neurones.

15.4 Characterization of the *KAL* Locus

The original clinical observation of pedigrees in which several affected males had a complex phenotype characterized by XKS and X-linked ichthyosis due to steroid sulphatase (STS) deficiency proved the starting point for mapping *KAL* (reviewed in Bouloux et al. 1993). A contiguous gene syndrome was postulated comprising codeletion of both *STS* and *KAL*, leading to the assignation of *KAL* to Xp22.3 close to *STS*. This locus was supported by data from linkage analysis (Meitinger et al. 1990). A deletion map was subsequently constructed from analysis of patients with Xp22.3 rearrangements and contiguous gene syndromes, leading to the assignment of a specific deletion interval encompassing the whole or part of *KAL*. Using positional cloning approaches two groups independently isolated the same candidate gene (*KALIG-1* or *ADMLX*, respectively; Franco et al. 1991; Legouis et al. 1991). Characterization of *KAL* revealed a 14-exon structure spanning approximately 210 kb of genomic DNA, with a centromerically oriented 5'-end. *KAL* escapes X inactivation and has a closely related but nonfunctional homologue (*KAL-Y*) on the Y chromosome (Yq11.2) which differs from *KAL* in not having exons 3, 8 and 9 and in minor degrees of sequence divergence in the remaining exons (del Castillo et al. 1992). The creation of a fusion gene, consisting of virtually the entire *KAL* but with the last exon and part of the last intron being derived from *KAL*-Y, has been demonstrated in a KS patient which results from abnormal pairing and precise recombination between *KAL* and *KAL*-Y and causing an X/Y translocation. Both the last splice junction and the stop codon sequences are identical to those of the normal *KAL* gene. However, the transcription and/or the stability of mRNA are affected by the translocation, implying that the 3' portion of *KAL* has functional importance and cannot be substituted by the corresponding region of *KAL-Y* (Guioli et al. 1992).

15.5 Spatiotemporal *KAL* Expression in Chick and Human (and Relationship to Phenotype)

Initial studies using reverse transcription polymerase chain reaction (RT-PCR) showed the presence of *KAL* mRNA in an 18-week-old human foetus as well as in adult tissues, including brain, muscle, kidney and liver (Franco et al. 1991). *KAL* transcripts were also found in embryonal cell carcinoma NT"/D1 and a lymphoblastoid cell line, indicating widespread expression both in neuronal and non-neuronal cells. The spatiotemporal expression of *cKAL* (the closely related chicken homologue of *KAL*) has been investigated using in situ hybridization. In the chick, expression of *cKAL* transcript was not above baseline during the early phase of olfactory system development, nor was *cKAL* mRNA detected in the developmental stages during which the olfactory epithelium differentiates from the placode to form olfactory sensory and GnRH neurones (Rugarli et al. 1993; Lutz et al. 1994). No signal was detected in the neuroepithelium of the presumptive bulb region at the stage when olfactory axons first reach the forebrain. It is only when the neuroepithelium of the presumptive olfactory bulb begins to differentiate into mitral cell precursors that *cKAL* is expressed in these cells. As the bulb begins to assume its characteristic laminar structure, *cKAL* transcript levels further increase in the mitral cells. This expression persists throughout life in chick. The lack of expression of *cKAL* in the olfactory epithelium as well as in the mesenchymal tissue between the bulb and epithelium strongly suggests that *cKAL* is not directly required for olfactory axon guidance from olfactory epithelium to the bulb. Rather, it appears to be required for aspects of cellular genesis, differentiation and synaptogenesis within the bulb itself.

Further proof that signals from the olfactory nerve are not required for expression of *cKAL* from the olfactory bulb has come from a study in which the olfactory placode was extirpated in a developing chick embryo (Lutz et al. 1994). Those embryos lacking an olfactory nerve had a histologically abnormal bulb which nevertheless expressed high-level *cKAL* mRNA, indicating that while development of proper olfactory-bulb architecture requires olfactory axon innervation, *cKAL* expression is independent of such developmental processes.

KAL transcripts have also been demonstrated in olfactory bulb granule cells, cerebellum (internal granular layer, Purkinje layer, and in lamina dissecans), dorsomedial hypothalamus and developing cerebral cortex (cortical plate) in a 19-week-old human foetus. However, in contrast to avian olfactory bulb, where *cKAL* is expressed in principal neurones (mitral and Purkinje cells), *KAL* is predominantly expressed in interneurones and glial cells (Lutz et al. 1994). *KAL* expression in human cerebellum may be related to the horizontal gaze evoked nystagmus and ataxia occasionally seen in patients with the syndrome (Schwankhaus et al. 1989). The occurrence of these abnormalities in genetically unrelated KS patients carrying point mutations or intragenic deletions at the *KAL* locus indicates a more generalized role of the gene during CNS as well as non-neuronal development (see below).

Using RT-PCR, we have found low-level *KAL* expression in a 45-day-old human embryo brainstem/spinal cord, mesonephros and metanephros (Duke et al. 1995). In contrast to the chick, in situ hybridization showed low-level *KAL* expression on the inner layer of the olfactory bulb, corresponding to mitral and granular cells; the highest signal was detected over the outermost layer of the bulb, which is constituted by the olfactory nerves. The presence of *KAL* transcript at 7 weeks in the epithelia of the mesonephros and metanephros, precursors of the adult kidney, support a role for *KAL* in renal development, as suggested by reports of unilateral and bilateral renal agenesis in XKS patients (Kirk et al. 1994). Phenotypically, mutants of *KAL* are also strongly associated with hereditary bimanual synkinesis (HBS, distal upper-limb mirror movements), an abnormality seen in >90% of XKS patients. Electrophysiological studies have revealed abnormal decussation of the pyramidal pathway, with significant numbers of corticospinal axons failing to cross the midline and, hence, projecting ipsilaterally down the spinal cord (Mayston et al. 1994). Previous hypotheses ascribing HBS in XKS to bilateral motor cortex activation have not been confirmed by positron emission tomography (PET) study. Either abnormal or disrupted *KAL* expression in brainstem/spinal cord during early development may explain the disrupted corticospinal pathways that underlie synkinesis.

15.6 KAL Protein

Several features of the predicted protein sequence suggest a function of KAL in neural development. The predicted protein (KALp; Swiss Protein database accession no: P23352) comprises 680 amino acids and contains a putative cleavable amino terminal leader peptide. It lacks both a *trans*-membrane domain and a putative phosphatidyl inositol anchorage site, implying that it is secreted. KALp contains a four-disulphide domain characterized by eight conserved cysteines forming four disulphide bonds. This core motif (whey acidic protein, WAP, domain) is a compact fold found in a number of proteins such as wheat germ agglutinin, neurotoxins and protease inhibitors (Franco et al. 1991). All known proteases inhibited by proteins containing this motif are soluble serine proteases. It is possible that this core could interact with a serine protease located on the cell membrane, examples of which include the plasminogen activator-like proteases that have specific binding sites on a variety of neurones and are believed to facilitate axonal elongation by regulating growth cone adhesion to specific matrix components.

The carboxy terminal two thirds of the protein contains two domains showing similarity with fibronectin III repeats first found in fibronectin, an extracellular matrix molecule. These repeats are also found in many other neural cell adhesion molecules as well as in receptor-linked protein kinases and phosphatases. (Phosphatidyl inositol-anchored cell adhesion molecules and also extracellular matrix proteins with fibronectin type III repeats such as fibronectin and tenascin have been implicated in neuronal migration and axonal growth and guidance.)

Furthermore, the importance of at least the first of these repeats is highlighted by the discovery in an XKS pedigree of a point mutation that results in the nonconservative amino acid substitution (from asparagine to lysine) within this repeat at position 267 (of SwissProt sequence P23352; Hardelin et al. 1993a). Zoo blot analysis of the original clone showed sequence conservation among several species, including monkey, cow, rabbit, sheep, but not the mouse or rat. Chick and quail homologues of *KAL* (c*KAL, qKAL*) have been isolated and have a 77% overall protein sequence identity with *KAL* (Legouis et al. 1993). Within the WAP domain and the fibronectin repeat regions, sequence identity lies in the 91%–94% range, emphasizing their functional importance. An additional similarity lies in the common hydrophobic character of the amino terminus, which suggests that the protein is extracellularly secreted in avians as well as in humans.

Although mutations in *KAL* patients were reported previously in several exons, no hot spots have yet been identified (Hardelin et al. 1992; 1993a, b). The screening strategy involved direct dideoxy sequencing of PCR-amplified exons using pairs of *KAL*-specific intronic primers that immediately flank each exon (except in the cases of exons 1 and 14 where only one such intronic primer is used; the other being derived from noncoding regions that flank the 5' or 3' coding sequences, respectively). The strategy concentrated on exonic point mutation and deletion detection. So far we have identified a wide spectrum of mutations: A total of five premature stop codons corresponding to amino acid positions Trp_{237}, Arg_{257}, Trp_{258}, Gln_{421}, and Arg_{423}; a single base pair (bp) deletion mutation at nucleotide sequence 981; a single bp insertion at nucleotide position 1166; an amino acid substitution corresponding to Asn_{267}; and a splice acceptor site mutation within intron 12. There are some XKS pedigrees in which detectable coding sequence mutations cannot be identified, implying that these patients carry mutations that cause promoter malfunction or defective splicing of the immature Kallmann RNA (P.-M. G. Bouloux, unpublished).

15.7 Current Hypothesis of KAL Protein Function

KALp is a secreted protein. Its homology with molecules important in axonal guidance, cellular adhesion, and antiprotease activity suggests that it may be the prototype of an entirely novel family of proteins. The spatiotemporal expression of KAL suggests that this protein could have any one of a number of potential functions, possibly acting as a locally secreted growth factor responsible for histogenesis/survival of the olfactory bulb or as a synaptogenic factor. It may also act as a chemotrophic molecule, influencing axonal patterning within the olfactory bulb and within the spinal cord affecting decussating pathways. Within the kidney, its distribution in the early ureteric bud and metanephric blastema is compatible with a role in the maintenance of epithelial integrity, acting possibly as a cell adhesion molecule. The characterization of the precise role of KAL in the nervous system must await the generation of the intact protein and/or a variant of it, and a bioassay system.

15.8 Recent Work on KAL Protein

It was proposed that in vitro generation of KALp, both glycosylated and nonglycosylated forms, may be used to study the effectiveness of antibodies to KALp (and subsequent functional studies). Our recent work has shown that:

1. The C-terminal part of the KALp may be generated in cell-free systems.
2. The expression of full-length KALp independently confirms the integrity of the previously predicted reading frame of *KAL*.

Subsequent to these studies, using the FOLDRNA programme, available on the University of Wisconsin Genetics Computer Group (version 7.0) package, the secondary structure formation of KAL RNA was predicted. This showed that the 5' coding region end of KAL RNA is especially prone to extensive irregular stem structure formation. These structures may possibly be inhibitory to translation initiation at the predicted start site at nucleotide position 90 of Genbank X60299 in rabbit reticulocyte lysate. As yet it is not clear whether this inhibition of expression in this system may be a part of the physiological regulation of *KAL* RNA or a limitation of the system, therefore requiring further experimentation. However, it may be possible that, once confirmed and quantitated, the low-level synthesis of KALp may be sufficient for future functional studies which will be required to elucidate the mode of action of this developmental protein.

Acknowledgments. We are grateful to Dr C Petit at the Pasteur Institute in Paris for the kind donation of amplimers for the XKS locus as well as a cDNA clone of XKS to enable some of the studies described to be performed.

References

Bouloux P-MG, Munroe P, Kirk JMW, Besser GM (1992) Sex and smell -an enigma resolved. J Endocrinol 133:323–326

Bouloux P-MG, Kirk JMW, Munroe P, Duke VM, Meindl A, Hilson A, Grant DB, Carter N, Betts D, Meitinger T, Besser GM (1993) Deletion analysis maps ocular albinism proximal to the steroid sulphatase locus. Clin Genet 43:169–173

del Castillo I, Cohen-Salmon M, Blanchard S, Lutfalla G, Petit C (1992) Structure of the X-linked Kallmann syndrome gene and its homologous pseudogene on the Y chromosome. Nature Genet 2:305–310

Duke VM, Winyard PJD, Thorogood PV, Soothill P, Bouloux P-MG, Woolf AS (1995) KAL, a gene mutated in Kallmann's syndrome is expressed in the first trimester of human development. Mol Cell Endocrinol 110:73–79

Franco B, Guioli S, Pragliola A, Incerti B, Bardoni B, Tonlorenzi R, Carrozzo R, Maestrini E, Pieretti M, Taillon-Miller P, Brown C, Willard HF, Lawrence C, Persico M, Camerino G, Ballabio A (1991) A gene deleted in Kallmann's syndrome shares homology with neural cell adhesion and axonal path finding molecules. Nature 353:529–535

Graziadei PPC, Monti Graziadei GA (1978) Continuous nerve cell renewal in the olfactory system. In: Jacobson M (ed) Development of sensory systems. Springer, Berlin Heidelberg New York, pp 55–83

Guioli S, Incerti B, Zanaria E, Bardoni B, Franco B, Taylor K, Camerino G (1992) Kallmann syndrome due to a translocation resulting in an X/Y fusion gene. Nature Genet 1:337–340

Hardelin JP, Levilliers J, del Castillo I, Cohen-Salmon M, Legouis R, Blanchard S, Compain S, Bouloux P-MG, Kirk JMC, Moraine C et al (1992) X chromosome-linked Kallmann syndrome: stop mutations validate the candidate gene. Proc Natl Acad Sci USA 89:8190–8194

Hardelin JP, Levilliers J, Blanchard S, Carel JC, Leutenegger M, Bouloux P-MG, Petit C (1993a) Heterogeneity in the mutations responsible for X chromosome-linked Kallmann syndrome. Hum Mol Genet 2:373–377

Hardelin JP, Levilliers J, Young J, Pholsena M, Legouis R, Kirk JMW, Bouloux P-MG, Petit C, Schaison G (1993b) Xp22.3 deletions in isolated familial Kallmann's syndrome. J Clin Endocrinol Metab 76:827–831

Kallmann FJ, Schonfeld WA, Barrerre SE (1944) The genetic aspects of primary euneuchoidism. Am J Ment Defic 48:203–206

Kirk JMW, Grant DB, Besser GM, Shalet S, Quinton R, Smith CS, White M, Edwards OME, Bouloux P-MG (1994) Unilateral renal aplasia in X-linked Kallmann's syndrome. Clin Genet 46:260–262

Legouis R, Hardelin JP, Levilliers J, Claverie JM, Compain S, Wunderle V, Millasseau P, Le Paslier D, Cohen D, Caterina D, Bouguerelet L, Delemarre-Van der Waal H, Lutfalla G, Weissenbach J, Petit C (1991) The candidate gene for the X-linked Kallmann syndrome encodes a protein related to adhesion molecules. Cell 67:423–435

Legouis R, Salomon M, Castillo I, Levilliers J, Capy L, Mornon JP, Petit C (1993) Characterization of the chicken and quail homologues of the human gene responsible for the X-linked Kallmann syndrome. Genomics 17:516–518

Lutz B, Kuratani S, Rugarli EI, Wawersik S, Wong C, Bieber FR, Ballabio A, Eichele G (1994) Expression of the Kallmann syndrome gene in human fetal brain and in the manipulated chick embryo. Hum Mol Genet 3:1717–1723

Mayston MJ, Harrison LM, Jobling L, Quinton R, Stephens JA, Bouloux P-MG (1994) Mirror movements in X-linked Kallmann's syndrome. Physiological Society abstract, pp 49–50

Meitinger T, Heye B, Petit C, Levilliers J, Golla A, Moraine C, Sippell WG, Murken J, Ballabio A (1990) Definitive localization of X-linked Kallman syndrome (hypogonadotropic hypogonadism and anosmia) to Xp22.3: close linkage to the hypervariable repeat sequence CRI-S232 [published erratum appears in Am J Hum Genet (1990) 47:883]. Am J Hum Genet 47:664–669

Rugarli EI, Lutz B, Kuratani SC, Wawersik S, Borsani G, Ballabio A, Eichele G (1993) Expression pattern of the Kallmann syndrome gene in the olfactory system suggests a role in neuronal targeting. Nature Genet 4:19–26

Schwankhaus JD, Currie J, Jaffe MJ, Rose SR, Sherins RJ (1989) Neurologic findings in men with isolated hypogonadotropic hypogonadism. Neurology 39:223–226

Schwanzel-Fukuda M, Pfaff DW (1989) Origin of luteinizing hormone releasing hormone neurons. Nature 338:161–164

Schwanzel-Fukuda M, Bick D, Pfaff DW (1989) Luteinizing hormone-releasing hormone (LHRH)-expressing cells do not migrate normally in an inherited hypogonadal (Kallmann) syndrome. Mol Brain Res 6:311–326

Schwanzel-Fukuda M, Pfaff DW, Crossin KL, Bouloux P-MG, Hardelin JP, Petit C (1996) Ontogeny and migration of LHRH neurons in early human embryos. Development (in press)

Schwob JE, Szumowski KE, Stasky AA (1992) Olfactory sensory neurones are trophically dependent on the olfactory bulbs for their prolonged survival. J Neurosci 12:3896–3919

16 The Polymorphisms of Gonadotropin Action: Molecular Basis and Clinical Implications

I. Huhtaniemi, P. Pakarinen, A.-M. Haavisto, C. Nilsson,
K. Pettersson, J. Tapanainen, and K. Aittomäki

16.1   Introduction 320
16.2   Immunological and Biological Measurements of Gonadotropins . 321
16.2.1 Microheterogeneity of Gonadotropins 321
16.2.2 Novel Sensitive Immunoassays and In Vitro Bioassays
        of Gonadotropins 322
16.2.3 The Clinical Value of Bio/immuno Ratio Measurements
        of Gonadotropins 325
16.3   Gonadotropic Genes 326
16.3.1 Mutations of Gonadotropic Genes 326
16.3.2 A Common Polymorphism in the LH β-Subunit Gene 327
16.4   Gonadotropin Receptor Genes 330
16.4.1 Activating and Inactivating Mutations
        of the Gonadotropin Receptor Genes 330
16.4.2 A Novel Inactivating Mutation of the FSHR Gene 332
16.5   Conclusions 336
References 337

16.1 Introduction

The genetic analysis of the pathogenesis of diseases has revealed that subfertility or infertility may also be hereditary. This is in contrast to the general assumption that infertility by nature cannot be an inherited condition. The currently available molecular biological methods enable detailed genetic analysis of mutations and polymorphisms, and astonishingly rapid progress has been made in this field. When genes involved in hormone action are affected, the consequences of the mutation determine whether hetero- or homozygocity is required for phenotypic alteration. Heterozygocity is sufficient in the case of gain-of-function mutations, whereas the loss-of-function mutations usually have to be homozygous. It is also possible, but still rarely proven, that a given mutation only affects the fertility of one sex. Due to their variable mode of inheritance and penetrance, the mutations affecting fertility stay in the population and in fact are more common than assumed.

Concerning gonadotropins, the key hormones of the hypothalamic–pituitary–gonadal axis, microheterogeneity due to variability in their carbohydrate structures has been known a long time. This phenomenon has been associated with alterations in their bioactivity and consequently with pathologies of gonadal function (Dufau and Veldhuis 1987; Beitins and Padmanabhan 1991; Tsatsoulis et al. 1991). Whether the variability of gonadotropin glycosylation has a genetic basis still remains unknown. Only few reports exist on genuine mutations in the gonadotropin subunit genes (see below). Another group of mutations affecting gonadotropin function can occur in their receptor genes. The structure of luteinizing hormone (LH) and follicle-stimulating hormone (FSH) receptor (R) genes was revealed a few years ago, and a number of constitutively activating and inactivating mutations in these genes are known today.

The purpose of this chapter is to summarize our findings on the molecular basis of heterogeneity of gonadotropins and their receptors, both with regard to their microheterogeneity at the level of glycosylation and to mutations affecting the protein structure. We describe methods to address their molecular basis and assess the physiological and pathophysiological consequences of these structural alterations.

16.2 Immunological and Biological Measurements of Gonadotropins

16.2.1 Microheterogeneity of Gonadotropins

The two gonadotropins, LH and FSH, are both composed of two peptide chains, α and β, which are coupled by disulfide bonds. The α-subunits are identical in LH and FSH, as well as in the two other glycoprotein hormones, human chorionic gonadotropin (hCG) and thyroid-stimulating hormone (TSH), and the hormonal specificity resides in the β-subunit. In addition, there are carbohydrate side chains in the gonadotropin subunits, two in the common α-chain, two in FSHβ, and one in LHβ. The carbohydrate side chains display a large variation in their sugar composition, called microheterogeneity, whose regulation is as yet incompletely understood. The differentially glycosylated forms of gonadotropins differ in their isoelectric points and they can be separated by isoelectric focusing and chromatofocusing, and, depending on the performance of the separation method used, up to tens of isoforms can be separated (Wide 1985; Keel and Grotjan 1989). The gonadotropins present in the pituitary gland and circulation are therefore a variable mixture of isoforms, the composition of which varies in various physiological and pathophysiological conditions, mainly by mechanisms so far unknown.

The variations in chemical composition of the carbohydrate moieties in gonadotropin isoforms are reflected by differences in their intrinsic biological activity. This has been observed by measuring ratios of the biological (B) to immunological (I) activities (i.e., B/I ratio) of the gonadotropin isoform fractions. Since the immunoreactivity largely monitors the mass of the hormone molecules, the B/I ratio monitors the intrinsic bioactivity of hormone molecules in a given isoform fraction. The B/I ratio of the different LH and FSH isoforms varies, and there are studies showing that the isohormone distribution and the average B/I ratio of gonadotropins vary in different physiological and pathophysiological conditions. Altered B/I ratios of LH have been detected, for instance, during endogenous and gonadotropin-releasing hormone (GnRH) evoked LH pulses, at puberty, after orchidectomy, during steroid hormone treatment, and during idiopathic infertility. The B/I ratio changes of FSH have been less extensively studied. Many of the changes have been considered diagnostic for altered pituitary–gonadal function (for reviews, see Dufau and Veldhuis 1987; Wang 1988; Beitins and Padmanabhan 1991; Tsatsoulis et al. 1991).

16.2.2 Novel Sensitive Immunoassays and In Vitro Bioassays of Gonadotropins

The majority of the B/I ratio changes have been documented by using conventional radioimmunoassay (RIA) for the detection of gonado-tropin immunoreactivity. Since these studies, a new generation of im-munoassays using monoclonal antibodies (Mab) and the immunometric assay principle, have reached the clinical diagnostics. The new assays have greatly enhanced specificity and sensitivity, up to 100-fold greater than with RIA (Lövgren et al. 1984; Pettersson and Söderholm 1990; Haavisto et al. 1993). When the RIA and immunometric assays are compared, the agreement is rather good at normal to high hormone concentrations, but RIA seems to overestimate low hormone levels. An

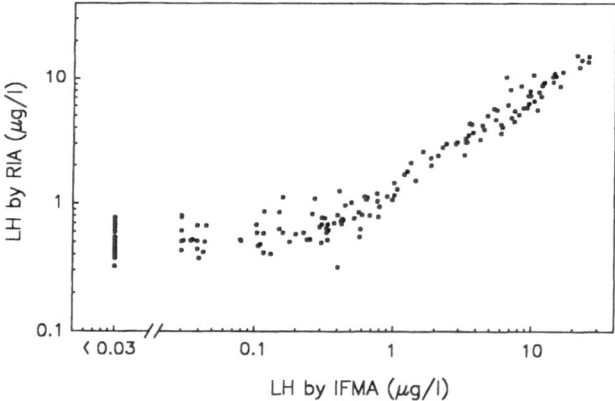

Fig. 1. Correlation of luteinizing hormone (*LH*) levels measured in a total of 165 serum samples from intact and castrated male and female rats and hypo-physectomized male rats using both immunofluorometric assay (*IFMA*; *x-axis*) and radioimmunoassay (*RIA*; *y-axis*). The correlation coefficient (*r*) at LH le-vels greater than 0.4 μg/l determined by IFMA (*n*=89) was 0.91; slope *y*=0.64*x* + 1.0). From Haavisto et al. (1993) with permission

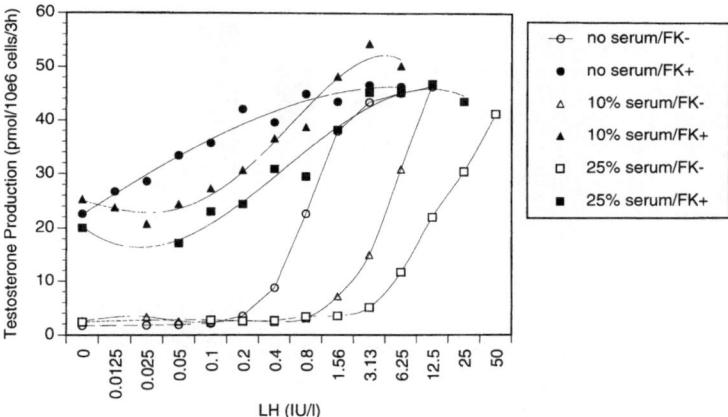

Fig. 2. Standard curves of the in vitro bioassays of luteinizing hormone (*LH*) in the presence and absence of 1.5 μmol/l of forskolin (*FK*) and different concentrations of LH-free human serum. Both the sensitizing effect of FK and desensitizing effect of serum on the LH dose-response are apparent. From Huhtaniemi et al. (1996) with permission

example of this problem with the linearity of the dose-response is shown in Fig. 1, where LH concentrations measured by RIA and immunofluorometric assay (IFMA) in rat serum are correlated (Haavisto et al. 1993). When the B/I ratio of the hormone is calculated, it is erroneously low at low hormone concentrations and automatically increases when the absolute concentration increases.

Some time ago, we started suspecting that the B/I ratio changes documented in the literature for LH are "contaminated" by the problems of conventional RIA in assessing accurately the low LH levels. We started reanalyzing the B/I ratios of LH in a variety of clinical conditions using a highly sensitive (<0.04 IU/l) and specific IFMA (Delfia, Wallac OY, Turku, Finland) for I-LH measurement. In addition, we were able to sensitize the in vitro bioassay of LH tenfold (down to 0.1–0.05 IU/l), by including a 1.5 μmol/l concentration of forskolin in the assay medium (Fig. 2) (Huhtaniemi et al. 1996). These improvements allowed us to measure LH levels in practically all human peripheral serum samples at the linear portion of the assay dose–response curves. We have

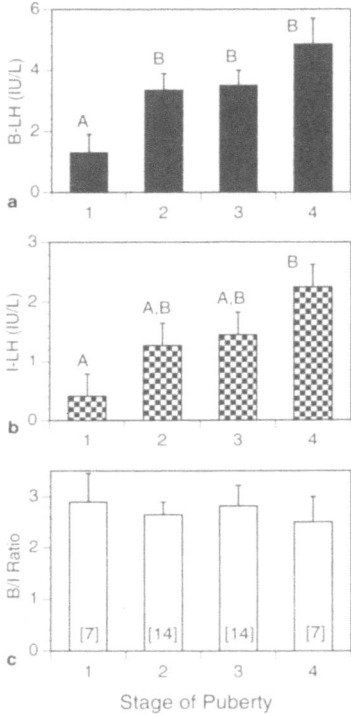

Fig. 3a–c. The mean (+ SEM) levels of biological luteinizing hormone (*B-LH*, **a**), immunological luteinizing hormone (*I-LH*; **b**), and the B/I ratios (**c**) in 14 peripubertal boys studied according to their stage of puberty (*1–4*). The number of subjects analyzed at each pubertal stage is presented in *brackets* at the *bottom of bars* in **c**. When different *letters* are *above the bars* these results differ significantly from each other (*p* < at least 0.05). From Huhtaniemi et al. (1996) with permission

measured the LH levels and B/I ratios, for instance during GnRH analog treatment (Jaakkola et al. 1990; Matikainen et al. 1992), during pulsatile LH secretion (Huhtaniemi et al. 1992), after surgical castration (Haavisto et al. 1990), and in patients with polycystic ovarian diseases (PCOD) (Ding and Huhtaniemi 1991). As the latest in this series we reassessed the B/I ratio changes of LH during pubertal progression of boys (Huhtaniemi et al. 1996). It has previously been shown that the B/I ratio of LH increases during pubertal progression (reviewed in Huhtaniemi et al. 1996), but when we measured B-LH with the sensitized in vitro bioassay and I-LH with IFMA, no change in the B/I ratio was found between stages G1 and G4 of puberty (Fig. 3).

16.2.3 The Clinical Value of Bio/immuno Ratio Measurements of Gonadotropins

On the basis of our recent findings, the B/I ratio of LH seems to be much more stable than previously shown. We consider therefore a sensitive and specific immunoassay of LH sufficient for clinical diagnostics. The same apparently applies to FSH, although fewer data on its B/I ratios are available, due to technical difficulties with reliable in vitro bioassay for this hormone. With the different clinical groups analyzed, we found only two conditions for which a genuine difference in the B/I ratio of LH could be documented: after surgical castration of men with prostatic carcinoma (Haavisto et al. 1990) and in women with PCOD (Ding and Huhtaniemi 1991). Some special conditions still remain for which the in vitro bioassay of gonadotropins can be recommended (Table 1).

The novel, sensitive immunoassays have been criticized for being "too specific." Because they use Mabs recognizing only specific antigenic epitopes of the antigen, there might be conditions where, due to the microheterogeneity of gonadotropins, a specific epitope is altered or blocked by the surrounding carbohydrate structures. In such a case the immunoassay is unable to detect all gonadotropic isoforms, or the stoichiometry of the detectable ones is distorted. Such conditions do exist, but as will be described below, this problem only applies to specific Mabs which can be identified. If the conditions and biological

Table 1. The different uses of in vitro bioassays of gonadotropins

1. Research on qualitative aspects of gonadotropins (structure vs. bioactivity relations)
2. Validation of biological relevance of immunoassays
3. Further exploration of clinical conditions with unexpected gonadotropin immunoassay results
4. Measurement of gonadotropins in exotic species

relevance of the assay are well characterized, this pitfall can be avoided. Undoubtedly, there will always be rare cases where the immunoassay result and the clinical picture of the patient do not match, and the in vitro bioassay is needed (Table 1). These cases are very interesting since they may reveal novel mutations in gonadotropic genes, which have so far remained largely unidentified.

In conclusion, we believe that the majority of the B/I ratio changes of LH, as documented in the past, are due to nonlinearity of the dose–response curve of conventional RIA measurements. When the LH activities are reassessed by using more sensitive and specific IFMA methods, most of the B/I ratio changes disappear. These findings also indicate that the diagnostic value of LH in vitro bioassay is less important than has been assumed previously.

16.3 Gonadotropic Genes

16.3.1 Mutations of Gonadotropic Genes

Only sporadic cases of mutations have so far been reported for gonadotropic genes. One inactivating mutation of the LHβ gene has been described where a single base substitution changes codon 54 from glutamine to arginine (Weiss et al. 1992). As a result, the LH formed maintained its immunological activity but was totally devoid of bioactivity, causing in the affected homozygous male absence of Leydig cells with lack of spontaneous puberty and infertility. In male heterozygotes, there was impaired androgen production and infertility. Female heterozygotes had normal sexual development and fertility.

Likewise, only one case of inactivating FSHβ gene mutation has so far been characterized at the molecular level (Matthews et al. 1993). In this case, there was a deletion in the FSHβ gene resulting in premature termination codon and translation of FSHβ protein that was unable to couple with the α subunit and to form bioactive hormone. The affected woman had primary amenorrhea with infertility, but exogenous FSH treatment resulted in successful pregnancy. Her mother, heterozygotic for the mutation, had had menstrual irregularity and infertility. In men, selective FSH deficiency has been previously reported to cause oligoazoospermia with normal testosterone production and virilization (Maroulis et al. 1977; Rabinowitz et al. 1979), but the molecular basis of the cases could not be solved at the time of these older reports. It is in fact surprising that so few mutations of the gonadotropic genes have thus far been identified, despite their likelihood in causing male and female sub- or infertility.

16.3.2 A Common Polymorphism in the LH β-Subunit Gene

In our studies on testing the suitability of various Mab combinations for LH measurement, we could not detect LH in a healthy woman with two children using one particular Mab combination (Pettersson et al. 1992). The antibody that did not detect her LH was directed against an antigenic epitope in the intact LH α/β dimer (assay 1). Interestingly, all other antibody combinations (α, β, and α/β specific) detected normal LH levels in her serum. Likewise, her LH bioactivity and B/I ratio (using a subunit specific IFMA for I-LH measurement, assay 2) were normal and in accordance with her normal fertility. Since her FSH and TSH levels were normal, we assumed that her LHβ subunit was abnormal in structure. The LH levels were also analyzed in her family members, and it turned out that her mother had similar nondetectable LH by assay 1, but her father and children displayed LH levels which by assay 1 were about 50% of that measured by the reference assay 2; hence, the ratio of LH with assay 1/assay 2 was about 0.5. This led us to the

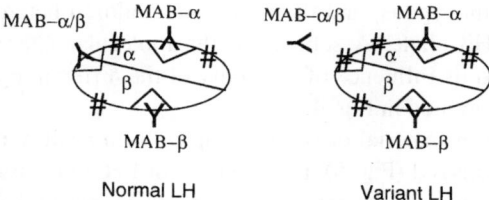

Normal LH   Variant LH

Fig. 4. Schematic presentation of the reason for aberrant immunoreactivity in individuals with the variant form of luteinizing hormone (*LH*) in two-site immunometric assays. Either the changes in the amino acid sequence and/or an extra carbohydrate chain in the LH β-chain block or eliminate the antigenic epitope present in the α/β LH dimer. Combination of monoclonal antibody (*MAB*) α/β and MAB-β was used in assay 1, and MAB-α and MAB-β in assay 2. #, carbohydrate chain

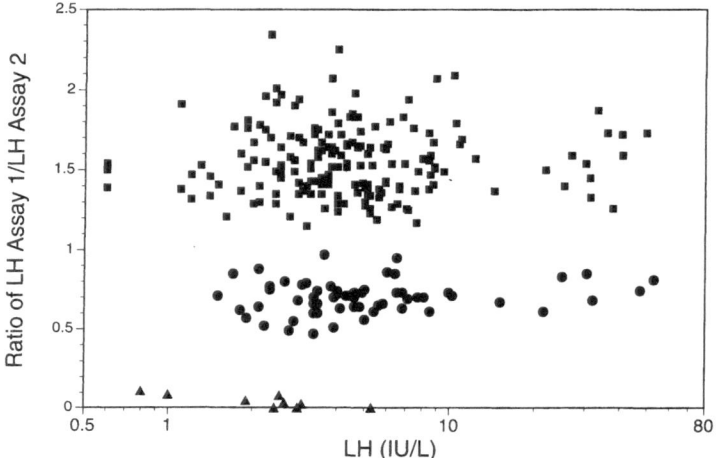

Fig. 5. The distribution of 249 normal subjects in the normal (*squares*), low (*circles*), and zero (*triangles*) ratio groups according to the results of the ratios of luteinizing hormone (*LH*) measured by assays 1 and 2. The LH level measured by assay 2 is shown on the *abscissa*. As no sex differences were detected, the male and female data are compiled. From Haavisto et al. (1995) with permission

conclusion that the aberrant LH form was genetic in nature, with a mendelian fashion of inheritance. Our subject and her mother were apparently homozygous, and the father and children heterozygous for the variant LHβ allele. A scheme of the molecular alteration of the variant LH and its influence of reactivity of the different epitopes with the Mabs is presented in Fig. 4.

When a larger material of serum samples from healthy Finnish volunteers was analyzed (Fig. 5), and the ratio of LH with assay 1/assay 2 was measured, the results fell clearly into three categories: (1) those between 1.0–2.0 (i.e., normal ratio individuals), (2) those at 0.5–0.75 (low ratio individuals), and (3) those with the ratio near 0 (0 ratio individuals). The combined frequency of the low and 0 ratio LH in the Finnish population was 28%, and the distribution followed the Hardy-Weinberg equilibrium.

We then sequenced the LHβ subunit gene of our subject with the 0 ratio LH and found two-point mutations, both resulting in amino acid change: Trp8 - Arg8 (*T*GG - *C*GG) and Ile15 - Thr15 (A*T*C - A*C*C). One of the mutations introduces an extra glycosylation signal (Asn-X-Thr) into the LHβ chain, which may introduce an oligosaccharide chain into Asn13. The same structure is present in the hCG β-chain where Asn13 is glycosylated. The aberrant immunoreactivity of the LH variant could be explained either by the two amino acid changes and/or the putative extra carbohydrate chain which could either alter or block, respectively, the antigenic epitope of the intact LH dimer (Fig. 4). Recently, Furui et al. (1994) from Japan reported on three infertile patients whose serum LH could not be measured with an immuno-radiometric assay kit using two Mabs, in the same fashion as in our measurements. It was of particular interest that the same two mutations in the LHβ chain were found in both Japanese and Finnish subjects. We know now that this LH polymorphism is widely distributed in different ethnic groups, varying from 9% to 29% in frequency (Rajkhowa et al., 1995; Nilsson et al., unpublished). The highest frequency is measured in Northern European populations and lowest in native Americans.

The homozygotes for the LH variant in our material are apparently healthy, with no reported infertility. In this respect our findings differ from those of Furui et al. (1994) who related the LH changes to the infertility detected in their three subjects. We have observed that the B/I ratio of the LH variant is higher than that of the wild-type hormone, but its half-life in circulation is shorter (Haavisto et al. 1995). Since the pulse frequency of the variant LH was normal, this results in overall LH action that is more potent at the receptor site, but shorter in duration. Such a change may have influence on LH action in the affected individuals, and we have so far collected some data indicating that this may indeed be the case. Men heterozygous for the LH variant have slightly but significantly lower serum concentrations of testosterone than men with wild-type LH (unpublished). Women with at least one variant LH allele have higher levels of serum testosterone, estradiol, and sex hormone-binding globulin, and the frequency of the variant allele is altered in certain subtypes of PCOD (Rajkhowa et al. 1995). Very recently, we have found that boys with variant LH have slower overall progression, gain of height, and gain of testis weight at puberty (Raivio et al., unpublished). These findings, especially in men, suggest that the overall bioactivity of the LH variant is lower than that of the wild-type hormone.

It is apparent on the basis of our observations that, although the subjects homo- or heterozygous for the variant LH allele are largely healthy, there may be subtle differences in LH action. Whether the fertility of the affected individuals is suppressed is not yet known. It is tempting to speculate that the variant LH allele could offer some kind of advantage to the affected individuals, thereby explaining the high frequency of the polymorphism. Although the pathophysiological significance of this finding is still open, it is very important for the clinical laboratory to be aware of this common polymorphic form of LH, which behaves aberrantly in several widely applied immunoassay systems.

16.4 Gonadotropin Receptor Genes

16.4.1 Activating and Inactivating Mutations of the Gonadotropin Receptor Genes

The gonadotropin receptor genes were cloned a few years ago from several species. They represent, together with the receptor for the third glycoprotein hormone, TSH, a special class of G protein-coupled receptors, spanning the plasma membrane seven times, with an unusually long extracellular domain (Segaloff and Ascoli 1993). They are encoded by long genes (> 70 kb), with 11 (LHR) or 10 (FSHR, TSHR) exons. The last long exon encodes the transmembrane and intracellular part which is about 50% of the size of the gene.

It was first disclosed with TSHR (Sunthornthepvarakul et al. 1995; van Sande et al. 1995; Utiger 1995), and soon thereafter with LHR (Fig. 6), that there are mutations in these genes that lead both to constitutively activated and inactivated forms of the receptors, explaining certain pathologies of thyroid and gonadal function. Concerning the gonads, the male-limited familial, gonadotropin-independent form of precocious puberty (testotoxicosis) was found to be due to a constitutively activating point mutation of the LHR gene (Kremer et al. 1993; Shenker et al. 1993). The first inactivating mutation of the LHR gene, causing male pseudohermaphroditism with Leydig cell hypoplasia, was discovered very recently (Kremer et al. 1995). Subsequently, a variety

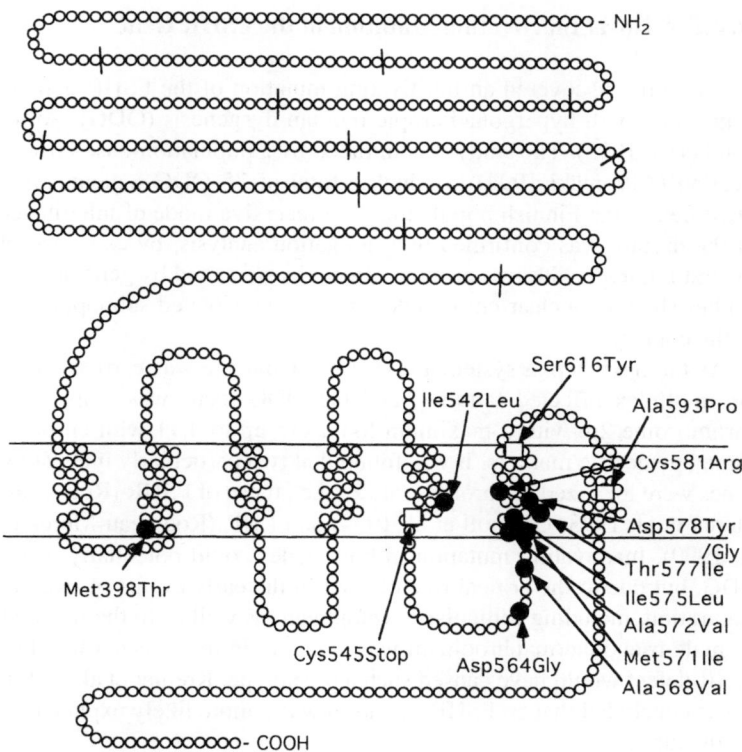

Fig. 6. The structure of the human LH receptor and locations of the activating (*black circles*) and inactivating (*open squares*) mutations so far detected. The *short lines* across the amino acid chain separate the 11 exons. The data are compiled from the following publications: Kremer et al. (1993); Shenker et al. (1993); Evans et al. (1995); Latronico et al. (1995); Kraaij et al. (1995); Kremer et al. (1995); Laue et al. (1995a–c); Yano et al. (1995)

of activating and inactivating mutations of the LHR gene have been described (Fig. 6). Very recently, one inactivating (see below) and one activating (Gromoll et al. 1996) mutation of the FSHR gene have been described.

16.4.2 A Novel Inactivating Mutation of the FSHR Gene

We recently discovered an inactivating mutation of the FSHR gene in connection with hypergonadotropic ovarian dysgenesis (ODG) (Aittomäki et al. 1995). The study was initiated by a population-based investigation (Aittomäki 1994) in which a total of 75 ODG patients were identified in the Finnish population. The recessive mode of inheritance of the disease was confirmed by segregation analysis, by existence of several kindreds with two or more affected sisters, and by genealogical studies showing a clear-cut founder effect in an isolated subpopulation of the country.

As the next step, a systematic search for linkage was carried out in the multiplex affected families, and the ODG locus was mapped to chromosome 2p, with a maximum lod score up to 4.71 with chromosome 2p-specific markers. It was found that two particularly interesting genes were localized to chromosome 2p, i.e., those of FSHR (Rousseau-Merck et al. 1993; Gromoll et al. 1994) and LHR (Rousseau-Merck et al. 1990). Inactivating mutation in both genes could potentially cause ODG, but due to the critical role of FSH in the early events of ovarian maturation, including follicular development, as well as to the fact that no male pseudohermaphroditism was apparent in the affected families (LHR defect would have caused such a phenotype, Kremer et al. 1995), it was concluded that an FSHR mutation was a more likely explanation for the disease.

Since most of the TSHR and LHR gene mutations have been discovered in the transmembrane region (see above), we first searched for mutation in exon 10 encoding this part of the molecule. Denaturing gradient gel electrophoresis (DGGE) of several overlapping polymerase chain reaction (PCR) products was used. Only a polymorphism not related to the disease phenotype was found in the intracellular tail of the receptor. We thereafter went on to screen the first 9 exons, encoding the extracellular part of the receptor protein by amplifying each of them using intron specific primers and sequencing the PCR products. During the course of the work we found out that it is also possible to amplify mRNA of the FSHR gene by using reverse transcriptase (RT)-PCR and RNA isolated from white blood cells as a template, a phenomenon termed illegitimate transcription (Chelly et al. 1989). Exons 6–9 were amplified in this way, and it was found that all affected individuals were

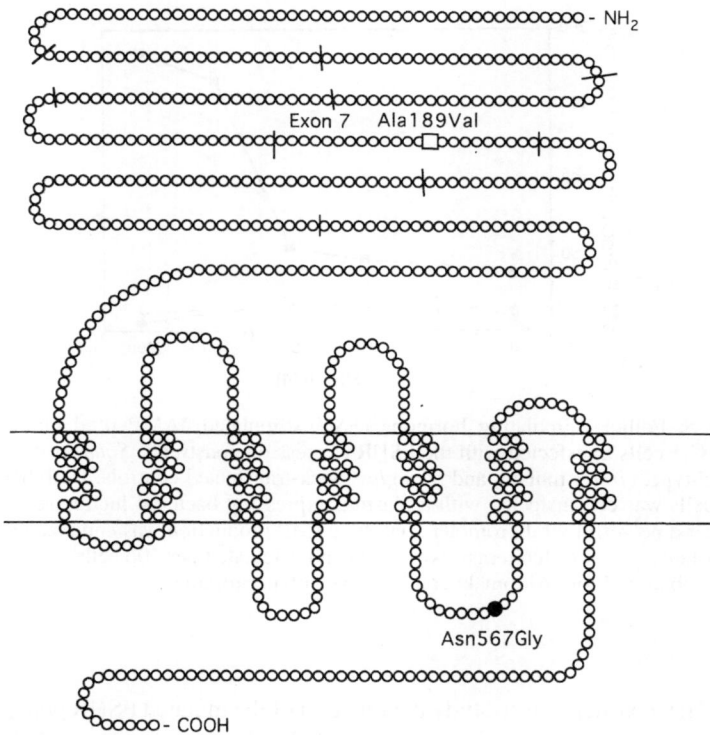

Fig. 7. The inactivating Ala189Val mutation (*open square*) in exon 7 of the FSHR gene detected in patients with hypergonadotropic ovarian dysgenesis (Aittomäki et al. 1995) and the activating Asn567Gly mutation (*black circle*) in the third intracellular loop detected in a hypophysectomized male with sustained spermatogenesis (Gromoll et al. 1996)

homozygous for a C to T transition in position 566 of exon 7 of the FSHR coding sequence, predicting a change of alanine 189 to valine (Fig. 7). When these data were compared with the linkage results, the disease haplotype segregated perfectly with the mutation. All affected individuals displaying the disease haplotype were homozygous for the mutation, and all parents that could be studied (obligatory heterozygotes) were heterozygous for the mutation.

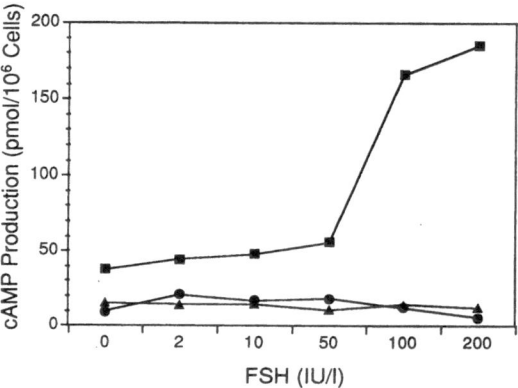

Fig. 8. Follicle-stimulating hormone (*FSH*)-stimulated cAMP production of MSC-1 cells transfected with the FSHR expression constructs. *Squares* denote wild-type, *circles* mutant, and *triangles* mock-transfected controls. Each batch of cells was cotransfected with a plasmid expressing bacterial luciferase gene under a powerful viral promoter, and the cAMP production was equalized to a constant amount of luciferase expression and calculated per 106 cells after a 3-h incubation. From Aittomäki et al. (1995) with permission

The next step was to study the function of the mutated FSHR gene, in order to prove its role in formation of the disease phenotype. When cDNA encoding the wild-type human FSHR protein was transfected into an immortalized murine Sertoli cell line (MSC-1), not expressing the endogenous FSHR gene, a three- to fourfold dose-dependent stimulation of cAMP production was observed with recombinant human (rh) FSH (Fig. 8). In contrast, when the transfection was performed using the mutated FSHR cDNA, rhFSH stimulation of cAMP was not observed. In accordance, when binding of ^{125}I-labeled rhFSH was measured in the same transfected cell lines, the binding measured in cells expressing the mutated receptor was only 3% of that measured in cells expressing the wild-type FSHR (Fig. 9). Interestingly, the equilibrium association constant of binding in both cases was similar (4.8–6.7×109 l/mol), which agrees well with the affinity measured for FSH binding in human testicular homogenates (Wahlström et al. 1983). It is therefore possible that the relatively minor alanine to valine mutation mainly affects the

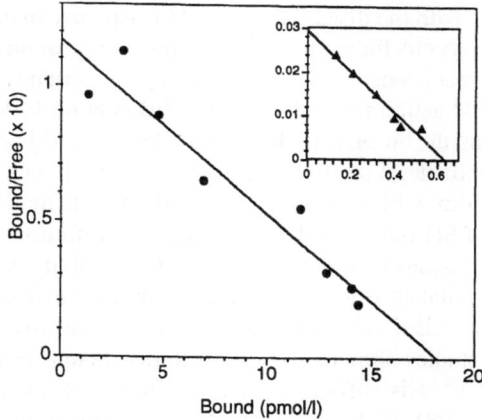

Fig. 9. Scatchard analysis of ^{125}I-labeled follicle-stimulating hormone (*FSH*) binding to transfected MSC-1 cells. *Circles* denote wild-type and *triangles* (*insert*) mutated FSHR expression constructs. In each case, 2×106 transfected cells were incubated in triplicate with increasing concentrations of labeled FSH in a total volume of 250 ml. The cells were cotransfected with luciferase (see Fig. 8). After appropriate corrections, the cell suspension transfected with the wild-type FSHR construct displayed 18.2 pmol/l, and that expressing the mutated construct 0.63 pmol/l of specific FSH binding. The equilibrium association constants (K_a) of FSH binding in the same cell preparations were 6.7 and 4.8×109 l/mol, respectively. From Aittomäki et al. (1995) with permission

trafficking of the receptor protein to the cell membrane or its rate of degradation.

Hence, we have identified a mutation in the FSHR gene which partly explains the pathogenesis of ODG. Many of the study subjects were derived from geographically defined subpopulations in Finland. The minimum frequency of ODG in females for the whole country was calculated as 1 in 8300, which translates into a carrier frequency of 1 in 45. According to our preliminary estimations, about 50% of the ODG cases in Finland are due to the C566T point mutation of the FSHR gene. If similar figures of frequency occur in other populations, ODG due to this mutation will turn out to be one of the most common recessive inherited diseases of mankind.

The families with the disease are bound to also have males heterozygous and homozygous for the disease. The phenotype of these men is of particular interest considering the ongoing uncertainty about the necessity of FSH action for male fertility (Zirkin et al. 1994). We have started analyzing the brothers of the affected females. Although no exact data are yet available, it seems that affected men both with normal and suppressed fertility will be detected. Since the FSHR mutation did not totally abolish FSH binding (about 3% was left with normal affinity), the possibility remains that the residual low FSH activity, together with normal LH-stimulated testosterone production, are sufficient to maintain spermatogenesis. Such a finding would not be surprising in light of the numerous studies showing that high intratesticular testosterone in the absence of FSH is sufficient for maintenance of spermatogenesis (Bremner et al. 1981; Zirkin et al. 1994). In the female the situation is apparently different, and normal FSH secretion is vital for normal follicular development. The severely suppressed FSH responsiveness of the females homozygous for the FSHR mutation is thus incompatible with normal ovarian function. LH action cannot compensate for the missing FSH action, since these two gonadotropins function in sequential fashion during the process of follicular maturation. It will be interesting to study whether massive doses of FSH could overcome therapeutically the subtotal FSHR failure and induce follicular maturation in the ODG patients.

16.5 Conclusions

The studies reviewed here have addressed the molecular heterogeneity of gonadotropins and their receptors at two levels, i.e., the microheterogeneity in carbohydrate structures and the polymorphisms and mutations in the genes.

The microheterogeneity of gonadotropins undoubtedly plays a role in their biological activity. There are some cases in which the intrinsic bioactivity of gonadotropins, reflecting alterations in the isohormone composition, varies according to the physiological and pathophysiological state of pituitary–gonadal function. More recent studies using immunoassays with increased sensitivity and specificity have shown that genuine alterations in the intrinsic bioactivity of gonadotropins (i.e., B/I ratio) are less common than previously demonstrated. However, such conditions do exist, and the next step in our understanding of the meaning of this phenomenon would be to learn more about the regulation of the glycosylation of gonadotropins.

Another topic of this review was the common variant of LH due to two point mutations in the LHβ gene. The polymorphism is unusually common, up to 30% frequency in the Finnish population. The variant form of LH differs clearly from wild-type hormone in its intrinsic bioactivity and half-life in circulation, which is why it is apparent that the overall LH action of the variant differs from that of the wild-type hormone. We have found slight alterations in the pituitary–gonadal function of individuals carrying the variant LHβ allele, but the clear clinical significance and possible correlations with pathologies of LH action remain to be established.

Finally, an inactivating mutation of the FSHR gene is described. The mutation explains a part of hypergonadotropic ovarian dysgenesis in females, but the phenotype of the affected males still remains to be studied. It will be interesting to find out to what extent the severe suppression of FSH action in these men affects their spermatogenesis. This disease will be of great importance in delineating the role of FSH in testicular function.

References

Aittomäki K (1994) The genetics of XX gonadal dysgenesis. Am J Hum Genet 54:844–851

Aittomäki K, Dieguez Lucena JL, Pakarinen P, Sistonen P, Tapanainen J, Gromoll J, Kaskikari R, Sankila E-M, Lehvaslaiho H, Reyes Engel A, Nieschlag E, Huhtaniemi I, de la Chapelle A (1995) Mutation in the follicle-stimulating hormone receptor gene causes hereditary hypergonadotropic ovarian failure. Cell 82:959–968

Beitins IZ, Padmanabhan V (1991) Bioactivity of gonadotropins. Endocrinol Metab Clin North Am 20:85–120

Bremner WJ, Matsumoto AM, Sussman AM, Paulsen CA (1981) Follicle-stimulating hormone and spermatogenesis. J Clin Invest 68:1044–1052

Chelly J, Concordet J-P, Kaplan J-C, Kahn A (1989) Illegitimate transcription: transcription of any gene in any cell type. Proc Natl Acad Sci USA 86:2617–2621

Ding Y-Q, Huhtaniemi I (1991) Preponderance of basic isoforms of serum luteinizing hormone (LH) is associated with the high bio/immuno ratio of LH
in healthy woman and in polycystic ovarian disease. Hum Reprod 6:346–
350

Dufau ML, Veldhuis J (1987) Pathophysiological relationships between the biological and immunological activities of luteinizing hormone. Baillieres
Clin Endocrinol Metab 1:153–176

Evans BAJ, Bowen D, Smith PJ, Gregory JW (1995) A mutation of the LH receptor gene in two siblings; one apparently normal and the other with familial precocious puberty. Abstracts of the 14th joint meeting of the British
Endocrine Society, no P262

Furui K, Suganuma N, Tsukahara SI, Asada Y, Kikkawa F, Tanaka M, Ozawa
T, Tomoda Y (1994) Identification of two point mutations in the gene coding luteinizing hormone (LH) β-subunit, associated with immunologically
anomalous LH variants. J Clin Endocrinol Metab 78:107–113

Gromoll J, Ried T, Holtgreve-Grez H, Nieschlag E, Gudermann T (1994) Localization of the human FSH receptor to chromosome 2p21 using a
genomic probe comprising exon 10. J Mol Endocrinol 12:266–271

Gromoll J, Simon M, Nieschlag E (1996) An activating mutation of the follicle-stimulating hormone receptor autonomously sustains spermatogenesis
in a hypophysectomized man. J Clin Endocrinol Metab (in press)

Haavisto A-M, Simberg N, Huhtaniemi I (1990) The bio/immuno ratio of
serum LH increases after orchidectomy in prostatic cancer patients and is
associated with decreased molecular weight and appearance of isohormones
with alkaline pI values. Biol Reprod 42:597–602

Haavisto A-M, Pettersson K, Bergendahl M, Perheentupa A, Roser J, Huhtaniemi I (1993) A supersensitive immunofluorometric assay for rat luteinizing hormone. Endocrinology 132:687–1691

Haavisto A-M, Pettersson K, Bergendahl M, Virkamäki A, Huhtaniemi I
(1995) Occurrence and biological properties of a common genetic variant
of luteinizing hormone. J Clin Endocrinol Metab 80:1257–1263

Huhtaniemi I, Ding Y-Q, Tähtelä R, Välimäki M (1992) The bio/immuno ratio
of plasma luteinizing hormone does not change during the endogenous secretion pulse; reanalysis on the concept using improved immunometric
techniques. J Clin Endocrinol Metab 75:1442–1445

Huhtaniemi I, Haavisto A-M, Anttila R, Siimes MA, Dunkel L (1996) Sensitive immunoassay and in vitro bioassay demonstrate constant bio/immuno
ratio of luteinizing hormone in healthy boys during the pubertal maturation.
Pediatr Res (in press)

Jaakkola T, Ding Y-Q, Kellokumpu-Lehtinen P, Valavaara R, Martikainen H,
Tapanainen J, Rsnnberg L, Huhtaniemi I (1990) The ratios of serum bioac-
tive/immunoreactive LH and FSH in various conditions with increased and

decreased gonadotropin secretion: reevaluation by an ultrasensitive immunometric assay. J Clin Endocrinol Metab 70:1496–1505

Keel BA, Grotjan HE Jr (1989) Microheterogeneity of glycoprotein hormones. CRC Press, Boca Raton

Kraaij R, Post M, Kremer H, Brunner HG, Grootegoed JA, Themmen APN (1995) A missense mutation in the second transmembrane segment of the luteinizing hormone receptor causes familial male-limited precocious puberty. Abstracts of the 77th annual meeting of the Endocrine Society, no P3–34

Kremer H, Mariman E, Otten BJ, Moll GW Jr, Stoelinga GB, Wit JM, Jansen M, Drop SL, Faas B, Ropers HH, Brunner HG (1993) Cosegregation of missense mutations of the luteinizing hormone receptor gene with familial male-limited precocious puberty. Hum Mol Genet 2:1779–1783

Kremer H, Kraaij R, Toledo SPA, Post M, Friedman JB, Hayashida CY, van Reen M, Milgrom E, Ropers H-H, Mariman E, Themmen APN, Brunner HG (1995) Male pseudohermaphroditism due to a homozygous missense mutation of the luteinizing hormone receptor gene. Nature Gen 9:160–164

Latronico AC, Anasti J, Arnhold IJP, Mendonca BB, Domenice S, Albano MC, Zachman K, Wajchenberg BL, Tsigos C (1995) A novel mutation of the luteinizing hormone receptor gene causing male gonadotropin-independent precocious puberty. J Clin Endocrinol Metab 80:2490–2494

Laue L, Chan W-Y, Hsueh AJW, Kudo M, Hso SY, Wu S-M, Blomberg L, Cutler GB Jr (1995a) Genetic heterogeneity of constitutively activating mutations of the human luteinizing hormone receptor in familial male-limited precocious puberty. Proc Natl Acad Sci USA 92:1906–1910

Laue L, Wu SM, Jelly DH, Cutler GB Jr, Chan WY (1995b) A novel constitutively activating mutation of the human luteinizing hormone receptor (hLHR) in an African American patient with "sporadic" male-limited precocious puberty. Abstracts of the 77th annual meeting of the Endocrine Society, no P3–36

Laue L, Wu SM, Kudo M, Hsueh AJW, Bourdony CJ, Cutler GB Jr, Chan WY (1995c) Heterogeneity of human luteinizing hormone receptor (hLHR) gene mutations in Leydig cell hypoplasia (LCH). Abstracts of the 77th annual meeting of the Endocrine Society, no P3–37

Lövgren T, Hemmilä I, Pettersson K (1984) Determination of hormones by time-resolved fluoroimmunoassay. Talanta 31:909–916

Maroulis GB, Parlow AF, Marshall JR (1977) Isolated follicle-stimulating hormone deficiency in man. Fertil Steril 28:818–822

Matikainen T, Ding Y-Q, Vergara M, Huhtaniemi I, Couzinet B, Schaison G (1992) Differing responses of plasma bioactive and immunoreactive follicle-stimulating hormone and luteinizing hormone to gonadotropin-releasing hormone agonist and antagonist treatments in postmenopausal women. J Clin Endocrinol Metab 75:820–825

Matthews CH, Borgato S, Beck-Peccoz P, Adams M, Tone Y, Gambino G, Casagrande S, Tedeschini G, Benedetti A, Chatterjee VKK (1993) Primary amenorrhoea and infertility due to a mutation in the β-subunit of follicle-stimulating hormone. Nature Gen 5:83–86

Pettersson K, Söderholm J (1990) Untrasensitive two-site immunometric assay of human lutropin by time-resolved fluorometry. Clin Chem 36:1928–1933

Pettersson K, Ding Y-Q, Huhtaniemi I (1992) An immunologically anomalous luteinizing hormone variant in a healthy woman. J Clin Endocrinol Metab 74:164–171

Rabinowitz D, Benveniste R, Lindner J, Lober D, Danniell J (1979) Isolated FSH deficiency revisited. N Engl J Med 300:126–128

Rajkhowa M, Talbot JA, Jones PW, Pettersson K, Haavisto A-M, Huhtaniemi I, Clayton RN (1995) Prevalence of an immunological LH β-subunit variant in a UK population of healthy women and women with polycystic ovary syndrome. Clin Endocr 43:297–303

Rousseau-Merck MF, Misrahi M, Atger M, Loosfelt H, Milgrom E, Berger R (1990) Localization of the human LH (luteinizing hormone) receptor gene to chromosome 2p21. Cytogenet Cell Genet 54:77–79

Rousseau-Merck MF, Atger M, Loosfelt H, Milgrom E, Berger R (1993) The chromosomal localization of the human follicle-stimulating hormone receptor gene (FSHR) on 2p21-2p15 is similar to that of the luteinizing hormone receptor gene. Genomics 15:222–224

Segaloff DL, Ascoli M (1993) The lutropin/choriogonadotropin receptor...4 years later. Endocr Rev 14:324–346

Shenker A, Laue L, Kosugi S, Merendino JJ Jr, Minegishi T, Cutler GB Jr (1993) A constitutively activating mutation of the luteinizing hormone receptor in familial male precocious puberty. Nature 365:652–654

Sunthornthepvarakul T, Gottschalk ME, Hayashi Y, Refetoff S (1995) Brief report: resistance to thyrotropin caused by mutations in the thyrotropin-receptor gene. N Engl J Med 332:155–160

Tsatsoulis A, Shalet SM, Robertson WR (1991) Bioactive gonadotropin secretion in man. Clin Endocrinol (Oxf) 35:193–206

Utiger RD (1995) Thyrotropin-receptor mutations and thyroid dysfunction. N Engl J Med 332:183–185

van Sande J, Parma J, Tonacchera M, Swillens S, Dumont J, Vassart G (1995) Somatic and germline mutations of the TSH receptor gene in thyroid diseases. J Clin Endocrinol Metab 80:2577–2585

Wahlström T, Huhtaniemi I, Hovatta O, Seppälä M (1983) Localization of luteinizing hormone, follicle-stimulating hormone, prolactin, and their receptors in human and rat testis using immunohistochemistry and radioreceptor assay. J Clin Endocrinol Metab 57:825–830

Wang C (1988) Bioassays of follicle-stimulating hormone. Endocr Rev 9:374–377

Weiss J, Axelrod L, Whitcomb RW, Crowley WF, Jameson JL (1992) Hypogonadism caused by a single amino acid substitution in the β subunit of luteinizing hormone. N Engl J Med 326:179–183

Wide L (1985) Median charge and charge heterogeneity of human pituitary FSH, LH and TSH. I. Zone electrophoresis in agarose suspension. Acta Endocrinol (Copenh) 109:191–189

Yano K, Saji M, Hidaka A, Moriya N, Okuno A, Kohn LD, Cutler GB Jr (1995) A new constitutively activating point mutation in the luteinizing hormone/choriogonadotropin receptor gene in cases of male-limited precocious puberty. J Clin Endocrinol Metab 80:1162–1168

Zirkin BR, Awoniyi C, Griswold MD, Sharpe RM (1994) Is FSH required for adult spermatogenesis? J Androl 15:273–276

Subject Index

acidic fibroblast growth factor 199
acrosomal contents 272
acrosome reaction 249
activating protein-1 175
adipocyte function 116
adipose tissue 105
adrenal 97
adrenal cortex 8
adrenocorticotropin 200
AKAP79 99
aldosterone 201
alternative upstream promoter 134
amenorrhea 326
AMPA receptors 99
anchoring proteins (AKAPs) 98
androgens 4, 167, 186, 326
androgen insensitivity 170
androgen production 8
androgen receptor 167
androgen resistance 179
andrology 288, 294
angiotensin-converting enzyme (ACE) 31
anterior pituitary 4
antigen-presenting cell 220
AP-1 family 175
apoptosis 85, 161
apoptotic 158
aromatase 188
association constant 334
asthenozoospermia 272

ATP 234
ATP-binding pocket 227
autophosphorylation 97, 233–234, 237, 241–242
autoregulatory loop 43
azoospermia 273, 302

B cell 232
B cell antigen receptor (BCR) 232
bandshift 44
Barnes maze 115
base substitution 326
basic FGF 199
behavior 101–102
blastocyst 279
blastula 278
Blk 233
bone marrow 97
brain 97
breast cancer 170
brown adipose tissue 116
BSA gradient 143

C subunit genes 96
c-FGR 229
c-kit receptor 144
c-Scr 228
c-Src molecules 239
C-terminal regulatory tail 224
C-terminal tail 228
c-yes 229

Ca^{2+} channels   99
Ca^{2+} influx   60
Ca^{2+} permeability   61
Ca^{2+} sensitive adenylyl cyclase
   101
Ca^{2+}/calmodulin-dependent protein
   kinase   35
calcineurin   99
calmodulin   34
calreticulin   173
calspermin   34
CaM kinase II   42
CaM kinase IV   35, 42
cAMP   18, 55, 70, 74–75, 96
cAMP response element   31, 99
cAMP-dependent protein kinase
   9, 96
cAMP-dependent steroidogenic
   response   21
capacitation   253
carbohydrate   321
carrier frequency   335
castration   324
catalytic domain   224, 228, 236
CD2   231
CD4   225, 231
CD45   237
CD5   231
CD8   225, 231
cDNA   30
cell cycle   276
cell cycle imbalance   276
cell death   150
cell divisions   279
centrosome   280
cGMP   56
chemoattraction   53
chimeric molecules   242
cholesterol   21
cholesterol dehydrogenase   193
cholesterol side chain cleavage
   15

chromatids   276
chromatin reorganization   45
chromatin structure   173
chromatoid body   130
chromosomes   276, 332
clinical andrology   298
clinical trials   288
clomiphene   300
coactivators   46, 174
collagenase   281
compartmentalized storage of
   mRNAs   130
compensatory mechanism   116
complex response elements   172
cone   57
congenital adrenal hyperplasia
   (CAH)   15, 200
congenital lipoid adrenal hyperplasia   22
cortex   97
cortisol   200
COS cells   241
CREB binding protein   33, 46, 99
CREM   33, 42, 74–76, 78, 80, 84
cryptorchidism   308
Csk   236
cumulus cells   249
cyclic nucleotide-gated (CNG) ion
   channels   56
cyclic nucleotide-signaling
   pathways   58
CYP11A   17, 20
CYP17   17, 20
cystic fibrosis   302
cystic fibrosis chloride channel
   100
cytochrome P450   1
cytoplasmic extracts   132
cytoskeletal elements   233
cytoskeleton   130
cytospin   144
cytotoxicity   242

DAX-1 9
deadenylation 125
dehydroepiandrosterone 186
deletion analysis 44
deletion mutation 314
denaturing gradient gel electro-
    phoresis 332
dentate granule cells 97
dephosphorylation 236, 238
depotentiation 109
developmental abnormalities 100
differential plating 143
differentiation 30, 99, 157, 220
dihydroprogesterone 186
dihydrotestosterone 186
dimerization 98
DNA 276
DNA degradation 152
DNA methylation 45, 278
DNA replication 276
DNA synthesis 277
DNase I digestion 41
Down's syndrome 134
Drosophila 126

egg-derived peptides 63
eggs 278
ejaculates 274
elongated spermatids 126, 272
embryogenesis 3, 277
embryonal long terminal binding
    protein (ELP) 2
embryonic lethality 104
embryonic stem (ES) cell 103
endometrium 186
enzyme histochemistry 198
epiblast 278
epididymal damage 296
epididymis 186, 278, 301
epitopes 325
Erk2 244
estradiol 329

estrogen receptor 175
estrogens 186, 300
eukaryotic cells 123
excitatory postsynaptic potential
    (EPSP) 109
exocytosis 249
expression 97
extra-embryonic tissues 277

facilitation 107
fat 97
fertile 116
fertilin 250
fertilisation 53, 272
fertility 294, 320
fetal germ cells 278
fetal gonad 279
fibronectin 313
fine needle aspiration 274
flow cytometry 158
follicle-stimulating hormone
    (FSH) 81, 274, 299, 320
follicular development 332, 336
footprint 44
formazan 146
forskolin 112, 323
free radicals 134
FTZ-F1 2
Ftz-F1-disrupted mice 9
fusion gene 310
Fyn 231, 237

gain-of-function mutations 320
gamete interaction 247
gametes 272
gametogenesis 278
gastrula 278
gastrulation 279
gene disruption 4
gene expression 80, 100
gene repression 168
gene transcription 168

genetic disorder   307
genomic imprinting   277
germ cell promoter sequences   127
germ cells   142, 273
germline   103
germline mutations   104
glial cells   97
glucocorticoid receptor   171
glucocorticoids   186
glutamic repeat   169
glycoprotein hormones   321
glycosylation   320
gonadal development   1, 8
gonadal function   320
gonadal sex   13
gonadotrope function   1
gonadotropic stimulation   273
gonadotropin releasing hormone
   (GnRH)   289, 298–299, 307,
   309
gonadotropin-releasing hormone
   receptor   6
gonadotropins   289, 298, 300, 308
gonads   8
granulocytes   232
granulosa cells   97
growth factor receptor   240
growth factor receptor PTKs   234
growth retardation   104
guanylyl cyclase   56

H19 allele   278
haploid cells   276
haploid gene expression   129
haplotype   333
Hardy-Weinberg equilibrium   328
Hck   232
hedgehog   100
hepatectomy   100
hereditary   320
hetero-oligomeric channels   61
heterodimerization   179

heterodimers   98
heterozygocity   320
hippocampal trisynaptic pathway
   106
hippocampus   97, 101
histones   276
HMG-1   172
homeostatic controls   103
homo-oligomeric channels   61
homologous chromosomes   277
homologous recombination   103
homozygocity   320
hormone response elements   171
horse serum   146
3β-HSD   187
human chorionic gonadotropin
   (hCG)   321
human conception   272
human growth hormone reporter
   gene   130
hydrophobic pocket   226
hyperactivation   272
hypergonadotropic ovarian dysgenesis   332
hypogonadism   289–290, 308
hypogonadotrophic hypogonadism
   9, 307
hypospermatogenesis   273
hypothalamic-pituitary-gonadal
   axis   320

ICER   76, 78, 83
ICSI   275
idiopathic hypogonadotropic hypogonadism   289
idiopathic infertility   290
illegitimate transcription   332
immature cells   273
immunofluorometric assay   323
immunometric assay   322
immunoprecipitation   127
immunoreactivity   321

imprinted genes 278
in situ hybridization 129
in vitro fertilization 300
infertility 295, 300, 320
inner mitochondrial membrane 21
insemination 300
insulin-degrading enzyme 172
insulin-like growth factor (IGF)-I
  199
interleukin-2 235, 237
intracellular calcium 280
intractable infertility 282
intracytoplasmic sperm injection
  275, 300
intron 38
isoelectric points 321
isoforms 321
isohormone 321

KAL gene 309
KAL mRNA 311
KAL protein 309
KAL-Y 310
kallikrein 298
Kallmann's syndrome 289, 307
KALp 315
Kennedy's disease 169
kidney 194
kinase domain 234
kit ligand 146
Klinefelters syndrome 275
knockout mice 6

laboratory models 289
Lck 231, 237
learning 102
leucocytes 274
leukocyte common antigen 237
Leydig cell hypoplasia 330
Leydig cells 4, 8, 198, 274
LHRH superagonist 207
locus 332

long-term depression (LTD) 101
long-term potentiation (LTP) 101,
  105
loss-of-function mutations 320
luteinizing hormone (LH) 300, 320
Lyn 232

macrophages 232
major histocompatibility (MHC)
  molecule 220
maldescended testes 295
male fertility 292
male germ cells 44, 124
male infertility 275, 297
male pronucleus 277
male pseudohermaphroditism 330
male sex steroids 167
malignant transformation 222
mammalian brain extracts 132
mammalian male germ cells 124
maternal genomes 277
maturation arrest 273
maturation factors 277
meiosis 30, 44
meiotic phase 272
metabolic regulation 105
metaphase 277
microheterogeneity 320
microinjection 275
microscopic epididymal sperm aspiration 275
microtubule association of transported mRNAs 133
microtubule-organising centre 280
microtubules 132
mineralocorticoids 186, 206
mitotic divisions 272
mitotic spindle 280
mitral cell dendrites 308
MMTV promoter 173
monoclonal antibodies 322

monoclonal antibody (mAb) 97.25
    51
Morris water maze   115
mossy fiber pathway   102, 106, 112
mouse sex-limited protein   172
mRNA localization   124
mRNA metabolism   125
mRNA processing events   123
mRNA transport and localization
    133
MTT   146
müllerian-inhibiting substance
    (MIS)   4
multicopy genes   279
multifactorial regulation   16
mutations   314
myometrium   186
myristylation   96, 225

NAD(H)   195
NADPH   195
neural development   313
neuronal stem cell   309
neurons   97
neurotoxins   313
NIH 3T3 fibroblasts   235
NIH3T3 cells   38
NK cells   238
nuclear extract   41
nuclear factor κB   177
nucleoproteins   276
nucleosomes   173
nucleus   30
null mutants   102, 104

obesity   117
olfactory axons   311
olfactory bulbs   307, 309, 314
olfactory epithelium   308
olfactory neurones   55, 308–309
olfactory placode   308
olfactory system   308

oligoasthenoteratozoospermia   302
oligoazoospermia   326
oligonucleotide   41
oligozoospermia   272
oncogenes   222
ooplasm   272
orphan nuclear receptor   1, 9
oscillogen   282
ovaries   4
overlay blots   99
ovum   272

p110   263
P450c17   18, 200
P450scc   18, 200
p75 promoter   176
p85   263
pachytene spermatocyte   142
palmitoylation   225
paternal genomes   277
paternal mRNAs   128
pathogenesis   320
penetrance   320
penetration   272
peptide mapping   132
percutaneous epididymal sperm as-
    piration   275
PH-20   249
phenotype   102, 334
phenotypic sex   13
phosphorylation   43, 72, 132, 178,
    220, 233, 236, 241
photoreceptor cells   57
PI 3-K   263
pituitary   97
pituitary gland   321
placebo   290
placenta   194
platelet-derived growth factor
    (PDGF)   199
platelets   232
point mutations   235, 314, 329

poly(A) binding protein (PABP) 126
poly(A) tail 124
polyadenylation 124
polycystic ovarian diseases (PCOD) 324
polymorphism 170
postmeiotic germ cells 34
postmeiotic male germ cells 124
postmitochondrial extracts from testis 128
precocious puberty 330
pregnancy 291, 296
preimplantation development 277
premature chromosome condensation 276
premature termination 326
preventive treatment 292
primordial prospermatogenic germ cells 272
proacrosin 249
probasin 172
progesterone 186
progesterone receptor 173
proliferation 220
promoters 37, 129
pronuclear membrane 277
pronuclei 272
propidium iodide 158
prostate 186
prostate cancer 170
prostatic carcinoma 325
protamines 31, 87, 125, 129, 276
protein kinase A 41, 70, 178, 228
protein kinase C 178
protein kinases 313
protein tyrosine kinases 220, 249
protooncogenes 222
pseudogene 96
pseudohermaphrodite 206
PTPase activity 237
putative olfactory receptors 61

pyramidal cells 97

R subunit genes 96
radioimmunoassay 322
rational treatment 292
receptor PTKs 252
renal agenesis 312
replication 100
reporter gene 37
repressor 45
reproductive medicine 288
reticulocyte lysates 131
retroposon 96
retrospective studies 292
retroviruses 222
RNA gel-retardation assays 132
RNA polymerase II 174
RNA synthesis 30
RNA-binding domains 126
RNA-binding proteins 127
rod 57
round spermatids 126, 272
Rous sarcoma virus 222, 239

Schaffer collateral pathway 102, 106
sedimentation velocity 143
semen 281
seminal fluid 297
seminiferous tubules 142, 272
separation 157
sequence elements 131
sequence-independent RNA-binding proteins 128
serine/threonine phosphorylation 233
serine/threonine-specific kinase 237
Sertoli cell conditioned medium (SCCM) 146
Sertoli cell line (MSC-1) 334
Sertoli cell preparation 145

Sertoli cells   44, 97, 142, 273
sex hormone   13
sex hormone-binding globulin   329
sex steroids   308
sexual differentiation   3
SF-1   4
SF-1-response element   8
SH2 domain   231, 236, 252
SH3 domain   231, 236
SH4 domain   225
short-term modifications   101
signal transduction   70
single-copy genes   134, 279
skin   186
smears   274
somatic cells   276
Sp1   19
sperm   58
sperm antibodies   297
sperm centrosome   280
sperm cytosolic oscillogen   277
sperm function   291
sperm motility   55, 104
sperm nuclear membrane   277
sperm nucleus   272
sperm-egg interactions   53
spermatic vein   296
spermatids   30, 83, 124, 142, 272,
    281
spermatocytes   30, 142
spermatogenesis   30, 126, 142,
    272, 308, 336
spermatogonia   272
spermatogonial stem cells   142
spermatozoa   30, 142, 272
spermatozoon   124, 272
spermiogenesis   83, 125
spermiogenic phase   272
spleen   97
splice variants   96
Src family   220, 222, 226

Src-homology 2 (SH2) domain
    224
Src-homology 3 (SH3) domain
    224
Src-like PTKs   224
STAPUT   144
steroid biosynthesis   100
steroid hormones   2
steroid hydroxylases   8, 15
steroidogenic acute regulatory pro-
    tein (StAR)   8, 22
steroidogenic factor 1 (SF-1)   1–2,
    16–17
steroidogenic pathways   15
stored mRNAs   124
striatum   97
subcellular localization   98, 130
subfertility   320
substitution therapy   289
Superoxide dismutase 1 (copper-
    zinc superoxid   134
Syk family   241
synaptic plasticity   105, 112
synaptic remodeling   101
synaptic transmission   101

T cells   99
T-cell activation   236
T-cell hybridoma   235
T lymphocytes   219
tamoxifen   300
targeted gene disruption   102, 117
targeting vectors   104
TCR signaling   231
telophase   277
teratozoospermia   272
testicular cords   4
testicular cytoplasmic factors   131
testicular sperm extraction   275
testis   4, 30, 97, 123, 197, 274
testis cDNA library   127

testis-brain RNA-binding protein
    (TB-RBP)   131
testis-specific mRNAs   125
testosterone   18, 168, 298, 329
testotoxicosis   330
therapeutic concepts   289
Thy-1   231
thymus   231
thyroid   330
thyroid hormone   2
thyroid-stimulating hormone
    (TSH)   321
tissue specific   97
tissue-specific expression   17
trafficking   335
transcription   30, 38, 123
transcription factor IIB (TFIIB)
    175
transcription factors   19, 46, 70,
    128, 168, 169
transcription initiation   174
transcriptional regulation   15
transcriptional repression   175
transfected cells   235
transforming growth factor
    (TGF)-β   200
transition proteins   87, 125, 129
translational arrest and activation
    130
translational control   130
translational repressors   128
translocation   263
transmembrane   330
transmembrane receptors   233
triglyceride stores   116
trypan blue   281
trypsin   281
tubular atrophy   275
tubular diameter   274
tubular lumen   274
tubular walls   274

type A spermatogonia   143
type B spermatogonia   142
tyrosine kinases   219
tyrosine phosphorylation   239, 261
tyrosine residues   233
tyrphostin   262

UV-crosslinking   131

v-Src   235
varicocele   296
velocity sedimentation   157
venereal diseases   294
ventral diencephalon   4
ventromedial hypothalamic nucleus
    6
viability   158
virilization   326
vitamin D   2
vitelline membrane   272
voltage-gated ion channels   99

water mazes   106
wheat germ agglutinin   313
Wilms tumor   278

Xenopus germ cell-specific
    transcription factor   128

Y chromosome   133
Yamaguchi's kinase   229
yolk sac   278
Yrk   233

Zap   241
zona fasciculata   199
zona glomerulosa   199
zona pellucida   249, 272
ZP3   249
ZRK   250

Ernst Schering Research Foundation Workshop

Editors: Günter Stock
Ursula-F. Habenicht

Vol. 1
Bioscience ⇌ Society
Workshop Report
Editors: D. J. Roy, B. E. Wynne, R. W. Old

Vol. 2
Round Table Discussion on Bioscience ⇌ Society
Editor: J. J. Cherfas

Vol. 3
Excitatory Amino Acids and Second Messenger Systems
Editors: V. I. Teichberg, L. Turski

Vol. 4
Spermatogenesis – Fertilization – Contraception
Editors: E. Nieschlag, U.-F. Habenicht

Vol. 5
Sex Steroids and the Cardiovascular System
Editors: P. Ramwell, G. Rubanyi, E. Schillinger

Vol. 6
Transgenic Animals as Model Systems for Human Diseases
Editors: E. F. Wagner, F. Theuring

Vol. 7
Basic Mechanisms Controlling Term and Preterm Birth
Editors: K. Chwalisz, R. E. Garfield

Vol. 8
Health Care 2010
Editors: C. Bezold, K. Knabner

Vol. 9
Sex Steroids and Bone
Editors: R. Ziegler, J. Pfeilschifter, M. Bräutigam

Vol. 10
Nongenotoxic Carcinogenesis
Editors: A. Cockburn, L. Smith

Vol. 11
Cell Culture in Pharmaceutical Research
Editors: N. E. Fusenig, H. Graf

Vol. 12
Interactions Between Adjuvants, Agrochemical and Target Organisms
Editors: P. J. Holloway, R. T. Rees, D. Stock

Vol. 13
Assessment of the Use of Single Cytochrome P450 Enzymes
in Drug Research
Editors: M. R. Waterman, M. Hildebrand

Vol. 14
Apoptosis in Hormone-Dependent Cancers
Editors: M. Tenniswood, H. Michna

Vol. 15
Computer Aided Drug Design in Industrial Research
Editors: E. C. Herrmann, R. Franke

Vol. 16
Organ-Selective Actions of Steroid Hormones
Editors: D. T. Baird, G. Schütz, R. Krattenmacher

Supplement 1
Molecular and Cellular Endocrinology of the Testis
Editors: G. Verhoeven, U.-F. Habenicht

Supplement 2
Signal Transduction in Testicular Cells
Editors: V. Hansson, F. O. Levy, K. Taskén

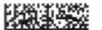